BASIC AND CLINICAL HEPATOLOGY

DEVELOPMENTS IN GASTROENTEROLOGY

VOLUME 2

Also in this series:

1. Peña AS, Weterman IT, Booth CC, Strober W, eds: Recent advances in Crohn's disease
ISBN 90-247-2475-9

Series ISBN 90-247-2441-4

BASIC AND CLINICAL HEPATOLOGY

edited by

P.M. MOTTA, M.D., Ph.D.

Department of Anatomy
Faculty of Medicine
University of Rome
Rome, Italy

and

L.J.A. DIDIO, M.D., D.Sc., Ph.D.

Department of Anatomy
Medical College of Ohio
Toledo, Ohio, U.S.A.

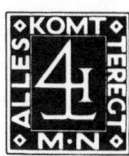

1982

MARTINUS NIJHOFF PUBLISHERS

THE HAGUE / BOSTON / LONDON

Distributors:

for the United States and Canada

Kluwer Boston, Inc.
190 Old Derby Street
Hingham, MA 02043
USA

for all other countries

Kluwer Academic Publishers Group
Distribution Center
P.O. Box 322
3300 AH Dordrecht
The Netherlands

Library of Congress Cataloging in Publication Data   CIP

Main entry under title:

Basic and clinical hepatology.

   (Developments in gastroenterology; v. 2)
   Includes index.
   1. Liver. 2. Liver – Diseases. I. Motta, Pietro M., 1942-   II. DiDio, Liberato J.A., 1920-   III. Series. [DNLM:
1. Liver. 2. Liver diseases.   W1 DE997VYB v. 2/WI 700 B3311]
QP185.B29   616.3'62   81-9545   AACR2

ISBN-13: 978-94-009-8218-5   e-ISBN-13: 978-94-009-8216-1
DOI: 10.1007/978-94-009-8216-1

CONTENTS

In Memoriam

Prof. Renato Locchi
Prof. Dr. J.-C. Wanson

FOREWORD

The liver has been an organ of mystery for centuries. Slowly but surely its secrets have been disclosed by both basic research and clinically oriented investigators whose current concepts have been brought together in this book by authors from five different countries.

Three major groups with many subgroups have made inroads into our better understanding of the liver. The first of these comprises the basic scientists whose study of single hepatocytes may provide the key to comprehension of mechanisms that will lead eventually to improvement in the morbidity and mortality associated with a variety of hepatic disorders.

The second group has been concerned with studies in depth of the liver's response to a variety of hormones, drugs, viruses, and infections. Both early and late results are their concern in the diagnosis and treatment of the individual patient.

A third group comprises the surgeons who have become increasingly aggressive in the removal of one or more segments of the liver. They have increased the scope of hepatic resection as a result of a better understanding gained from studies of various segments of the liver. They have accepted the term, segmentectomy, and have extended feasible procedures to include trisegmentectomy. Indeed, transplantation of the liver has been successfully accomplished.

The clinician has become increasingly reliant on the roentgenologist for assistance in localizing tumors of the liver and providing information with regard to its blood supply by angiogram. Fewer hepatic common ducts require surgical reexploration since calculi can be removed technically by the roentgenologist, absorbed by the new solvents, or removed via an incised ampulla of Vater with use of a special flexible scope passed orally.

Those interested in basic research should be aware of the problems encountered by the clinician. It is just as important for the clinician to be knowledgeable regarding basic science studies on the individual liver cell. Such studies are often the cornerstone of subsequent developments in the successful diagnosis and treatment of patients.

Such a multifaceted organ as the liver doubtless has many more unsolved mysteries that continue to challenge the basic scientist, but the combined efforts of all these groups have begun to bring long-time liver problems under control.

The authors have succeeded together in building a storehouse of current knowledge about the liver. The basic scientist as well as the clinician should find this book invaluable.

Robert M. Zollinger, M.D.
Professor and Chairman Emeritus
The Department of Surgery
The Ohio State University

CONTRIBUTORS

BERNAERT, Denise. Laboratory of Cytology and Experimental Cancerology, Free University of Brussels, Rue Héger Bordet 1, B–1000 Brussels, Belgium.

BLAKEMORE, William S. Department of Surgery, Medical College of Ohio, C.S. 10008, Toledo, Ohio 43699, U.S.A.

BUDD, G. Colin. Department of Physiology, Medical College of Ohio, C.S. 10008, Toledo, Ohio 43699, U.S.A.

BUSACHI, Carlo A. Department of Medicine, University of Bologna, Policlinico S. Orsola, I–40138 Bologna, Italy.

CARAMIA, Felice G. Department of Pathology, Faculty of Medicine, Policlinico Universitario Umberto I°, Viale Regina Elena 324, I–00161 Rome, Italy.

CHRISTOFORIDIS, A. John. Department of Radiology, Medical College of Ohio, C.S. 10008, Toledo, Ohio 43699, U.S.A.

DEMEULENAERE, Leo H.F. Department of Internal Medicine, St.-Andriesziekenhuis, B–8080 Tielt, Belgium.

DIDIO, Liberato J.A. Department of Anatomy, Medical College of Ohio, C.S. 10008, Toledo, Ohio 43699, U.S.A.

FRATI, Luigi. Department of Pathology, Faculty of Medicine, Policlinico Universitario Umberto I°, Viale Regina Elena 324, I–00161 Rome, Italy.

FUJITA, Tsuneo. Department of Anatomy, Niigata University School of Medicine, Asahi-Machi, Niigata 951, Japan.

JONES, Albert L. Departments of Medicine and Anatomy, and the Liver Center, University of California, San Francisco, California, U.S.A.

LASCHI, Renzo. Department of Clinical Electron Microscopy, University of Bologna, Policlinico S. Orsola, I–40138 Bologna, Italy.

MARTIN, Donald C., Jr. Department of Surgery, Medical College of Ohio, C.S. 10008, Toledo, Ohio 43699, U.S.A.

METZ, Jürgen. Department of Anatomy III, University of Heidelberg, Im Neuenheimerfeld 307, D–6900 Heidelberg, F.R.G.

MODESTI, Andrea. Department of Pathology, Faculty of Medicine, Policlinico Universitario Umberto I°, Viale Regina Elena 324, I–00161 Rome, Italy.

MOSSELMANS, Roger. Laboratory of Cytology and Experimental Cancerology, Free University of Brussels, Rue Héger Bordet 1, B–1000 Brussels, Belgium.

MOTTA, Pietro M. Department of Anatomy, Faculty of Medicine, University of Rome, Viale Regina Elena 289, I–00161 Rome, Italy.

MURAKAMI, Takuro. Department of Anatomy, Okayama University Medical School, Okayama 700, Japan.

NISHI, Masayo. Department of Internal Medicine III, Niigata University School of Medicine, Niigata 951, Japan.

OHTANI, Osamu. Department of Anatomy, Okayama University Medical School, Okayama 700, Japan.

PENASSE, Willy. Laboratory of Cytology and Experimental Cancerology, Free University of Brussels, Rue Héger Bordet 1, B–1000 Brussels, Belgium.

PICCOLI, Mario. Department of Pathology, Faculty of Medicine, Policlinico Universitario Umberto I°, Viale Regina Elena 324, I–00161 Rome, Italy.

TORRISI, Maria R. Department of Pathology, Faculty of Medicine, Policlinico Universitario Umberto I°, Viale Regina Elena 324, I–00161 Rome, Italy.

VAN WAES, Leen I.M. Department of Gastroenterology/Hepatology, Academic Hospital of the Free University of Brussels, Laarbeeklaan 101, B–1090 Brussels, Belgium.

WANSON, Jean-Claude.† Laboratory of Cytology and Experimental Cancerology, Free University of Brussels, Rue Héger Bordet 1, B–1000 Brussels, Belgium.

PREFACE

Recent technological and scientific advances from the subcellular to the macroscopic levels of organization discussed during the Symposium of the Pan American Congress of Anatomy, held in São Paulo, Brazil, in 1977, were the primum movens that prompted the editors to present in this monograph the major basic achievements and clinical applications of new knowledge on hepatology. Although limited by the relatively concise text, this comprehensive approach corresponds to what may be called modern hepatology, as the subject matter in each chapter concentrates on innovations and recent contributions as well as on pure and applied data based on theoretical, practical, and even speculative aspects of recent knowledge of the liver. Experimental details, case reports, and controversial interpretations have been avoided to give place to new findings that have gained acceptance by the majority of investigators and practitioners dealing with hepatology.

Basic and Clinical Hepatology is intended to serve general practitioners, surgeons, specialists, investigators, and students. This publication compiles data from scientific articles, review papers, and textbooks. We have attempted to summarize basic, clinical, and surgical information and, at the same time, point out gaps in present knowledge as well as the need for further research. This approach favors the presentation of new trends in the study of the liver and has consequently led to the exclusion of traditional well-established information. Contributions obtained by means of new techniques utilized in transmission and scanning electron microscopy, with or without freeze-fracture, as well as those made with the remarkable tools that have been developed for use in radiology have been included. These techniques have enabled pathologists and clinicians to better understand the anatomy and physiology of the liver, both normal and diseased; to help with interpretation of clinical and experimental findings; and to offer a sound basis for surgical treatment of ailments of the human liver.

Although the use of the Nomina Anatomica, Nomina Embriologica, and Nomina Histologica was recommended, there are some departures from the official nomenclature, and in these instances the terminological change is justified.

We are grateful to Mr. John Flukas for his skillful editorial cooperation, and to Dr. Silvia Correr who offered many constructive suggestions while checking and carefully reading most of the text. Special thanks are due to Mr. Jeffrey K. Smith for his effort and encouragement during all the stages of the preparation of this volume.

We regret to add a sad note relating to the deaths of Prof. Renato Locchi and Prof. Dr. J.-C. Wanson, in whose memories this book is dedicated.

Finally, we would like to mention the pioneering interest of Prof. Z. Fumagalli in the modern correlation between basic and applied study on the liver, as evidenced by his sponsorship of special reports on the subject during the Italian Congress of Anatomy in Messina (1958).

In a publication of this magnitude and diversity, some errors and omissions may be found. The editors ask the reader's indulgence and, additionally, hope that corrections and comments will be forwarded to them.

P.M. Motta (Rome, Italy)
L.J.A. DiDio (Toledo, Ohio, USA)

1. SEGMENTS OF THE LIVER: THE ANATOMICAL BASIS FOR PARTIAL HEPATECTOMY

L.J.A. DiDio

1. THE CONCEPT OF ANATOMICOSURGICAL SEGMENTS OF THE LIVER

The etymology of the word *segment* gives an indication of the cause for the confusion that has surrounded subdivision of the liver, and may help in the understanding of the concept of anatomical and surgical territories of viscera.

The term *segment* originates from the Latin *segmentum* (a section, a piece cut off, a fragment, a cutting) and it is related to *secare* (to cut).

In biology, segment designates any of the portions, divisions, sections, or territories into which a body, an organ, or a viscus is separable by imaginary, natural, artificial, or arbitrarily established boundaries. In geometry, it is a part of a figure; for example, a circle or sphere, marked off by a line or plane, as a part of an area limited by an arc and its chord. It is also defined as a piece cut along the radii of a circular area. In embryology, segments may mean metameres or serially homologous structures, such as the repetition of similar parts of annelids, somites, or myotomes. In spite of there being good reasons to use the word zone instead of segment [1] worldwide adoption of the latter overrides any possible change.

In anatomy and in surgery, a segment is defined as a territory of an organ or viscus having an independent function, supply, or drainage, and as susceptible to anatomical identification and surgical separation or removal.

The best-known examples are the bronchopulmonary, the renal [2–5], the splenic [6–12] segments and, more recently, the gastric [13] and the cardiac segments [14].

Anatomicosurgical visceral segments are independent territories of parenchymatous organs, now extended to hollow organs, that provide the natural and essential background for systematic surgical removal of portions of anatomical structures. Recognized, classified, and described in the lungs, kidneys, spleen, liver, stomach, and heart, among other viscera, the anatomicosurgical segments have a common denominator and organ differences.

The common denominator is the complete, or almost complete, independence in certain divisions or subdivisions of each organ of their blood supply and drainage as well as their ducts or canals (or bronchi, for example), where present. The vascular and ductal elements constitute the segmental pedicle analogous to that of each lobe (lobar pedicle) and that of the entire viscus. At least in some organs, the lymph drainage and nerve supply also follow the other components of the segmental pedicle. The independence between segments can be complete or incomplete, the latter being related to the presence of anastomoses between vessels of adjacent segments. These anastomoses are, however, small in size and/or in number, and are located at the limits between segments. These intersegmental limits are recognizable as avascular or paucivascular zones, i.e., areas or lines, at which level surgical incisions are made for removal of the segment. Segmental independence can be permanent or temporary. Temporary independence, which is observed for example as lines or zones of ischemia when the blood supply is cut, need be sufficiently long for the performance of the segmentectomy. The normal, dynamic anatomy of the segment is modified and eventually altered by the surgical reduction or obliteration of the blood supply, drainage, or the flow of the contents of bronchi, renal calyces, or bile ducts, as the case may be, and thus facilitates the removal of a portion of the organ.

The differences among the organs stem from the

morphological and functional features of each vis-cus. Accordingly, the 'segmenta hepatis' differ mor-phologically from the segments of other viscera but, similar to these, they constitute the anatomical basis for partial resection of the organ.

2. PORTO-BILIO-ARTERIAL (PORTAL) SEGMENTS AND HEPATIC (DRAINAGE) VENOUS SEGMENTS

The segments of the liver are defined as subdivisions of its parenchyma, based on the arterial and portal supply as well as on the biliary and venous drain-age. The segments, however, are not separated by septa of connective tissue.

The historical background of the segments of the liver is relatively short. In fact, the anatomy of the segments has been known for many years but application of this knowledge for surgical purpose is recent, especially in comparison to the chronol-ogy of the identification and classification of seg-ments in other organs. Although known for a long time, it is obvious that the practical importance of the anatomy of the segments depended upon ad-vances in the technology related to surgery and pathology.

Traditional division and nomenclature of the liver were based on its surface morphology and anatomical relationships, and were directed by descriptive guidelines: right, left, quadrate, and caudate lobes, the latter comprising in turn the caudate and papillary processes.

The new or segmental division of the liver takes into account primarily the tridimensional arrange-ment of vascular (blood supply and drainage, lymph drainage) and ductal (biliary drainage) com-ponents as well as the nerve supply of the surgically removable independent territories of the liver. The hepatic angio-architecture shows very well that these segments are separate, supplied by isolated pedicles, and their independence allows for the performance of partial hepatectomy [15].

The characteristics of the segmental division of the liver are (a) the individual supply and drainage of each territory, (b) the constant pattern in the arrangement of vascular, ductal, and nerve ele-ments, (c) the presence of eight porto-bilio-arterial segments intertwined with four hepatic segments,

(d) the hepatic veins bridging the limits between porto-bilio-arterial segments, and (e) the permanent or temporary independence of the segments and, when temporary, at least of sufficient duration for the performance of the surgical procedure, such as partial hepatectomy, single or multiple segment-ectomy.

The most demonstrable background for recog-nition of liver segments was found in the intra-parenchymatous distribution of the portal vein, of the hepatic artery, of lymph vessels and nerves, and of the arrangement of the biliary ducts, which happen to run together (ordinarily an element representative of each component). On the other hand, the rootlets and roots of the hepatic veins, as expected, follow a course separate from the men-tioned elements. The major trunks of the hepatic veins occupy intersegmental positions and each drains adjacent porto-bilio-arterial segments.

3. HEPATON, LOBULE, SEGMENT, LOBE

For practical and mnemonic purposes, the seg-mental arrangement of the liver can be considered as the magnification of the oversimplified classic liver lobule. This lobule is, according to Elias, an ephemeral expression of a field of pressure gradient [16]. In addition, one can extrapolate the topog-raphy of the vascular, ductal, and nerve elements of the hepaton (the supracellular morphological and functional unit of the liver) to the entire organ in order to better understand the framework in which the segments and their pedicles are arranged. (Analogous to nephron, neuron, and osteon, a he-paton represents the minimum amount of paren-chyma able to function as the entire liver.) In fact, a section through a hepatic lobule or acinus as well as a stereoscopic diagram of hepatic structure show that (a) branches of the portal vein, (b) radicles of the biliary tree, (c) branches of the hepatic artery, (d) lymphatic vessels, and (e) nerve elements run together in angles of each polyhedral lobule; where-as the small central vein, a rootlet or a tributary of the hepatic (formerly called suprahepatic) vein, occupies the center (as implied in the name), the core, or the axis of the lobule (Fig. 1).

Considering the elements (artery and bile duct) that are located in the angles of the hepatic lobule as

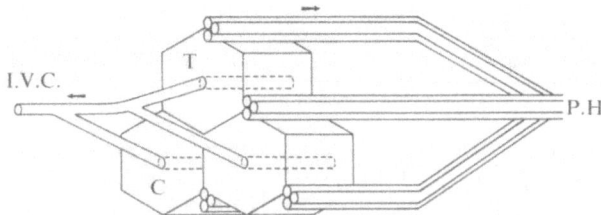

Figure 1. Simplified diagram of three liver lobules that illustrate portal triads (T), the elements of which unite and lead ultimately to the porta hepatis (P.H.), while the central veins (C) join and lead ultimately to the inferior vena cava (I.V.C.). The location of the triads and of the central veins reminds one of the different arrangement of porto-bilio-arterial (portal) segments and of hepatic venous segments as well as their interdigitation.

satellites or 'comitantes' of the portal branches, the name portal triad (or tetrad or pentad, if one also counts the lymphatic and/or nervous elements) can be applied. Disregarding for purposes of simplification the lymphatic and nervous components, the *portal triad* is made up of a branch of the portal vein (representative of *vasa publica*), a branch of the hepatic artery (representative of *vasa privata*), and a rootlet of the bile ducts (the interlobular bile ductule). A comprehensive name for all these structures could, therefore, be 'porto-bilio-arterial' elements (the so-called Glissonian system) or, simply, 'portal' elements, as they seem to follow, or to be followed by, the portal ramification or distribution in the parenchyma of the liver.

It is apparent that the arrangement of the porto-bilio-arterial elements does not coincide with that of the hepatic venous elements. In fact, these two sets of elements interdigitate, an arrangement that explains why the hepatic veins are intersegmental, that is, located on the boundaries of the porto-bilio-arterial segments, draining adjacent segments.

By comparing the liver (portal and hepatic) segments and other known visceral segments, one notices that to a certain extent the position of the central veins (or their corresponding larger vessels) is equivalent to that of the intersegmental veins of the lungs and of the kidney while the segmental pedicles of the spleen stand alone by not resembling the other parenchymatous organs in this respect. Another exclusive feature of liver segmentation resides in the different location of the segmental pedicles; the porto-bilio-arterial segments have pedicles at the level of the hilum or porta hepatis, whereas the hepatic venous segments are drained by veins directed toward the inferior vena cava. Final-

ly, one or more segments are contained in the traditional lobes of the liver.

Carrying the microscopic image to the entire liver and primarily utilizing plastic injection and corrosion specimens, it is easy to visualize and understand the different topography of the porto-bilio-arterial elements and of the hepatic venous elements. As pointed out, this difference leads to the identification of 'portal' (porto-bilio-arterial) segments and 'hepatic venous' segments, and to the recognition that the segmental pedicles do not contain all the elements relating to each segment: the porto-bilio-arterial elements of a segment have to be reached from the hepatic hilum, while the hepatic vein(s) draining the segment will be found at the limit between segments, which can be better identified when one (or more) vascular element(s) of the segmental pedicle is temporarily or permanently ligated.

4. HISTORICAL BACKGROUND OF SEGMENTATION OF THE LIVER

A brief survey of the literature shows that several descriptions, implicit or explicit, of the segments of the liver have been published with a number of classifications and variable nomenclature, and with the use of a wide variety of techniques that have given rather consistent results. The most commonly known are contained in papers, theses, books, or monographs [1, 15, 17–19, 20–45].

Comparison between the descriptions of liver segmentation presented by the authors mentioned above indicated that the variations, oscillating around a medium, which is the most frequent type, can be explained by observation of different samples of the population. The average pattern, however, was found and can be utilized as a basis for study and practical application [1], especially in surgery and pathology.

5. NOMENCLATURE AND NUMBERING OF THE SEGMENTS OF THE LIVER

The variable terminology used by the investigators is explained by the fact that the segments were studied in situ, in the isolated liver, in the ana-

4

tomical position for description, or in another position, considering the middle of the organ or the sagittal plane of the human body as the major reference.

The International Anatomical Nomenclature Committee [46] recognized that there is not yet complete agreement among authorities on segmentation. It is hoped that a recommendation will be prepared by the committee for adoption of a terminology that will satisfy the majority. Toward this goal, the following nomenclature, numbering of segments, and naming of fissural planes and elements of segmental pedicles will serve as a subsidy to the Committee.

Previous excellent contributions on the subject by several authors, already quoted, were compared and correlated, and were again compared and correlated with the traditional morphological division. It was found that the correlations were conducive to an average or prevailing pattern in the intrahepatic distribution of the elements of the hepatic pedicle and of the venous drainage of the liver toward the inferior vena cava. In fact, it became evident that Couinaud's system of liver segmentation was the natural culmination of the pioneering work done or developed by the investigators mentioned above, as is demonstrated in his comprehensive monograph [33]. This conclusion was drawn on the basis of the confirmation of Couinaud's system of division and subdivision of the liver by several authors [1, 30, 35, 36, 39, 44, 45, 47, 48].

In our former department of anatomy (Faculty of Medicine, University of Minas Gerais, Belo Horizonte, Brazil), Nogueira [35, 36] was able to duplicate Couinaud's findings in 52 specimens and we reproduced his results in eight preparations in the department of anatomy of the Medical College of Ohio [45]. Based on our own experience and on the data of other investigators, we recommend the adoption of Couinaud's classification with slight modification and a few additions to the terminology and numbering of the hepatic venous segments (Fig. 2).

The portal (porto-bilio-arterial) segments are numbered clockwise with Roman numerals from I to VIII. The hepatic venous segments (venous drainage segments) interdigitate with the portal segments and are numbered clockwise in Arabic

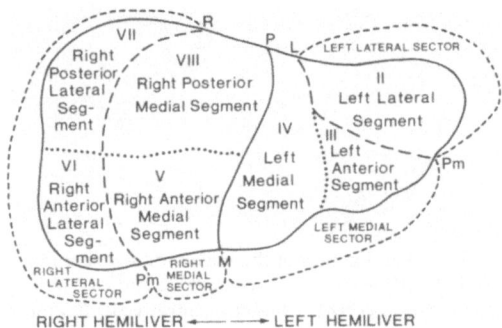

Figure 2. Diagram of the diaphragmatic aspect of the human liver showing the division into halves, sectors, and segments, based on the porto-bilio-arterial or, simply, portal distribution, according to Couinaud [33]. M-cystic fossa and P-fossa of the inferior vena cava, united by a line – MP – indicating the *median* fissural plane, on the surface of the liver; R and Pm, posterior and anterior extremities of the right paramedian fissural plane (broken line, long dashes – RPm); L and Pm, posterior and anterior ends of the left paramedian fissural plane (broken line, long dashes – LPm); dotted lines indicate intersegmental fissural planes. The limits of the sectors are indicated by broken lines (small dashes), external to the periphery of the liver. RPmMP, right medial sector; LPmMP, left medial sector. The dorsal segment (1 or I) is not visible.

numerals from 1 to 4, looking at the diaphragmatic aspect of the liver in situ from an anterosuperior view (the numbering is counterclockwise when looking at the visceral aspect of the liver).

The *portal segmentation* ordinarily presents the following pattern. The liver is divided into halves, that is, *right hemiliver* and *left hemiliver*, by a middle plane that runs from the middle of the cystic fossa to the left side of the fossa of the interior vena cava, except for the caudate lobe or dorsal sector, which remains undivided to constitute a segment (Fig. 3). Each hemiliver is subdivided into *sectors* by paramedian planes. (The adjective paramedian is used in

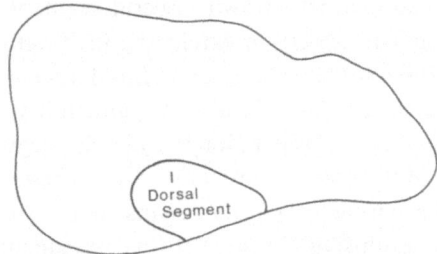

Figure 3. Diagram of the visceral aspect of the liver, reflected superiorly, to show the location of the dorsal segment I of the porto-bilio-arterial segmentation or dorsal segment 1 of the hepatic venous drainage segmentation (the territory is the same in either subdivision) and corresponds to the former caudate lobe.

relation to the isolated liver and not in relation to the median sagittal, or simply sagittal, plane of the body.) Each sector is further subdivided into eight portal *segments* by certain planes of separation, as illustrated (Figs. 2 and 3).

The *hepatic venous segments* correspond to the four independent territories drained by the hepatic veins into the inferior vena cava and are separated by fissural planes (Fig. 4).

The segment that is represented by the traditional caudate lobe is the only one where there is coincidence and not interdigitation of the two systems (Figs. 3 and 4). It is called the dorsal segment and is the only territory that corresponds at the same time to a portal segment (I) and to a hepatic venous segment (1).

The segments of the liver (Figs. 2–5) may be classified, named, and numbered as shown in Table 1.

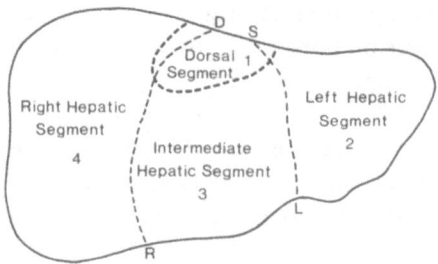

Figure 4. Diagram of the diaphragmatic aspect of the liver, showing the boundaries between the four hepatic venous segments (of blood drainage). The dorsal segment 1 is seen by transparency. The broken lines indicate the fissural planes: dorsal, to separate the homonymous sector and segment (caudate lobe); left (SL), and right (DR) fissural plane.

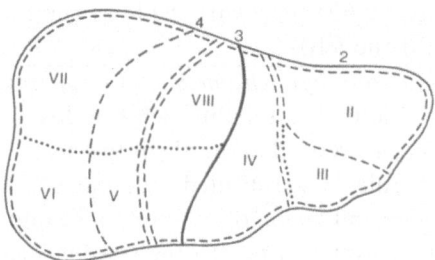

Figure 5. Diagram of the diaphragmatic aspect of the liver showing all the segments except dorsal segment 1 or I. The portal segments (II–VIII) are superimposed on the hepatic venous segments (2, 3, 4) or vice versa, to show their interdigitation and other relationships.

6. FISSURAL PLANES

The planes of separation, incision, or cleavage are called fissural planes because they are seen after vascular injection of a plastic substance, followed by corrosion, or after permanent or temporary surgical obliteration of a vessel. While a fissure, therefore, is a cleft (anatomically visible), a fissural plane is a cleavage or a potential plane of separation that may correspond to a limit or boundary of pathological lesions and may be artificially made.

The *fissural planes* of portal segmentation are (Figs. 2–4):

1) Median, main, or principal fissural plane between the hemilivers. The term *median* could be replaced by *central* if one wishes to avoid possible confusion with the median plane of the body. This

Table 1.

A. Portal (porto-bilio-arterial) segmentation

Left hemiliver	Dorsal sector[a] ...	dorsal segment (I): invisible on the diaphragmatic aspect
	Left lateral sector[a] ...	left lateral segment (II)
	Left medial sector ...	left anterior segment (III)
		left medial segment (IV)
Right hemiliver	Right medial sector ...	right anterior medial segment (V)
	Right lateral sector ...	right posterior medial segment (VIII): invisible on the visceral aspect
		right anterior lateral segment (VI)
		right posterior lateral segment (VII)

B. Hepatic venous segments (segments for blood drainage)

Dorsal hepatic venous segment (1)
Left hepatic venous segment (2)
Intermediate hepatic venous segment (3)
Right hepatic venous segment (4)

[a] Unisegmental sectors; the other sectors are bisegmental.

plane makes a 60° angle with the horizontal (opening toward the left).

2) *Right* and *left paramedian*, to separate the medial and lateral sectors, in each hemiliver. If the word *central* were chosen, then the term paramedian should be substituted by *paracentral*. The terms *medial* and *lateral* refer again to the middle of the isolated liver and not to the (median) sagittal plane of the body. The *right paramedian plane* has the anterior extremity at a point in the inferior margin of the liver situated between the median fissural plane and the right hepatic 'angle' (one-third from the latter). From this point, the plane runs 6 cm from and parallel to the right liver margin, then curves toward the left and ends at its posterior extremity (behind the termination of the right hepatic vein, on the right side of the inferior vena cava). This plane makes a 50° angle with the horizontal (opening toward the right). The *left paramedian plane* has the anterior extremity at a point in the inferior margin of the liver located midway between the round ligament and the left hepatic 'angle'. Its posterior extremity is situated to the left of the termination of the left hepatic vein. This plane almost transversely cuts the left lobe of the liver since it is curved, having the concavity toward the left and posteriorly; it has a transverse anterior portion and a sagittal posterior portion.

3) *Dorsal*, to separate the dorsal sector, which constitutes the segment (I) that corresponds to the traditional caudate lobe.

4) *Intersegmental*, between the following segments:

a) Left lateral segment (II) and left anterior segment (III) separated by the intersegmental plane, represented by the transverse portion of the left paramedian fissural plane (which is curved and not straight as the right paramedian fissural plane).

b) Left lateral segment (II) and left medial segment (IV), separated by the sagittal portion of left paramedian fissural plane.

c) Left anterior segment (III) and left medial segment (IV), separated by the left intersegmental fissural plane, which is the anterior continuation of the sagittal portion of the left paramedian fissural plane.

d) Left medial segment (IV) and right anterior medial segment (V), separated by the anterior portion of the median fissural plane.

e) Left medial segment (IV) and right posterior medial segment (VIII), separated by the intersegmental plane, represented by the posterior portion of the median fissural plane.

f) Right anterior medial segment (V) and right anterior lateral segment (VI), separated by the anterior portion of the right paramedian fissural plane.

g) Right anterior medial segment (V) and right posterior medial segment (VIII), separated by the medial portion of the transversal intersegmental fissural plane.

h) Right anterior lateral segment (VI) and right posterior lateral segment (VII), separated by the lateral portion of the transversal intersegmental fissural plane.

i) Right posterior lateral segment (VII) and right posterior medial segment (VIII), separated by the intersegmental fissural plane, represented by the posterior portion of the right paramedian fissural planes.

The four hepatic venous segments are separated by hepatic venous *fissural planes* (Fig. 4), which are the right, the left, and the dorsal:

a) The *dorsal*, to separate from the remaining liver the dorsal segment (1) that coincides with the portal segment (I).

b) The *left*, between the left hepatic venous segment (2) and the intermediate hepatic venous segment (3).

c) The *right*, between the intermediate hepatic venous segment (3) and the right hepatic venous segment (4).

The *dorsal fissural plane* can be divided into a right and a left portion as it separates the dorsal segment from the right and the left hemiliver.

The left hepatic fissural plane corresponds to the insertion of the falciform ligament on the diaphragmatic aspect and to the left longitudinal sulcus of the visceral aspect of the liver. Its anterior and posterior extremities correspond, respectively, to the insertion of the round ligament and to the dorsal termination of the sulcus of the ductus venosus. It is perpendicular to the visceral aspect of the liver, separates the left hepatic venous segment (traditional left lobe) from the intermediate hepatic venous segment, and is located midway between the left and the intermediate hepatic veins.

The *right hepatic fissural plane*, situated midway between the intermediate and the right hepatic veins, separates the intermediate from the right hepatic venous segment. It is slightly curved with the concavity toward the left. Its posterior extremity is found between the terminations, in the inferior vena cava, of the right and intermediate hepatic veins. Its anterior extremity corresponds most frequently to a point midway between the cystic fossa and the right anterior angle of the liver or, in other words, it is located between the anterior extremities of the median and the right paramedian fissural plane.

7. DESCRIPTION OF THE SEGMENTS AND SEGMENTAL PEDICLES

7.1. *Portal segmentation* (Fig. 6)

I) The *dorsal segment* is seen only on the visceral aspect of the liver. It corresponds to the caudate lobe and includes the deep hepatic parenchyma, behind the hilum; that is, between the portal vein and the inferior vena cava. It has boundaries with the left medial (IV), right posterior medial (VIII), and right posterior lateral (VII) segments. The old caudate lobe constitutes at the same time a portal segment (I) and a hepatic venous segment (1) from the standpoint of vascularization. The elements of its segmental *pedicle* are (a) three veins from the left branch of the portal vein; (b) one or two arteries from the left branch of the hepatic artery; (c) biliary ducts leading to the right and left roots of the hepatic duct; and (d) dorsal hepatic veins draining into the inferior vena cava, in the intermediate or in the left hepatic vein.

II) The *left lateral segment* is seen as an oval territory on visceral and diaphragmatic aspects of the liver in the extreme left of the organ. The *pedicle* of the left lateral segment is made up of (a) the homonymous vein (or angular vein) of the portal vein; (b) the homonymous artery, originating with the artery of segment III from a common trunk given off by the left branch of the hepatic artery; (c) the segmental biliary duct, which joins that of

segment III to form a large duct that in turn becomes the left root of the hepatic duct; (d) segmental veins that drain into the left hepatic vein.

III) The *left anterior segment*, triangular in shape, appears on both aspects of the liver. Its *pedicle* is formed by (a) two branches of the vein of the left medial segment (IV) from the portal vein (left branch); (b) the segmental artery, from the left branch of the hepatic artery; (c) the segmental biliary duct that leads into the left root of the hepatic duct; (d) segmental veins draining into the left hepatic vein.

IV) The *left medial segment*, rectangular in shape, appears on both aspects of the liver, but is seen only partially in the visceral aspect since the posterior half is covered by segment I. Its *pedicle* contains (a) several branches of the vein of the left medial segment (IV), in turn a branch of the portal vein (left branch); (b) the segmental artery, a collateral given off by the left branch of the hepatic artery; (c) the segmental biliary duct empties in the trunk formed by the confluence of the ducts of segments I and II; (d) the left root of the intermediate hepatic vein and its affluents.

V) The *right anterior medial segment* is seen in both aspects of the liver as a quadrangular territory. Its *pedicle* comprises (a) a group of veins, which are the anterior branches of the vein of the right medial sector, in turn a branch of the portal vein (right branch); (b) the segmental arteries originated from the artery of the right medial sector; (c) the biliary ducts that lead to the biliary duct of the right medial sector; (d) segmental veins that drain into the right root of the intermediate hepatic vein and a few that are tributaries of the right hepatic vein.

VI) The *right anterior lateral segment* is visible on both aspects of the right anterior 'angle' of the liver. Its *pedicle* consists of (a) one or more branches of the vein of the right lateral sector, a branch of the portal vein (right branch); (b) segmental arteries originated from the artery of the right lateral sector; (c) segmental biliary ducts which join those of segment VII to form the biliary duct of the right lateral sector; (d) the roots and affluents of the right hepatic vein. In 20% of the cases, Nogueira [35] observed that the right root of the intermediate hepatic vein contributes to the drainage of this segment.

8

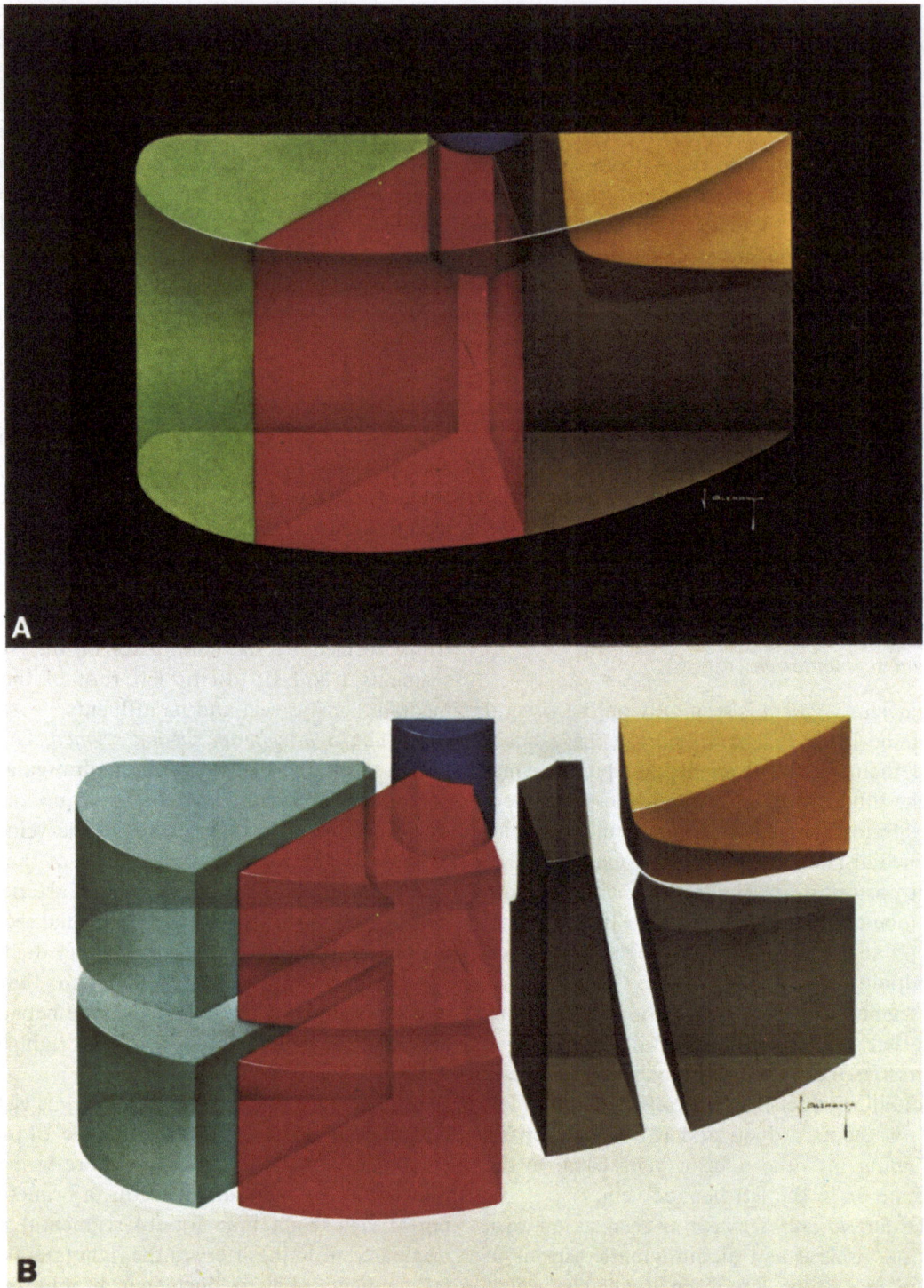

Figure 6. Ideal diagrams of the sectors and segments of the liver in transparent colors to give their approximate arrangement. In diagrams *A–C*, colors indicate the following: *blue*, dorsal sector, segment 1 or I or caudate lobe; *yellow*, left lateral sector or segment II; *brown*, left medial sector, made up of segments III and IV (left anterior and left medial, respectively); *red*, right medial sector, made up of segments V and VIII (right anterior medial and right posterior medial, respectively); *green*, right lateral sector, made up of segments VI and VII (right anterior lateral and right posterior lateral, respectively). The sectors are made up of one or more segments.

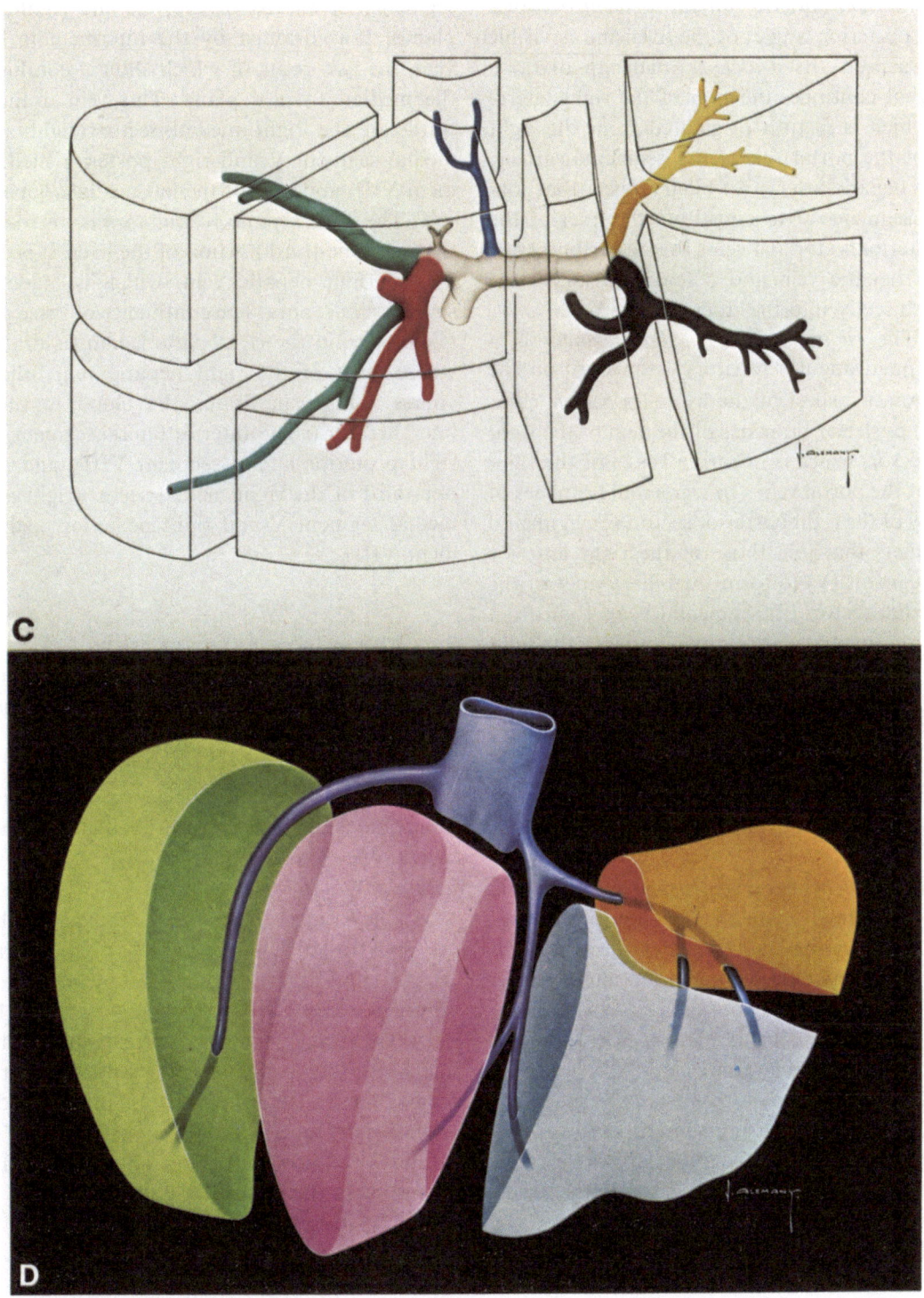

In diagram *D*, colors indicate the following: *yellow*, left lateral sector; *light blue*, left medial sector; *red*, right medial sector; *green*, right lateral sector; *dark blue*, inferior vena cava and hepatic veins (left, intermediate, and right). The hepatic veins are intersegmental and drain adjacent portal segments. Portal segments interdigitate with hepatic venous segments. Courtesy of Professors J.G. Dangelo, C.A. Fattini, and C.E.D. Nogueira, Federal University of Minas Gerais, School of Medicine, Belo Horizonte, Minas Gerais, Brazil.

10

VII) The *right posterior lateral segment* occupies the right posterior 'angle' of the liver and is visible on both aspects. Its *pedicle* is made up of (a) a branch that continues the vein of the right lateral sector, which is in turn originated from the right branch of the portal vein; (b) a segmental artery, from the hepatic artery; (c) biliary ducts that join those of segment VI to constitute the duct of the right posterior sector; (d) veins that are tributary of the right hepatic vein and a few accessory veins draining directly into the inferior vena cava.

VIII) The *right posterior medial segment* is a roughly quadrangular territory, seen only on the diaphragmatic aspect of the liver. Its *pedicle* comprises (a) posterior branches of the vein of the right medial sector, which is in turn a vessel of the right branch of the portal vein; (b) segmental branches of the artery of the right posterior sector; (c) segmental biliary ducts that join those of the right anterior medial segment (V) to form the biliary duct of the right medial sector; (d) segmental veins that drain into the intermediate hepatic vein and into the right hepatic vein.

7.2. Hepatic venous segmentation (Fig. 6)

The hepatic venous segments are the territories drained by the homonymous veins.

1) The *dorsal hepatic venous segment* (1) is the same as the dorsal segment (I) of the portal segmentation. It is the only segment in which the vascular elements coincide and do not interdigitate. It is not visible on the diaphragmatic aspect of the liver. Its veins are small and, in most cases, one vein drains into the inferior vena cava.

2) The *left hepatic venous segment* corresponds to the old left lobe. The left hepatic vein is formed by two roots (right and left) at the level of the left lateral segment (III). This vein drains the traditional left lobe, which includes segments II and III, and part of segment IV. The left hepatic vein or its roots cross the left paramedian fissural plane, instead of following the plane, and cannot be used as a landmark. Contrary to this vein, the right and intermediate hepatic veins are the main reference for the recognition of the respective fissural plane.

3) The *intermediate hepatic venous segment* is separated from the left and right hepatic venous segments by means of the left and right fissural planes. It is drained by the intermediate hepatic vein, the two roots of which show a confluence in the median fissural plane. This vein drains two-thirds of the right medial sector (right anterior medial segment V and right posterior medial segment VIII, and part of the left medial segment IV).

4) The *right hepatic venous segment* is located in the right one-third portion of the liver. It is drained by the right hepatic vein, which is made up of several small roots. The confluence of these rootlets takes place in the right paramedian fissural plane, where most of the right hepatic vein follows its course. This vein drains the blood of the right lateral sector (right anterior lateral segment VI and right posterior lateral segment VIII), and at least one-third of the right medial sector (right anterior medial segment V and right posterior medial segment VIII).

8. COMPARISON BETWEEN THE MORPHOLOGICAL AND THE SEGMENTAL DIVISIONS OF THE LIVER AND THEIR FISSURAL PLANES

In comparing the boundaries of the traditional morphological lobes of the liver and portal segments, one observes that:

a) The formerly designated left hepatic lobe corresponds to the left lateral sector (left lateral segment II) plus a portion of the left medial sector (left anterior segment III), i.e., segments II and III.

b) The former right lobe corresponds to the right hemiliver (four segments) plus a portion of the left medial sector (segment IV). In other words, the former right lobe includes segments VIII, VII, VI, V, and IV, except for the portion of segment IV that corresponds to the former quadrate lobe.

c) The former caudate lobe corresponds to the dorsal sector; that is, the dorsal segment (I and 1).

d) The former quadrate lobe, as mentioned above, corresponds to a portion of the left medial sector or of the left medial segment (IV), seen from the visceral aspect.

The comparison between the hepatic venous segments and the portal sectors or segments can be made on each aspect of the liver.

a) *Diaphragmatic aspect* (Fig. 5). The left hepatic venous segment (segment 2) comprises the left lateral sector (segment II) and the left anterior segment (segment III) of the left medial sector.

The intermediate hepatic venous segment (segment 3) contains part of the left medial sector (that is, only segment IV of the latter), plus part of the right medial sector (that is, the medial portions of the right medial anterior segment V and of the right medial posterior segment VIII).

The right hepatic venous segment (segment 4) corresponds to a portion of the right medial sector (lateral portions of the right medial anterior segment V and of the right medial posterior segment VIII), plus the entire right lateral sector (segment VI plus segment VII).

In summary, the right and left hepatic venous segments include the entire respective portal sector plus segments of other sectors, whereas the intermediate hepatic venous segment corresponds only to portal segments.

b) *Visceral aspect*. Segment 1 corresponds to the dorsal sector, which is the dorsal segment I. Segment 2 has the same extension as described for the diaphragmatic aspect. Segment 3 corresponds to a portion of the right medial sector (part of segment V) and to a part of the left medial sector (segment IV). Segment 4 includes the right lateral sector (segments VI and VII) and part of the right medial sector (part of segment V).

Comparison between the old hepatic lobes and the hepatic venous segments shows that:

a) The caudate lobe corresponds to the dorsal segment 1.
b) The old left lobe is represented by segment 2.
c) The old right lobe contains segments 3 and 4.
d) The quadrate lobe includes less than the left half of segment 3.

Comparison between the fissural planes of the portal and hepatic venous segments indicates that the dorsal fissural plane is the same in both types of segmentation: it separates the dorsal sector (segment 1 or segment I) from the rest of the liver.

According to Couinaud [33] and Couinaud and Nogueira [37], on the diaphragmatic aspect of the liver, the left hepatic fissural plane coincides only partially with the left paramedian fissural plane. The coincidence occurs in the sagittal tract of the left paramedian fissural plane; that is, in the posterior sagittal intersegmental fissural plane, which separates segment II and the posterior portion of segment IV. Anteriorly, the left hepatic fissural plane coincides with the left anterior sagittal intersegmental fissural plane (between segments III and IV).

The right hepatic fissural plane is located midway between the right paramedian and the medial fissural plane.

On the visceral aspect, the left hepatic fissural plane coincides with the anterior and posterior left sagittal intersegmental fissural planes; it corresponds to the left longitudinal sulcus, between segments II and III on one side and segment IV on the other.

In the visceral aspect, the right hepatic fissural plane is situated between the right paramedian and the median fissural plane.

9. APPLIED ANATOMY OF THE SEGMENTATION OF THE LIVER

Since the liver is uniform in structure and function, its segmentation is less relevant physiologically than pathologically, clinically, and surgically. A successful hepatectomy [49], which included removal of the right hemiliver and a portion of the left hemiliver (segment IV), performed after several isolated reported cases [50], provided evidence that such a large resection of the liver was compatible with human survival. Up to 80% of the parenchyma can be removed with little alteration in hepatic function [51].

Circumscribed pathological processes, or those incipient lesions that can be diagnosed early, may be eliminated by ablation of the segment or segments in which they are localized, thus preserving the healthy portion of the hepatic parenchyma. Knowledge of the segmental localization of lesions ultimately leads to conservative surgical repair instead of mutilating surgery, restricting resection as much as possible to the limits of the lesion and maximally respecting the function of the organ with minimum sacrifice of parenchyma.

In subsegmental hepatectomy, a wedge resection (that is, removal of a portion of the parenchyma smaller than a segment and without anatomic dissection planes) can be performed for biopsy and in cases of benign tumors or cysts [50].

Preferential localization of pathological processes in the liver had been known for a long time and related, for instance, to the streams of blood in the portal vein leading more to the left or to the right lobe (of the old division). More specifically, degeneration of hepatic lobes limited to a territory of the main branches of the portal vein had been observed [52]. This relationship was experimentally confirmed [53] by injecting radioactive phosphorus in various tributaries of the portal vein and in the jugular vein of animals.

Recognition of segments, based on the intra-parenchymatous distribution of vessels and biliary ducts in independent territories having their own pedicles, led to the performance of typical or 'réglées' segmentectomies [54].

Hemostasis is produced by preventive ligation of the pedicle of the segments to be removed. In one case of resection of the left lobe (segments II and III) because of a malignant cholangioma, Alves [55] had to keep the entire hepatic pedicle ligated for 9 min without causing any damage to the patient.

After segmental pedicle ligation, the liver is sectioned along the fissural planes. At the level of the fissural planes, there is change in color and the incision along the margin of discoloration, resulting from the occlusion of the hepatic artery, is practically bloodless. The corresponding hepatic veins or tributaries that cross the limits of the segments are clamped and ligated. The denuded surface of the liver can be covered, when possible, by a flap of the falciform ligament [50].

Resection of the liver may follow the portal, the hepatic venous segmentation, or both. Ligation of vessels precedes parenchyma resection.

9.1. Partial hepatectomy based on portal (porto-bilio-arterial) segmentation can be performed by using hilar or fissural via to approach the pedicle. The hilar access is the most usual except to approach the pedicle of the right medial sector (segments V and VIII). In this case, and in those showing tumors and adhesions that make access

difficult, the fissural approach is the alternate route. The cleavage line follows, for example, the median fissural plane, allowing direct access to the portal pedicle that is to be ligated.

The fissural planes between portal segments are practically avascular, from the surgical standpoint, except for the presence of the hepatic veins deep in the parenchyma. The latter must naturally be preserved, limiting ligation to their tributaries belonging to the segment intended for removal.

As examples of surgical interventions that are based on portal segmentation, one can cite

a) Right or left hemihepatectomy.
b) Sectoriectomy, which comprises one or more of the following:
   right lateral,
   right medial,
   left medial,
   left lateral and dorsal.
c) Segmentectomy: of the eight segments, according to Couinaud, only the right anterior medial (V), the right posterior medial (VIII), and the right posterior lateral (VII) cannot be individually resected, and are thus anatomical units and not anatomicosurgical units.
d) Intermediate hepatectomy: ablation of both medial sectors, considered impractical.
e) Extended hemihepatectomy: hemihepatectomy plus ablation of a sector of the opposite side.
f) Extended sectoriectomy: resection of a sector plus an adjacent segment.
g) Associated segmentectomy: resection of two segments belonging to different sectors.

9.2. Partial resection of the liver based on the hepatic venous segmentation is divided into simple and multiple segmentectomies.

Simple segmentectomies are (a) dorsal hepatic venous segmentectomy (ablation of segment 1): (b) left hepatic venous segmentectomy – corresponding to the 'left lobectomy' of the old terminology, to associate segmentectomy (II and III), the first that was performed (segment 2); (c) intermediate hepatic venous segmentectomy (resection of segment 3); (d) right hepatic venous segmentectomy (ablation of segment 4).

Multiple segmentectomies are those in which more than one segment is removed.

9.3. Mixed hepatectomies correspond to resection of a liver territory following a portal fissural plane and a hepatic venous fissural plane.

The limitations imposed on surgery and the application of the views from medical practice show that partial hepatectomy can be performed in a number of anatomicosurgical segments that are less than the described anatomical segments.

Segmentectomy may be used for biopsy, for removal of localized benign tumors, for trauma, and for cysts [50, 51].

The applicability to humans of segmental orthotopic liver transplantation, shown feasible in mammals, has been discussed in view of biliary atretic infant treatment and hepatic resections in cases of tumors or as emergencies in trauma [56].

REFERENCES

1. DiDio LJA (1958) Il problema delle zone vascolari epatiche nei rapporti con la patologia e chirurgia del fegato. Monit Zool Ital [Suppl] 67: 1–33
2. Graves FT (1954) The anatomy of the intrarenal arteries and its application to segmental resection of the kidney. Br J Surg 42:132–139
3. DiDio LJA (1955) Macro and microscopic data on the vena renalis sinistra in man. The venous renal segments [in Portuguese]. Chairmanship thesis, Univ São Paulo, Brazil
4. DiDio LJA (1956) Applied anatomy of the renal veins. The importance of the mesenterico-aortic forceps. The vascular renal segments [in Portuguese]. An Fac Med Univ Minas Gerais Belo Horizonte 16: 51–202
5. DiDio LJA (1961) Anatomicosurgical vascular segments of the human kidney. Anat Rec 139: 299
6. Neder AM (1958) Anatomical study of the splenic venous segments and on their drainage in man [in Portuguese]. Fac Med Univ Minas Gerais Belo Horizonte 18:265–310
7. Zappalá A (1958) Anatomical study of the terminal division of the arteria lienalis. Arterial segments of the spleen [in Portuguese]. PhD dissertation, University of Minas Gerais, Belo Horizonte, Brazil
8. Zappalá A (1959) Contribution to the anatomy of the splenic vessels and segments. Anatomical data in man and experimental in dogs for partial splenectomy [in Portuguese]. Chairmanship thesis, University of Recife, Brazil
9. Zappalá A (1963) The anatomical basis for segmental resection of the spleen [in Portuguese]. An Fac Med Univ Recife 23:7–36
10. Campos-Christo MB (1960) Splenectomies partielles réglées: à propos de 3 cas opérés. Presse Med 68:485–486
11. Campos-Christo MB (1963) Anatomical and experimental bases for partial spleenectomies [in Portuguese]. Rev Bras Cir 46:80–90
12. Pina JAE (1979) Arterial territories of the spleen. Lisboa: Univ Nova de Lisboa
13. Guerra AJ (1976) Contribution to the study of the vascular territories of the human stomach in adults [in Portuguese]. In: Proceedings 11th Brazilian Congress of Anatomy, Niteroi, Rio de Janeiro, Brazil, pp 184–186
14. DiDio LJA, Rodrigues H (1978) Anatomical study of the arterial segments in the human heart [in Portuguese]. In: Proceedings 5th Pan American Congress of Anatomy, São Paulo, Brazil, p 144
15. Couinaud C (1952) Hépatectomies gauches lobaires et segmentaires. J Chir 68:697–715
16. Elias H (1955) Liver morphology. Biol Rev Cambridge Philos Soc 30:263–310
17. Rex H (1888) Beiträge zur Morphologie der Saugerleber.

Morphol Jahrb Anat Entwicklungsgesch 14:517–616
18. Hjortsjö CH (1948) Die Anatomie der intrahepatischen Gallengänge beim Menschen, mittels Röntgen- und Injektionstechnik studiert nebst Beiträgen zur Kenntnis der inneren Lebertopographie. Lunds Univ Arsskr Avd 2 44: 1–112
19. Hjortsjö CH (1951) The topography of the intrahepatic duct systems. Acta Anat (Basel) 11:599–615
20. Elias H, Petty D (1952) Gross anatomy of the blood vessels and ducts within the human liver. Am J Anat 90:59–111
21. Elias H (1953) Functional morphology of the liver. Res Serv Med 37:1–25
22. Healey JE, Schroy PC (1953) Anatomy of the biliary ducts within the human liver. AMA Arch Surg 66:599–616
23. Healey JE, Schroy PC, Sorensen RJ (1953) The intrahepatic distribution of the hepatic artery in man. J Int Coll Surg 20:133–148
24. Couinaud C (1954) Lobes et segments hépatiques. Presse Med 62:709–712
25. Elias H (1954) Segments of the liver. Surgery 36:950–952
26. Healey JE (1954) Clinical anatomic aspects of radical hepatic surgery. J Int Coll Surg 22:542–549
27. Gans H (1955) Introduction to hepatic surgery. Amsterdam: Elsevier
28. Gans H (1955) The intrahepatic anatomy and its repercussion on surgery. Arch Chir Neerl 7:131–146
29. Gans H, Bax HR (1955) Partial resection of the liver in early carcinoma of the gall-bladder. In: Proceedings Congrés International de Chirurgie, Copenhagen, pp 1–13
30. Pinheiro LCSF (1955) Das Hepatectomias Regradas. Rio de Janeiro: Editora Grafica Seleções Brasileiras, 171 pp
31. Hjortsjö CH (1956) The intrahepatic ramification of the portal vein. Lunds Univ Arsskr Avd 2 52:1–30
32. Hjortsjö CH (1957) Leverns Segmentering. Uppsala: Lunds Universitet
33. Couinaud C (1957) Le Foie: études Anatomiques et Chirurgicales. Paris: Masson et Cie
34. Goldsmith NA, Woodburne RT (1957) The surgical anatomy pertaining to liver resection. Surg Gynecol Obstet 105:310–318
35. Nogueira CED (1958) Pesquisas sôbre as *Venae Hepaticae* em relação aos planos divisores dos territorios anatomocirurgicos no Homen. PhD dissertation, Surgery, Fac Med Univ Minas Gerais, 95 pp
36. Nogueira CED (1958) Bases anatomicas das hepatectomias regradas. Rev Assoc Med Minas Gerais 9:191–193
37. Couinaud C, Nogueira CED (1958) The suprahepatic veins in man. Acta Anat (Basel) 34:84–110
38. Elias H (1964) Zur chirurgischen Anatomie der Leber. Verh Anat Ges 59. Vers München (1963); Ergeb Anat Anz 113:235–252
39. Michailov SS, Kagan JJ, Archipowa SE (1966) Anatomische

14

Untersuchungen über den Segmentaufbau der menschlichen Leber. Anat Anz 119:317–336

40. Platzer W, Maurer H (1966) Zur Segmenteinteilung der Leber. Acta Anat (Basel) 63:8–31
41. Elias H, Sherrick JC (1967) Morphology of the liver. New York: Academic
42. Elias H (1970) Surgical anatomy of the liver. Recent Results Cancer Res 26:116–136
43. Healey JE (1970) Vascular anatomy of the liver. Ann NY Acad Sci 170:8–17
44. Mikhailov GA (1970) Individual variations in hepatic lobes, segments and vessels. In: Proceedings 9th International Congress of Anatomy, Leningrad, pp 1–5
45. DiDio LJA (1978) The anatomical background for partial hepatectomy. In: Proceedings 5th Pan American Congress of Anatomy, São Paulo, Brazil, pp 198–204
46. International Anatomical Nomenclature Committee (1977) Nomina Anatomica. Amsterdam: Excerpta Medica, 4th edn
47. Mancuso M, Natalini E, Del Grande G (1955) Contributo alla conoscenza della struttura segmentaria del fegato in rapporto al problema della resezione epatica. Policlinico Sez Chir 62, apud Couinaud

48. Mancuso M, Natalini E, Del Grande G (1955) Anatomia e tecnica chirurgica dell'exeresi tipica lobare e segmentaria del settore sinistro del fegato. Policlinico Sez Chir 64:127–150
49. Lortat-Jacob TC, Robert HG, Henry C (1952) Un cas d'hépatectomie droite réglée. Mem Acad Chir 78:244–250
50. Schwartz SI (1964) Surgical diseases of the liver. New York: McGraw-Hill
51. Schwartz SI (1979) Principles of surgery. New York: McGraw-Hill, 3rd edn
52. Hoche ML (1925) Sur l'existence de territoires distincts dans le domaine de la veine porte hépatique. CR Soc Biol 92:717–718
53. Hahn PF, Donald D, Grier RC (1945) Portal circulation: physiologic bilaterality. Am J Physiol 143:105–107
54. Patel J, Couinaud C (1952) Les bases anatomiques des hépatectomies réglées. In: Proceedings 16th International Congress Surgeons, Copenhagen, pp 1–18. Bruxelles: Impr Méd Sci
55. Alves JR (1957) Das Hepatectomias. Rev Bras Cir 34:23–31
56. Smith B (1969) Segmental liver transplantation from a living donor. J Pediatr Surg 4:126–132

2. FINE STRUCTURE OF HUMAN LIVER CELLS

F.G. CARAMIA, M. PICCOLI, A. MODESTI, M.R. TORRISI, and L. FRATI

1. INTRODUCTION

Electron-microscopic investigation of the liver is a subject of more than ordinary interest and there are still numerous studies regarding the functions and morphology of the hepatocyte. The cellular components that have received the most attention, however, in the last decade have been the surface areas of the hepatic membranes and the Golgi apparatus.

By combining morphological and chemical techniques, Bolender et al. [1] have reported that the ER (endoplasmic reticulum) membranes show differences with respect to the amount of marker-enzyme activity. Thus, the generally accepted hypothesis that the liver lobule consists of heterogenous hepatocytes with respect to their structure and function has been confirmed. The Golgi apparatus has been extensively studied with the electron microscope and several detailed observations of cytochemical activity on isolated Golgi fractions have been presented. These investigations show, for example, that the Golgi apparatus participates in the secretion of most of the serum proteins; they provide evidence for a sequential progress of secretory products through the various components of the Golgi apparatus.

The nonparenchymal cells of the liver also possess characteristics that suggest different functional roles. Recently it has been reported that Kupffer and endothelial cells bind and internalize rapidly different iodinated glycoproteins; thus, endothelial cells are more active than Kupffer cells, and endothelial cells recognize a different set of glycoproteins than do the hepatocytes.

The liver consists of at least four different cell types of which the hepatocytes represent the major component (70%). The hepatocytes, all basically similar in their appearance, have a polygonal shape with five or more surfaces structurally and functionally different (Figs. 1, 2, and 8) [2]. The hepatocyte surfaces show two distinct regions: (1) Those exposed to the perivascular Disse space and there to the lumen of bile canaliculi, both studded with numerous microvilli (see also chapter 3). (2) The bile canaliculus is separated by remainder of the surface of adjoining hepatocytes by two bands of tight junctions that segregate the canaliculus content from the narrow intercellular cleft and from the perisinusoidal space of Disse (Figs. 8 and 9). In addition to the parenchymal cells, three categories of nonparenchymal cells have been described: the lining endothelial cells, the Kupffer cells, and the fat-storing cells.

2. HEPATOCYTES

2.1. Nucleus

The nucleus of the liver cell is generally a spheroid body within the cell (Fig. 1). It is delimited by a thin membrane consisting of two layers (outer and inner membranes) with an internal space of 100 Å. The membrane is largely fenestrated, and gaps (pores) of 40–100 μm in size are suitable for rapid exchanges between nucleoplasm and cytoplasm. Various opinions can be found on the function of these gaps and, because of the presence or absence of an occlusive pore's material, the function of exchange can be stressed or not. Actually there is no evidence of any identified macromolecular compound that crosses preferentially out of the nucleus through these gaps. Occasionally, RNA-containing material has been observed as granules crossing the pores.

The outer leaflet of the membrane is closely

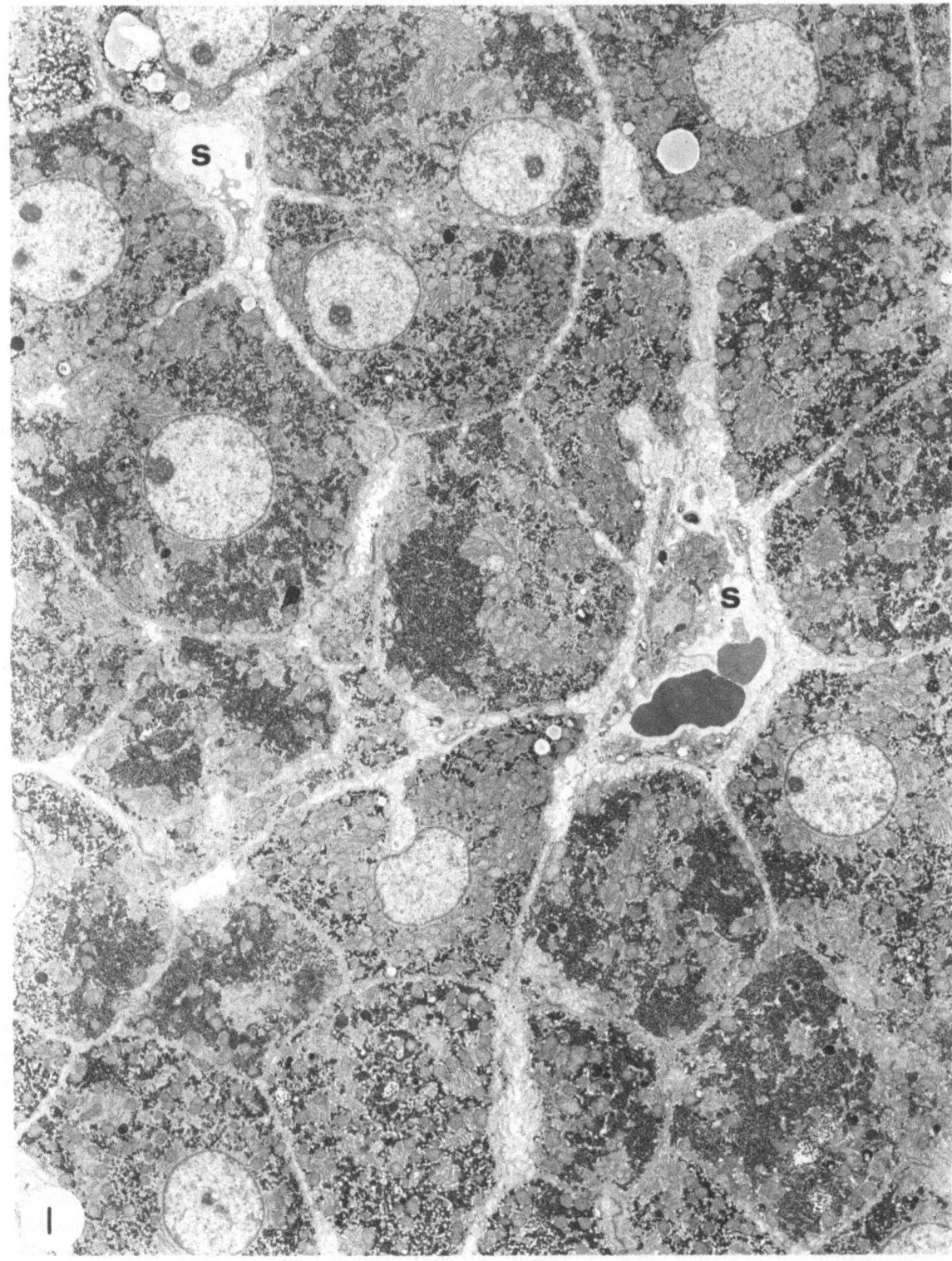

Figure 1. Low-power micrograph of part of a human hepatic lobule. The polygonal liver cells show five or six sides, of which either one or two contact the Disse space around visible sinusoids (S). Most of the remaining sides are in contact, along part of their length, with the extensions of the Disse space, interrupted at intervals by bile canaliculi; ×2800.

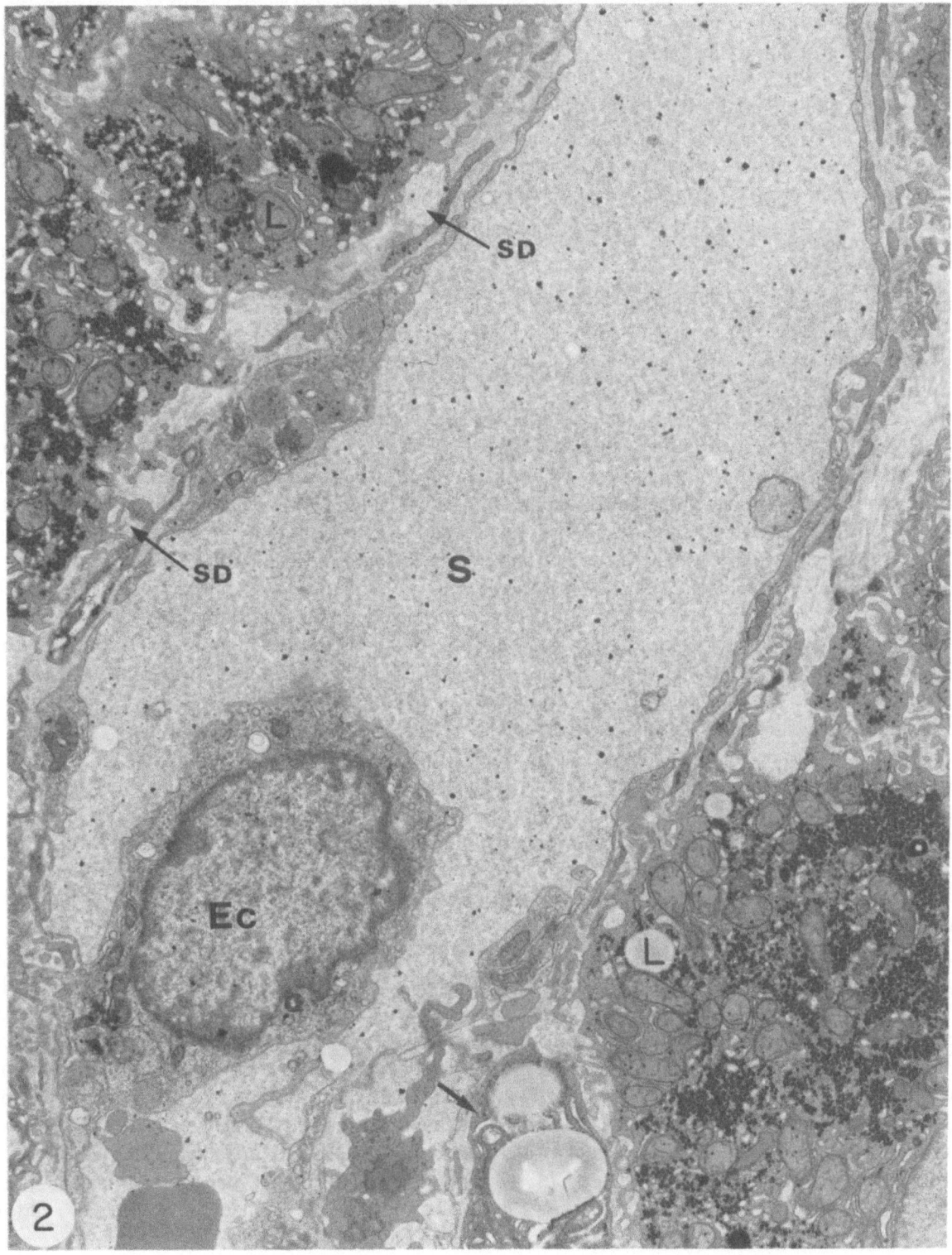

Figure 2. Human liver cells bordering on a sinusoid (S). Numerous irregularly oriented microvilli extend into the perisinusoidal space of Disse (SD). The perivascular space itself contains microvilli and reticular fibers. A fat-storing cell (arrow) in the Disse space and a sinusoid-lining cell (endothelial cell) (Ec) are also shown; L, lipid; × 6000.

related to the cytoplasmic membranes and an exchange between the perinuclear space and the endoplasmic reticulum is thus made.

Large intranuclear glycogen bodies were found in both diabetic and nondiabetic patients [3]. Periportal hepatocytes in biopsies can show rounded glycogen bodies, of monoparticulate type, without a limiting membrane [4].

2.2. Nucleolus

Usually eccentrically placed in the nucleus, the nucleolus of liver cells has a regular spherical or oval shape and varies greatly in size and density from one hepatocyte to another (Fig. 1). It is recognized to be the site of the synthesis of ribosomal RNA. Electron-microscopic studies have shown that the nucleolus is made up of four principal parts: the fibrillar and granular components, the nucleolar chromatin, and the amorphous matrix [5]. At high magnification, the fibrillar and granular components (nucleolonema) form a network of anastomosing strands in which condensed chromatin can be present to coalesce with the chromatin located adjacent to the nuclear envelope. In the meshes of the nucleolonema, a fibrillar substance of somewhat lower density called *amorphous matrix* is frequently associated with the fibrillar or granular components. Such material varies in density from very low to great, and is stained less intensely after pepsin digestion [6]. The sucrose density gradient sedimentation analysis has revealed that the fibrillar and granular components of the nucleolus contain 6S and 28S RNA [7].

2.3. Cytoplasmic inclusions

Inclusions, such as glycogen, pigments, and iron-containing granules, can be observed in the cytoplasm. The glycogen (Figs. 3 and 5–7) is usually in the form of isodiametric particles, rather irregular in outline, occurring individually or in aggregates (α-rosettes) of smaller units (β-particles). In the liver, the glycogen is very abundant, scattered in rosettes or small clusters of various sizes throughout the cytoplasm, and stains more intensely than other particulate cytoplasmic components. In the human liver, it is noteworthy that glycogen aggregates, which seem to vary with animal species,

appear as uniform small rosettes (α-particles) interspersed between membranes of the SER. Although studies on the biosynthesis of glycogen have not definitively established which cytoplasmic organelles are involved, the close morphological relationship with smooth membranes suggests that the SER may be of importance in regulating the glycogen metabolism, especially during periods of active synthesis [8].

Actually in the cytoplasm of hepatocytes, many metabolic events can be evidenced by the ultrastructural analysis. For example, lipoprotein particles (i.e., very low density lipoproteins, VLDL), which are packaged by the Golgi apparatus into vacuoles, move to the cell membrane and are secreted (exocytosis) into the Disse space [9, 10].

The morphological identification of such components in the cytoplasm can explain the metabolic pathways and their compartmentalization. In fact it was recently seen that lipoproteins may undergo transformations inside the GERL (Golgi endoplasmic reticulum lysosome system), an organelle considered a specialized hydrolase-rich region of the endoplasmic reticulum that forms secretory vacuoles to be transported to the Disse space [11].

2.4. Plasma membranes

The plasma membranes of liver cells, besides the normal function of cell-delimiting membranes, exert the specific function of hepatocytes, such as exchanges with bile canaliculi or with plasma space. Recent studies have revealed specific biochemical functions of plasma membranes, and the use of appropriate staining methods have shown differences between the sinusoidal and bile canalicular membranes, which are stained for nucleoside phosphatase and alkaline phosphatase (AMP and glycophosphate as substrates) or for nucleoside phophatase (ATP substrate), respectively. Because plasma membranes contact either bile canaliculi, intercellular Disse spaces, or related extensions (plasma spaces), attention has been drawn to the ultrastructural aspects of hepatocytes toward various functional spaces.

Numerous and tortuous microvilli are present in both sinusoidal and bile canalicular membranes, thus increasing the surface for the various functions (uptake or secretion) (Figs. 8, 9, and 11). Pino-

19

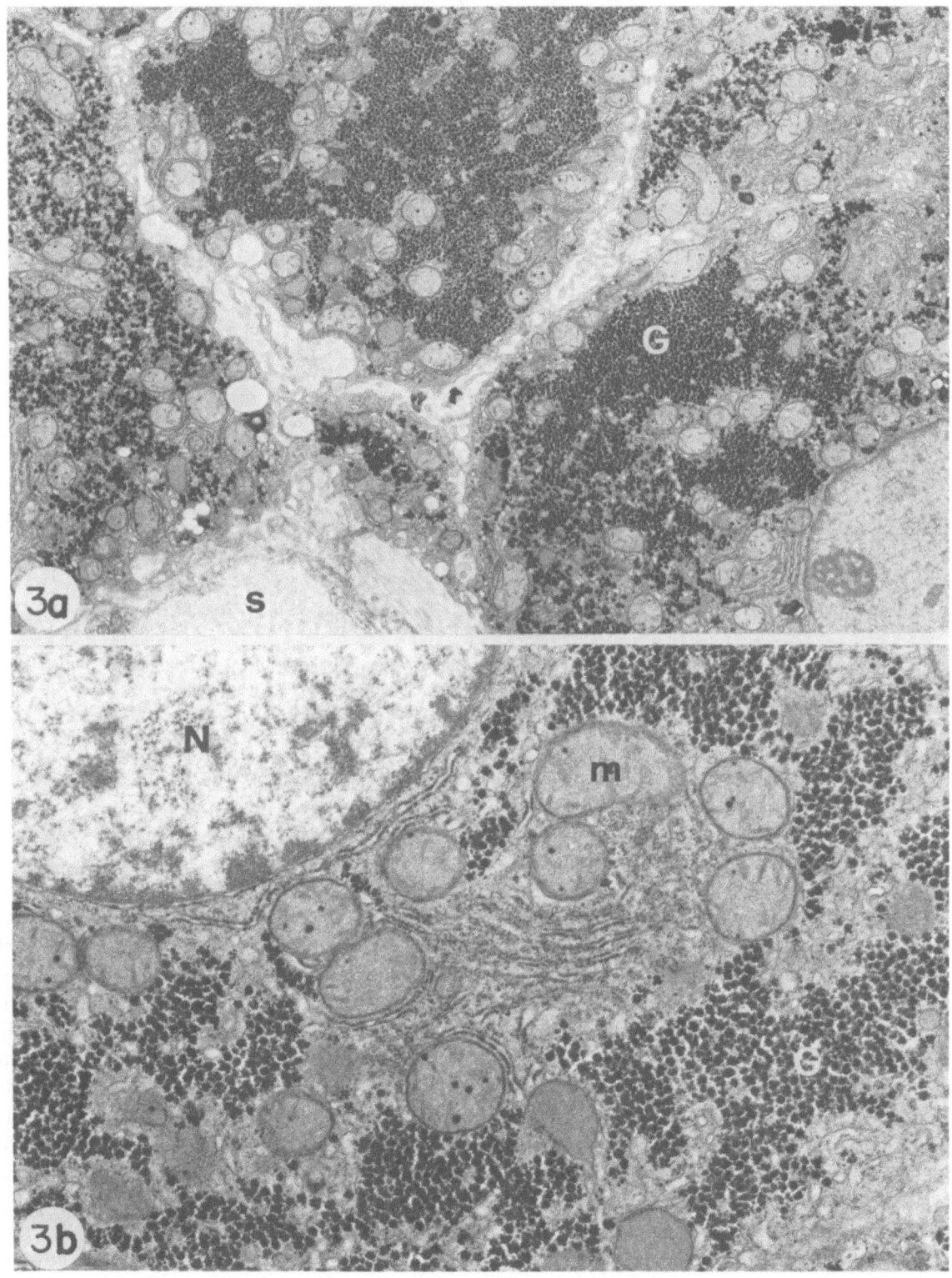

Figure 3a and b. Glycogen in the human liver is usually in the form of rosettes of uniform size. They can be found isolated (alpha-particles) in close relation with the agranular endoplasmic reticulum or concentrated in large masses from which other cytoplasmic organelles are excluded. N, nucleus; G, glycogen; m, mitochondria; S, sinusoid; (*a*) × 5000; (*b*) × 19,500.

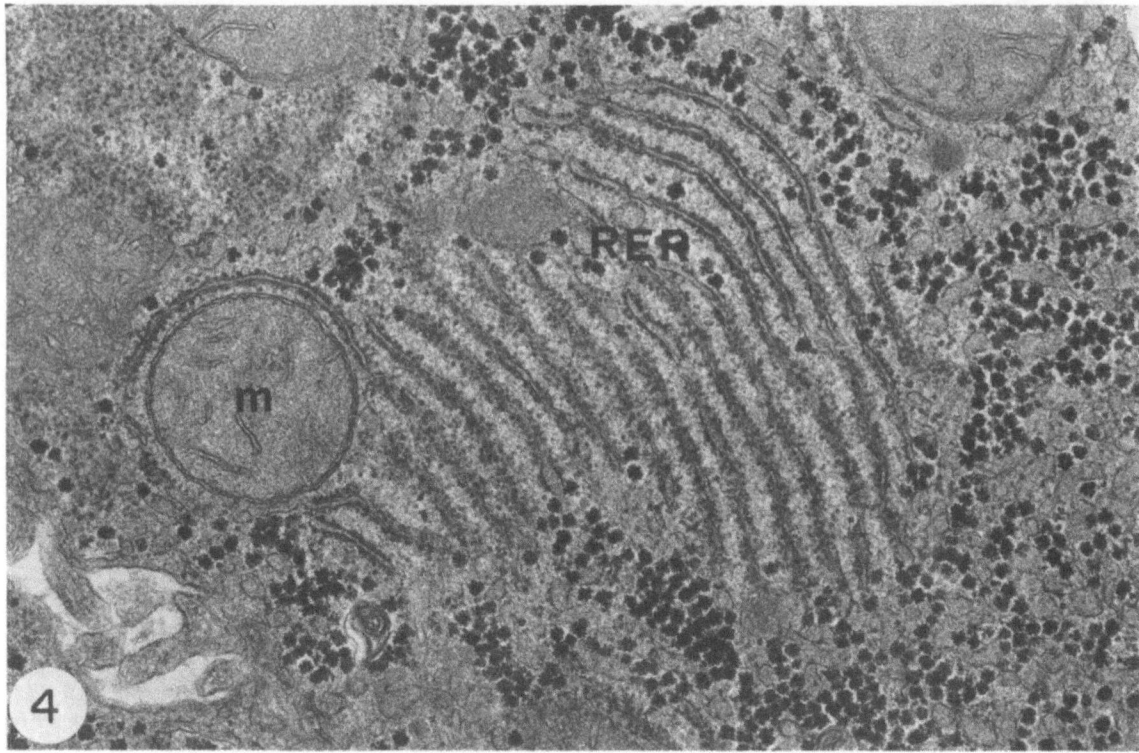

Figure 4. Part of two adjacent cells. In close proximity to the intercellular space, tubular elements of granular reticulum (RER) roughly parallel to one another can be seen. It consists of thin ribosome-associated membranes enclosing a narrow central space, the cisternae. The mitochondria (m) in the liver cells tend to be close to the areas of RER. Human liver; ×34,000.

cytotic invaginations on the sinusoidal border and microfilaments around bile canalicular membranes can be evidenced just near the cell border. This latter image, first described by Biava [12], represents the fine dissolution of SER and Golgi vesicles into the material related to bile secretions. The lateral surface, except for the part delimiting the bile canaliculi, is smooth and an intercellular space of about 100–250 Å is generally observed. Adjacent hepatocytes possess tight junctions near the bile canaliculi; external leaflets of neighboring plasma membranes are here fused, whereas intermediate junctions are often observed next to the tight junctions. An intercellular space, in which is present a hepatocyte secretory material, is delimited by the adjacent plasma membranes, which are wavy or continue in a parallel and straight configuration, forming desmosomes [13]. Parallel layers of cytoplasmic condensed material and fine fibrils complete the classic desmosome structure. Sternlieb [14] has described mitochondrion–desmosome complexes in human hepatocytes, with a mitochondrion

placed on either side of the desmosome (mirror-like).

2.5. Mitochondria

In the hepatocytes, they are spherical or rod-shaped organelles provided with numerous cristae, which play an essential role in generating energy from substrates that can be oxidized. Liver mitochondria usually near the endoplasmic reticulum or the nucleus can be concentrated along the sinusoidal surface and should be considered as structures functionally related to the energetic processes (Figs. 3, 7, and 8) [15]. Extranuclear circular DNA and procaryotic-type ribosomes (70S) have been recently found in the mitochondrial matrix, thus indicating an autonomous genetic control of protein synthesis. This finding is suggestive of a few autonomous functions of these organelles, which participate in the life of the cell, but can respond with self-conditioned reactions to an outer stimulus. Ultrastructural findings seem to support the occurrence

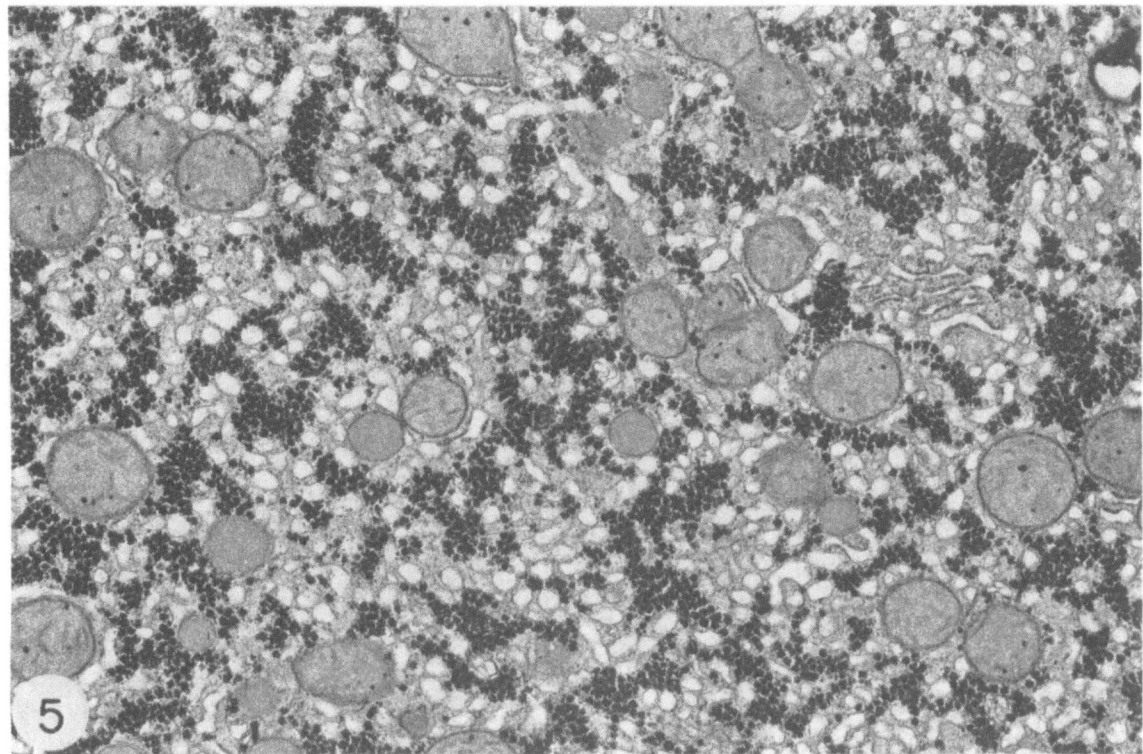

Figure 5. Agranular endoplasmic reticulum concentrated in areas of glycogen. In this micrograph, it appears as isolated circular and short segments of branching tubules, much more extensive than usual. Most of them have light centers similar to the long cisternal profiles of the granular form. Human liver; × 14,500.

of mitochondria multiplication not dependent on cell division. Giant mitochondria [4] and isolated rod-shaped mitochondria can show a narrowing that seems to prepare a division of the organelle. Because both the biochemical studies and the ultrastructural findings on the duplication of mitochondrial DNA up to now are not conclusive, the question is still unresolved.

In human hepatocytes, mitochondria are larger and more numerous in the periportal zone, whereas in centrolobular hepatocytes they are less numerous than in the peripheral area [4, 15].

2.6. Endoplasmic reticulum

Endoplasmic reticulum appears as a network of membranes, which can be organized in vesicles, sacs, and cisternae with or without ribosomes in the outer surface. Both the rough endoplasmic reticulum (RER) and the smooth one (SER) are often in continuity (Figs. 4–7). RER predominates in periportal hepatocytes, whereas centrolobular cells

show SER more developed than RER [16].

Near mitochondria and along the sinusoidal surface, the RER is often disposed in parallel arrays. Its lumen is slightly electron dense and no particles, except ribosomes, are evidenced. However, endoplasmic reticulum can increase many fold in response to any external stimulation, and during phenobarbital treatment a twentyfold membrane accumulation has been described [1, 17].

This phenomenon reverses itself after the end of treatment, at a rate similar to that found during the induction. These data suggest a great mobility in the dimension of both RER and SER, in response to different metabolic situations. In the developing human liver, proliferation of membranes is regulated by growth functional demands: initially an increase in membrane density in each hepatocyte occurs, and cell size also increases. The endoplasmic reticulum proliferation is accompanied by development of enzyme activity and ribosome accumulation. Actually, ribosomes, which can be well observed as free ribosomes in cytoplasm or attach-

22

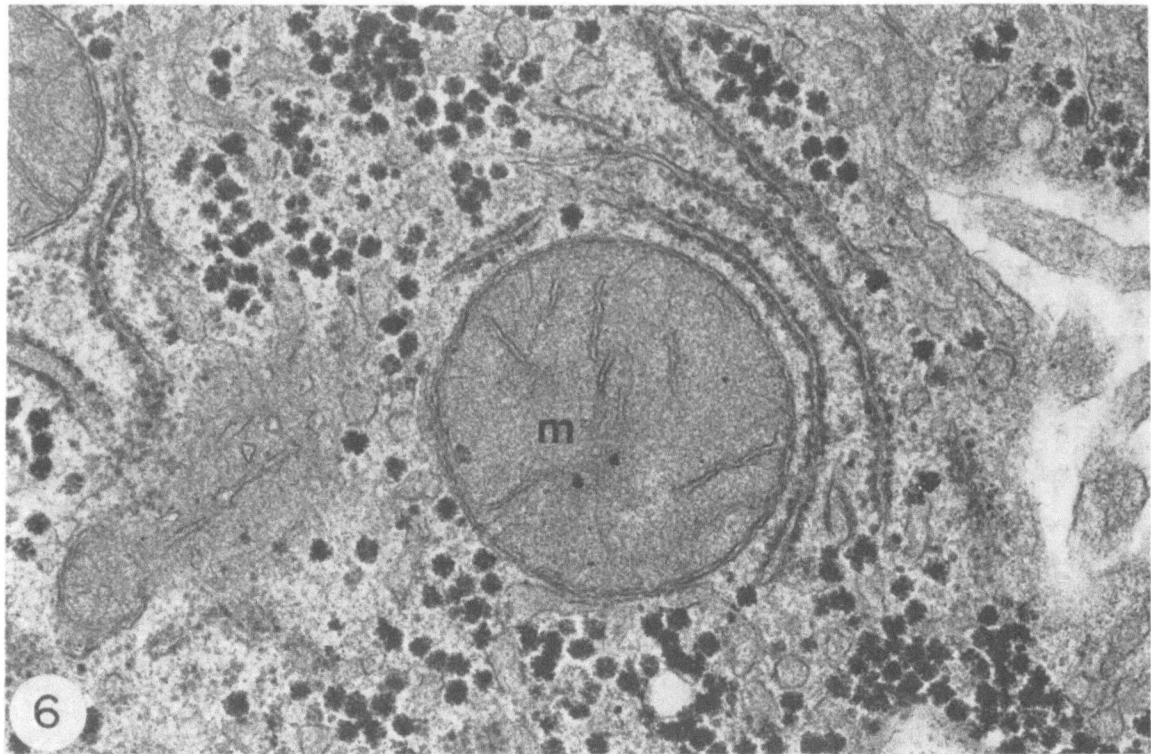

Figure 6. The mitochondria (m) of human liver cells have usually an oval or round shape with few cristae in a homogeneous matrix that contains two or three mitochondrial granules. Tubular profiles of the granular reticulum frequently wrap around mitochondria, but at all points stand off from its surface at a uniform distance; × 51,500.

ed to the outer membranes of ER, consist of large and small subunits (60S and 30S, respectively). The large subunit is attached to the ER, whereas the small one is assembled following mRNA engagement. When mRNA is engaged and protein synthesis starts, polysomes can be observed. In vitro studies of protein synthesis by following sedimentation on sucrose gradients of both ribosomes and polysomes have shown a close relationship between the start of the process and the conversion of ribosomes in larger complexes.

It is now clear that synthesis of hepatic proteins, such as albumin, occurs in rough endoplasmic reticulum and that the ultrastructural findings of ribosomes in the transition area between RER and SER cannot modify this general opinion. On the other hand, SER function is related to the storage of proteins and to their secretion; in fact a moderately electron dense material is evidenced in the lumen of SER, which is more enlarged and abundant in the centrolobular than in the periportal cells. Depending on the functional state of the cell,

SER appears in cross sections as a tubular structure interposed among glycogen rosettes; in the stimulated liver, vesicles take the place of tubules and rounded invaginations are observed in longitudinal sections.

Enzymes involved in the metabolism of lipids and carbohydrates, and in the transformation of drugs, hormones, etc., have been found in the SER; bilirubin, glucuronide transferase, glucose-6-phosphatase, drug-metabolizing enzymes, and lipid-synthesis-related enzymatic activities are located in the SER.

2.7. Golgi apparatus

In liver cells, the Golgi apparatus is situated around the bile canaliculi and in the perinuclear area (Fig. 9). The Golgi complex usually shows three or four cisternae or saccules roughly disposed in a parallel array with the slightly concave form of a disk. The saccules are constantly dilated at their lateral extremities. They may contain a finely granular ma-

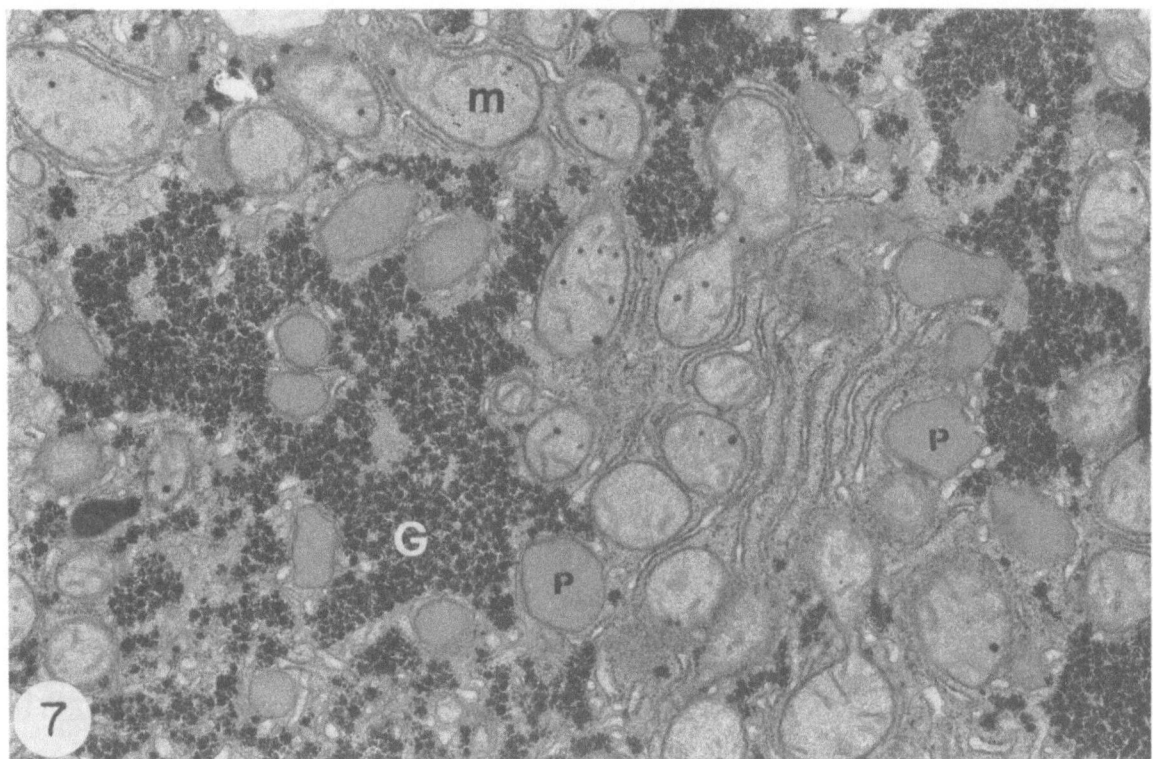

Figure 7. This cytoplasmic area of a human hepatocyte shows the typical appearance of microbodies (P). Smaller than mitochondria, these organelles are surrounded by a single membrane and display a matrix of medium density. G, glycogen; m, mitochondria; ×16,000.

terial that has been considered to be very low density lipoprotein (VLDL). The inner or concave aspect is full of vesicles or anastomosing tubules of various sizes that are more electron opaque than the VLDL particles. This area of the Golgi apparatus is considered a special system of endoplasmic reticulum (ER), called GERL by Novikoff [18]. GERL elements can also be dilated with lipoprotein (LP) particles, which show a greater electron opacity than the VLDL particles seen in the dilated element of the Golgi apparatus. LP-filled dilatations of GERL appear to be continuous with the smooth membranes of ER that, in turn, continue with rough ER [11].

Cytochemical studies in rat hepatocytes have shown that all components of GERL and the other LP-containing vacuoles display AcPase activity, whereas the VLDL-containing vacuoles show no AcPase activity but do display TPPase activity. These observations demonstrate that the liver cells, like other cell types, possess two different populations of lipoprotein-containing vacuoles such as the

VLDL packaged in the Golgi zone and the LP particles found in the dilated regions of GERL.

2.8. Lysosomes

Lysosomes can be well evidenced in both hepatocytes (Figs. 8 and 9) and Kupffer cells (Fig. 10), and different enzymatic activities have been recognized by using biochemical methods. The enzymes of lysosomes (hydrolytic acid enzymes) have been characterized also by either histochemical (light-microscopic) or electron-microscopic analysis. Only four enzymatic activities have been found with this latter method: acid phosphatase, aryl-sulfatase, esterase, and β-glucuronidase. Glucosaminidase-activity staining is positive in Kupffer cells, but not in hepatocytes; acid phosphatase and β-glucuronidase activities are higher in periportal than in centrolobular hepatocytes [4]. This more intense enzymatic activity is related to enlarged bodies similar to those found in Kupffer cells.

Lysosomes are delimited by a single membrane

24

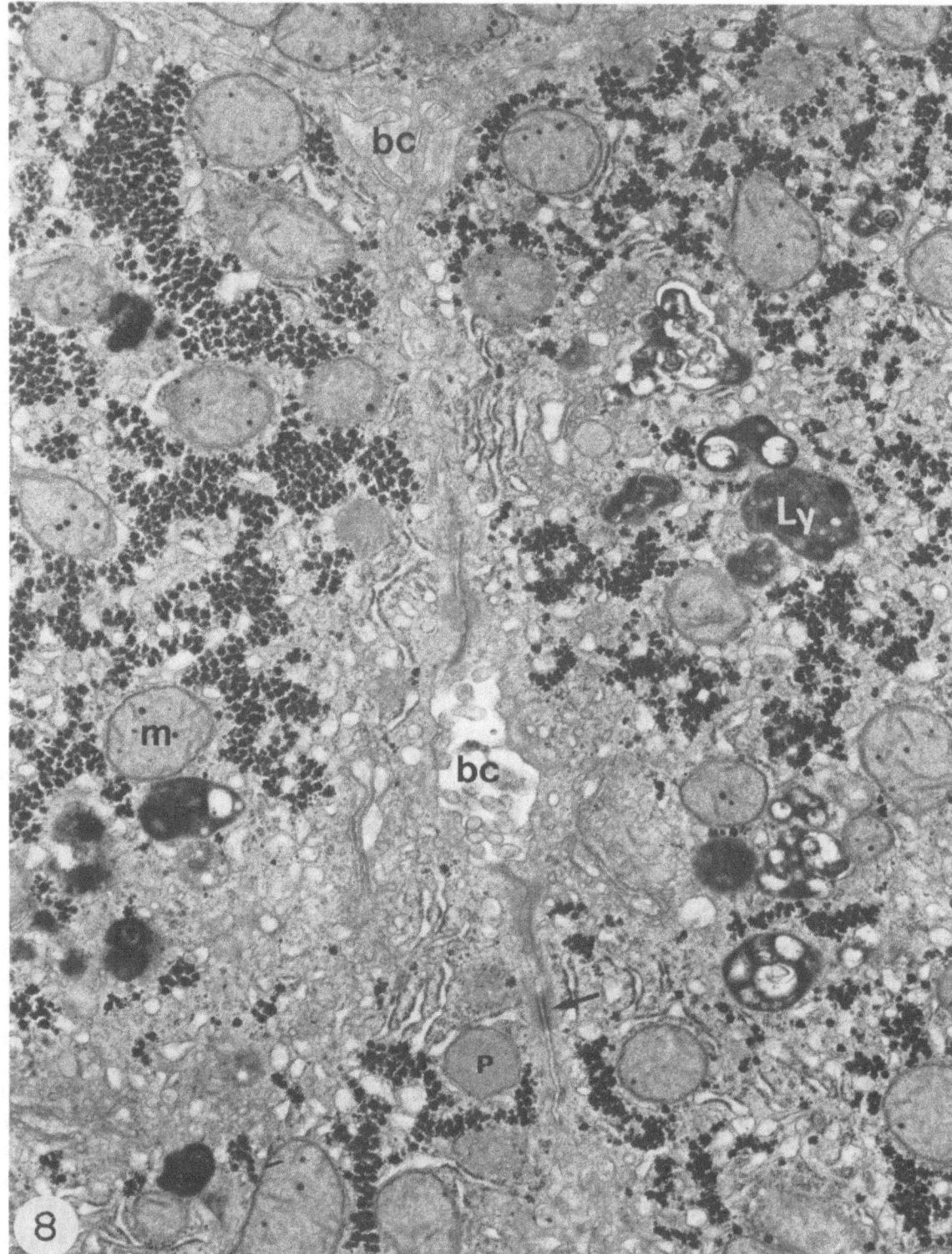

Figure 8. Pericanalicular regions of three opposing human hepatocytes. Two bile canaliculi (bc) are filled with microvillous profiles in more or less random directions from the surface of the hepatic cells. The lumen is separated from the narrow intercellular space by a junctional complex (*maculae occludentes, zonulae adhaerentes,* and *desmosomes*) at each lateral margin of a canaliculus (arrow). Around the canaliculi, typically a Golgi complex, membrane-bound dense bodies identified as lysosomes (Ly) and microbodies (P) can be seen. They are irregular in shape and consist of an agglomeration of large or small dense granules dispersed in a fine granular matrix of lower density. Others may contain concentrically arranged membranes intermingled with dense spherical granules of various sizes; × 19,000.

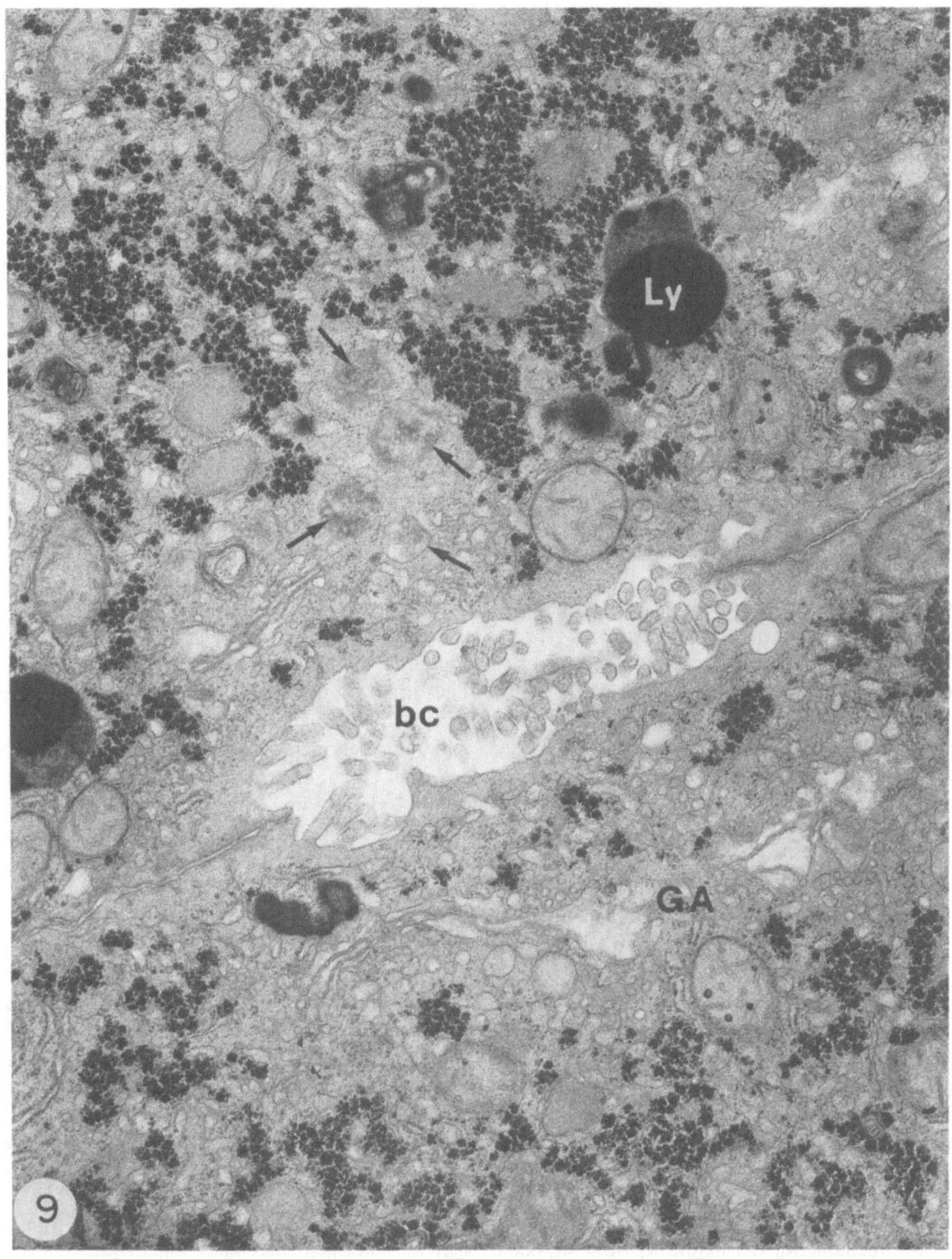

Figure 9. Two Golgi complexes (GA) adjacent to the bile canaliculus (bc). They consist of curved parallel arrays of saccules forming stacks. Many vesicles of various sizes are present on both concave and convex surfaces. The arrows indicate four apparent vacuoles containing LP particles related to the Golgi complex. Ly, lysosome. Human liver; × 19,500.

and contain a moderately electron dense material (primary lysosomes). Secondary lysosomes (lipofucsin-positive granules), autophagic vacuoles, as well as multivesicular bodies are normally found in hepatocytes.

Lipofucsin-positive lysosomes are membrane-limited bodies with clumps of high-density material, globules of lipid material and, as the third component, an amorphous and light-density matrix. These residual bodies seem to be related to the heme oxidation and are more abundant in the peribiliary area. Heterophagocytosis can be observed in the cell area facing the Disse space, especially when foreign material is assumed and phagosomes are fused with lysosomes to form heterolysosomes. Residual bodies are more frequently eliminated in the area of the Disse space, but iron particles are reused by the hepatocyte or liberated into the bile canaliculus or the blood [15].

Hemosiderin granules with iron-core particles of about 70 Å are probably residual bodies derived by proteolytic digestion of ferritin proteins, digestion which can be incomplete because of the low specificity of lysosome hydrolases. Biopsies frequently show autophagic vacuoles, which contain cytoplasmic organelles, such as mitochondria, endoplasmic reticulum, glycogen, and ferritin. Because autophagic vacuoles increase in number after administration of glucagon, cAMP, and epinephrine [19], and these substances, such as cAMP, are related to genetic expression, this phenomenon could be associated with a metamorphosis [15].

Autophagic vacuoles are often double-membrane limited, thus indicating that they are derived from the endoplasmic reticulum. Only after the fusion with lysosomes and the hydrolase activation do autophagic vacuoles appear surrounded by a single membrane (Fig. 8).

Multivesicular bodies (MVB) are membrane-limited bodies of uncertain origin, similar to those seen near the Golgi apparatus, but distributed in all cytoplasm. They are characterized by the presence of a light electron-dense material having a texture and small vesicles or smooth tubular structures. No data are available on the nature of their content, except that they are acid phosphatase positive.

2.9. Microbodies

Smaller than mitochondria, this class of cytoplasmic organelles was first described in the proximal convoluted tubule of the kidney [20] and later in liver cells, where they are rather numerous [21]. They consist of a moderately electron opaque, finely granular matrix limited by a single smooth membrane (Fig. 7). Their size and shape varies considerably within the same cell. In normal cells, most microbodies are circular or ovoid and are commonly located at the boundary between granular endoplasmic reticulum and areas containing agranular reticulum or glycogen.

Unlike the hepatic cells of different species of animals, the microbodies of human liver cells lack a distinct dense core or nucleoid. The microbodies are more abundant during fetal and early postnatal development, in the regenerating liver, and after the administration of certain chemical agents (chlofibrate). Microbodies are rich in several enzymes such as uricase and catalase, an enzyme capable of reducing H_2O_2 to water [21–23]. They may also contain *d*-amino acids and hydroxyacid oxidase. The origin of these organelles have not yet been completely defined. The observation that different cell organelles, including the endoplasmic reticulum and the Golgi apparatus, are found in a close spatial relationship with microbodies led some authors to suggest that these organelles originate from other membranous elements [24, 25].

3. KUPFFER CELLS

Between the endothelial cells lining the sinusoidal wall and hepatocytes, Kupffer cells are found to have a variable and stellate shape, with a surface characterized by amoeboid protrusions (Fig. 10). They have the same relation to parenchymal cells as endothelial cells, but are not continuous with their fenestrated sinusoidal wall and lack basement membrane.

The Kupffer cells have an elongated cytoplasm that in some instances may extend into the perisinusoidal Disse space or between two adjacent hepatocytes, but often span the sinusoidal lumen [2]. Their exact topographical relationship has been clarified by scanning electron microscopy (see

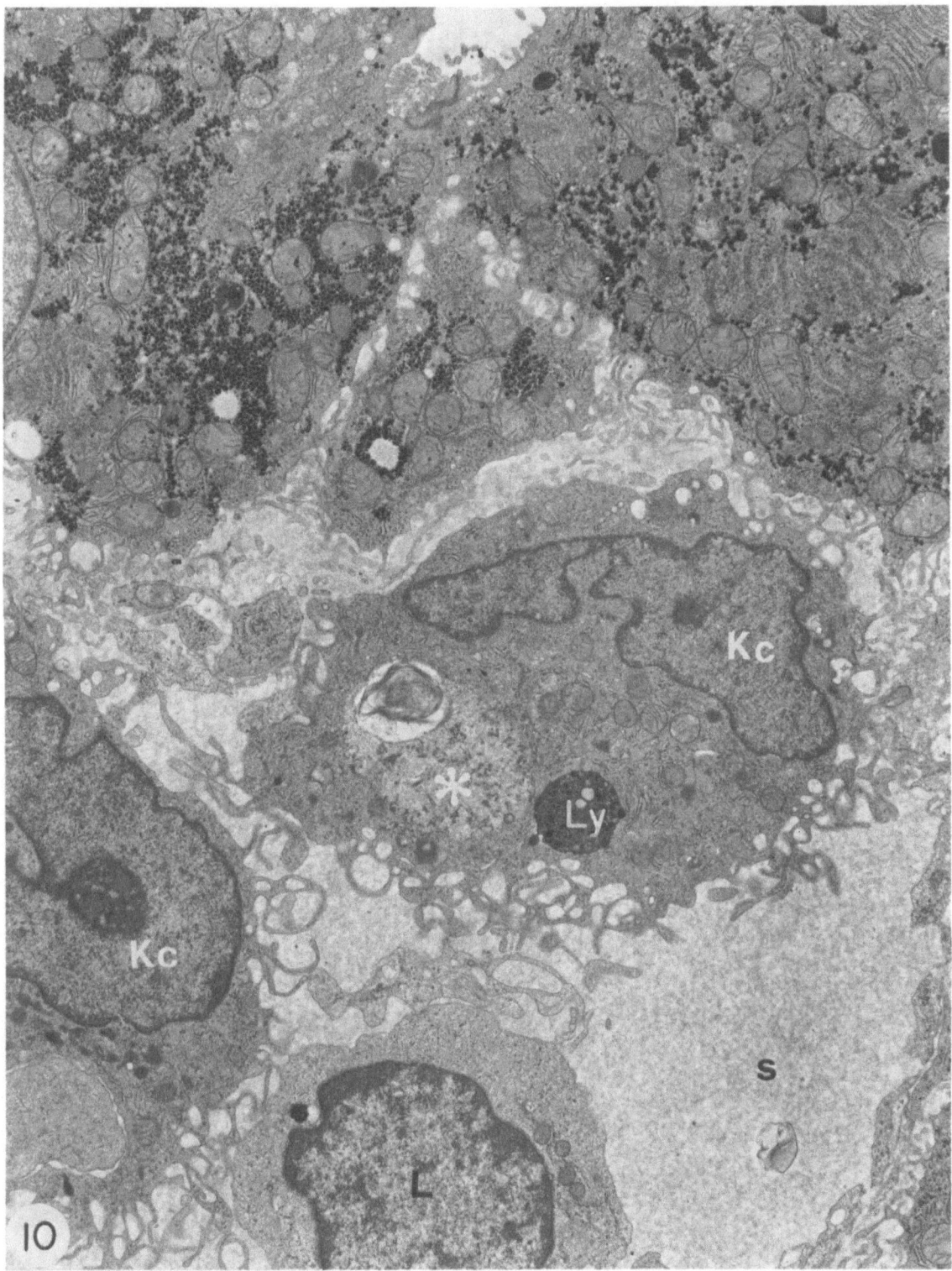

Figure 10. Two Kupffer cells (Kc) with numerous elongated cytoplasmic processes of variable thickness and length protruding into the lumen of a sinusoid (S). Their microvilli are apparently intermingled with those of the parenchymal cells. The nuclei are large and irregularly shaped with a prominent nucleolus. In the abundant cytoplasm, phagocytosed materials (asterisk) and dense bodies (lysosomes) (Ly) are noted. A lymphocyte (L) is also present in the sinusoid. Human liver; ×7800.

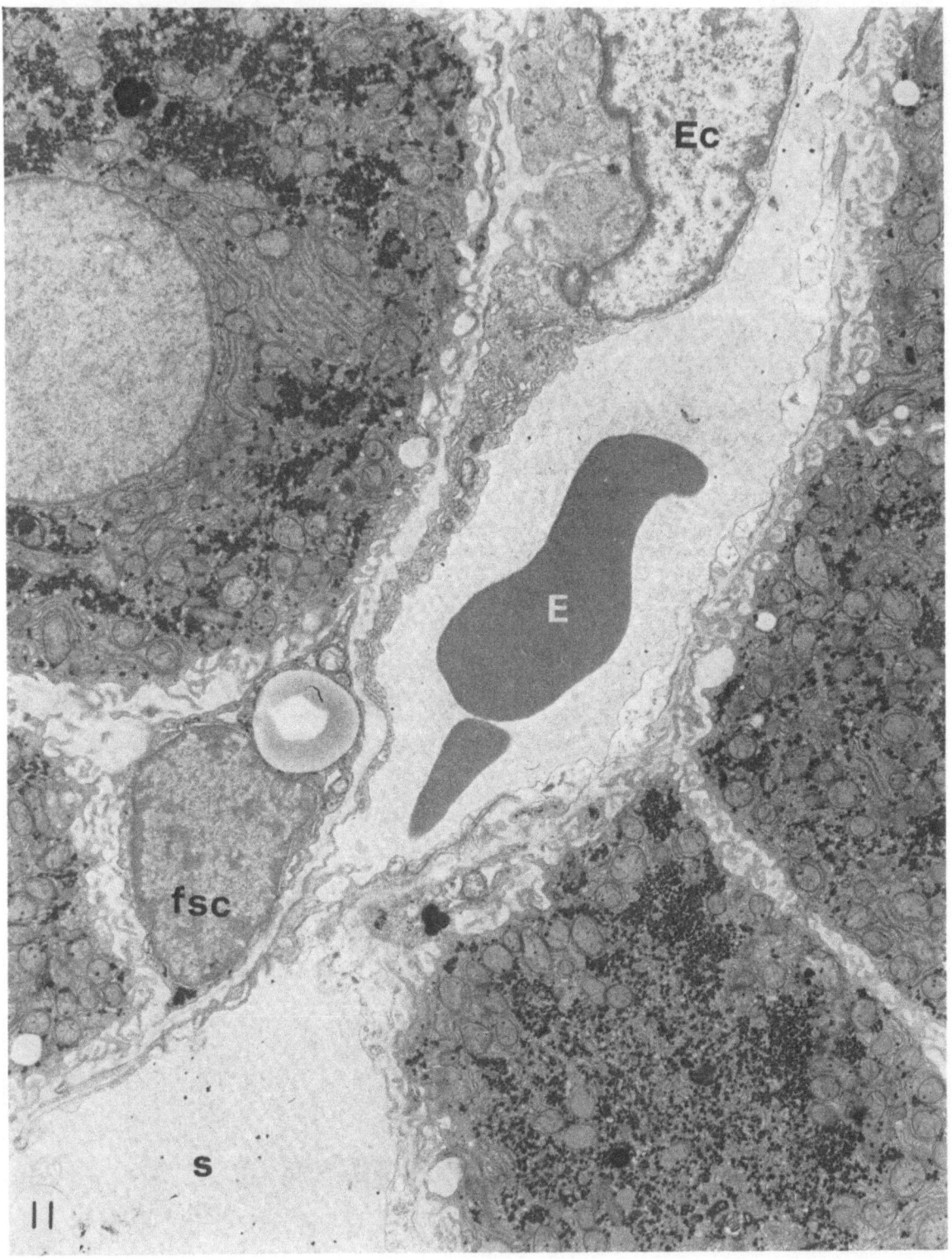

Figure 11. Disse space containing a fat-storing cell (fsc). It is closely related to both sinusoidal lining and parenchymal cells. Its cytoplasm contains a single large drop of lipid with a clear center surrounded by a dense band and dilated RER cisternae. Ec, endothelial cell; S, sinusoid; E, erythrocyte. Human liver; ×5000.

chapter 3). They differ from the endothelial-lining cells into which they have an irregular and elongated nucleus with prominent nucleolus, and their cytoplasm possesses numerous mitochondria and a large endoplasmic reticulum. Kupffer cells may contain particulate material, lysosomes, lucent vacuoles, and phagocytotic material but do not show fat droplets, as do the fat-storing cells.

Cytochemical studies have shown the presence in Kupffer cells of acid phosphatase and of a peroxydatic activity, making them members of the reticulolendothelial system [26]. In addition, recent studies provide evidence that these hepatic cells are not self-sustaining, but derive from a bone marrow precursor [27].

4. FAT-STORING CELLS

Named 'Sternzellen' by von Kupffer [28], fat-storing cells by Ito and Nemoto [29], interstitial cells by Suzuki [30, 31], and lipocytes by Bronfenmajer et al. [32], these cells are found predominantly in the peripheral zone of the lobule outside the sinusoid, where collagen bundles are often seen. In the human liver, they show a fairly simple profile (a stellate appearance is rather exceptional) that frequently is oval, although their form varies depending on the number and size of lipid droplets (Fig. 11). Their cytoplasm thins out into processes that extend along the Disse space or the intercellular space of two adjacent hepatocytes [2]. Nevertheless, the cytoplasmic processes never penetrate the endothelium which always separates them from the sinusoidal lumen. The fat-storing cells are quite different from the phagocytic Kupffer cells: they have a relatively large oval or spherical nucleus and a scanty cytoplasm containing a variable number of lipid droplets pushing aside the nucleus and other organelles or mitochondria and dilated cisternae of RER. Sometimes, glycogen granules can be noted around lipid droplets or aggregated near the nucleus. The Golgi complex is poorly developed.

Different studies have shown that the lipid droplets contain vitamin A [33] and that they increase in number after the administration of excess vitamin A [34].

REFERENCES

1. Bolender RP, Paumgartner D, Muellener D, Losa G, Weibel ER (1980) Integrated stereological and biochemical studies on hepatocytic membranes. IV. Heterogeneous distribution of marker enzymes on endoplasmic reticulum membranes in fractions. J Cell Biol 85:577–586
2. Motta PM (1977) The three-dimensional fine structure of the liver as revealed by scanning electron microscopy. Int Rev Cytol [Suppl 6]:347–399
3. Caramia FG, Chergo GF, Menghini G (1967) A glycogen body in liver nuclei. J Ultrastruct Res 19:573–585
4. Ma MH, Biempica L (1971) The normal human liver cell. Am J Pathol 62:353–370
5. Bernhard W, Granboulan N (1968) The nucleus. In: Dalton AJ, Haguenau F (eds) Ultrastructure in biological systems, vol 3. New York: Academic, p. 81
6. Schoelf GI (1964) The effect of actinomycin D on the fine structure of the nucleolus. J Ultrastruct Res 10:224–243
7. Narayan KS, Steele WJ, Busch H (1966) Evidence that the granular and fibrillar components of nucleoli contain 28 and 65 RNA, respectively. Exp Cell Res 43:483–492
8. Margolis RN, Curnow RT (1980) Observations on the role of SER in hepatic glycogen metabolism. J Cell Biol 87:203a
9. Chapman MJ, Mills GL, Taylaur CE (1973) The effect of a lipid-rich diet on the properties and composition of lipoprotein particles from the Golgi apparatus of guinea pig liver. Biochem J 131:177–185
10. Jackson RL, Morrisett JD, Gotto AM (1976) Lipoprotein structure and metabolism. Physiol Rev 56:259–316
11. Novikoff PM, Yam A (1978) Sites of lipoprotein particles in normal rat hepatocytes. J Cell Biol 76:1–11
12. Biava GG (1964) Studies on cholestasis: a re-evaluation of the fine structure of human normal bile canaliculi. Lab Invest 13:840–864
13. Matter A, Orci L, Rouillier C (1969) A study on the permeability barriers between Disse's space and the bile canaliculi. J Ultrastruct Res [Suppl 11]:1–71
14. Sternlieb I (1969) Mitochondrion-desmosome complexes in human hepatocytes. Z Zellforsch 93:249–253
15. Tanikawa K (1979) Ultrastructural aspects of the liver and its disorders, 2nd edn. Tokyo: Igaku-Shoin
16. De La Iglesia FA, Sturgess JM, McGuire EJ, et al (1976) Quantitative microscopic evaluation of the endoplasmic reticulum in developing human liver. Am J Pathol 82:61–70
17. Bolender RP, Weibel ER (1973) A morphometric study of the removal of phenobarbital induced membranes from hepatocytes after cessation of treatment. J Cell Biol 56:746–761
18. Novikoff AB (1976) The endoplasmic reticulum: a cytochemist's view. Proc Natl Acad Sci USA 73:2781–2787
19. Rosa F (1971) Ultrastructural changes produced by glucagon, cyclic 3'5'AMP and epinephrine on perfused rat liver. J Ultrastruct Res 34:205–213
20. Rhodin JAG (1958) Anatomy of kidney tubules. Int Rev Cytol 7:485–534
21. De Duve C, Baudhuin P (1966) Peroxisomes: microbodies and related particles. Physiol Rev 46:323–357
22. Hruban Z, Rechcigl M Jr (1969) Microbodies and related particles. Morphology, biochemistry and physiology. Int

Rev Cytol [Suppl 1] 1:1–296 (includes 879 references)

23. Leighton F, Poole B, Lazarow PB, De Duve C (1969) The synthesis and turnover of the rat liver peroxisomes. I. Fractionation of peroxisome proteins. J Cell Biol 41:521–535

24. Essner E (1967) Endoplasmic reticulum and the origin of microbodies in fetal mouse liver. Lab Invest 17:71–87

25. Tsukada H, Mochizuki Y, Konishi T (1968) Morphogenesis and development of microbodies of hepatocytes of rats during pre- and postnatal growth. J Cell Biol 37:231–243

26. Aschoff L (1924) Morphologie des reticulo-endothelialen Systems. In: Kraus F, et al (eds) Ergebnisse Innere Medizin und Kinderheilk. Berlin: Springer

27. Gale RP, Sparkes RS, Golde DW (1978) Bone marrow origin of hepatic macrophages (Kupffer cells) in humans. Science 201:937–938

28 Von Kupffer C (1876) Ueber Sterzellen der Leber. Briefliche Mittheilung an Prof. Waldeyer. Arch Mikrosk Anat 12: 353–358

29. Ito T, Nemoto M (1952) Über die Kupfferschen Sternzellen und die 'Fettspeicherungszellen' ('fat-storing cells') in der Blutkapillarenwand der menschlichen Leber. Folia Anat Jpn 24:243–258

30. Suzuki K (1958) A silver impregnation method in histology [Abst] [in Japanese]. Takeda Pharmaceutical Ind. Osaka No. 310–320

31. Suzuki L (1963) The end apparatus of the vegetative nervous system [Abst]. In: Proceedings 16th General Assembly of the Japan Medical Congress, Osaka 4:13–28

32. Bronfenmajer S, Schaffner F, Popper H (1966) Fat-storing cells (lypocytes) in human liver. Arch Pathol 82:447–453

33. Hirosawa K, Yamada E (1973) The localization of the vitamin A in the mouse liver as revealed by electron microscope radioautography. J Electron Microsc 22:337–346

34. Wake K (1974) Development of vitamin A-rich lipid droplets in multivesicular bodies of rat liver stellate cells. J Cell Biol 63:683–691

3. SCANNING ELECTRON MICROSCOPY OF THE MAMMALIAN LIVER

P.M. Motta, T. Fujita, and M. Nishi

1. INTRODUCTION

Scanning electron microscopy (SEM) is a necessary complementary approach for any biomedical study having a morphological basis [1–3]. Correlated with the use of conventional electron microscopy (TEM), SEM not only enables the examination of different cell surfaces, but also provides clear information of the actual three-dimensional microorganization of tissues and organs [3–5].

Refinements in SEM have progressed sufficiently to provide readily interpretable and reproducible images of three-dimensional features and spatial arrangements of single cells within tissues, and even parenchymal organs, such as the liver, can be easily prepared and studied by correlated SEM and TEM [6, 7].

This chapter reviews the fine surface morphological characteristics of liver components. The information presented is based mainly on the livers of laboratory mammals. Human liver tissues, arising from surgical and/or biopsy specimens, were used only when histological examination indicated normal morphology.

In addition, other specimens (experimental and pathological) obtained from animals and human biopsies were observed by using SEM and correlated with normal results in order to determine whether or not they could be of value in routine diagnostic problems.

Detailed descriptions of methods used for preparing liver tissues can be readily obtained from recently published research papers [6–10].

2. MICROARCHITECTURE OF THE LIVER: LIVER LOBULES

The rich vascular supply of the liver, with its nutritive (hepatic arteries) and functional (portal veins) components, forms a complex three-dimensional glandular architecture that is arranged in liver units called lobules and/or acini [11–13]. The smallest portion of liver tissue capable of autonomous function appears to be the so-called *acinus hepaticus* [13].

Liver acini cannot be easily defined by any anatomical mark. Acini are irregular hepatic areas supplied by a terminal branch of the hepatic artery and portal vein, and are drained by a terminal branch of the bile duct. In some cases the territory of an acinus may overlap zones belonging to adjacent acini [13].

The hepatic lobules previously considered to be the classic liver glandular units are more easily detected and by morphology represent portions of liver parenchyma clustered around a central vein (lobule of Kiernan) [11] or portal triad (lobule of Mall) [12] (Fig. 1a).

When the perfused liver parenchyma is sectioned with a razor blade or is gently fractured with jeweler's forceps after critical-point drying, the SEM reveals good images of the three-dimensional microarchitecture of lobules and/or acini [6, 7].

Because the liver tissues are somewhat plastic and dependent upon portohepatic pressure gradients [14], liver lobules can be more easily studied by using SEM in hepatic tissues where experimental and/or physiopathological conditions are more accurately retained [6, 7]. Further, in these situations, SEM observations of blood vascular casts add significantly to the elucidation of some confusing aspects of the microangio-architecture of the

P.M. Motta and L.J.A. DiDio (eds.), Basic and clinical hepatology, pp. 31–50. All rights reserved.
Copyright © 1982 Martinus Nijhoff Publishers, The Hague/Boston/London.

32

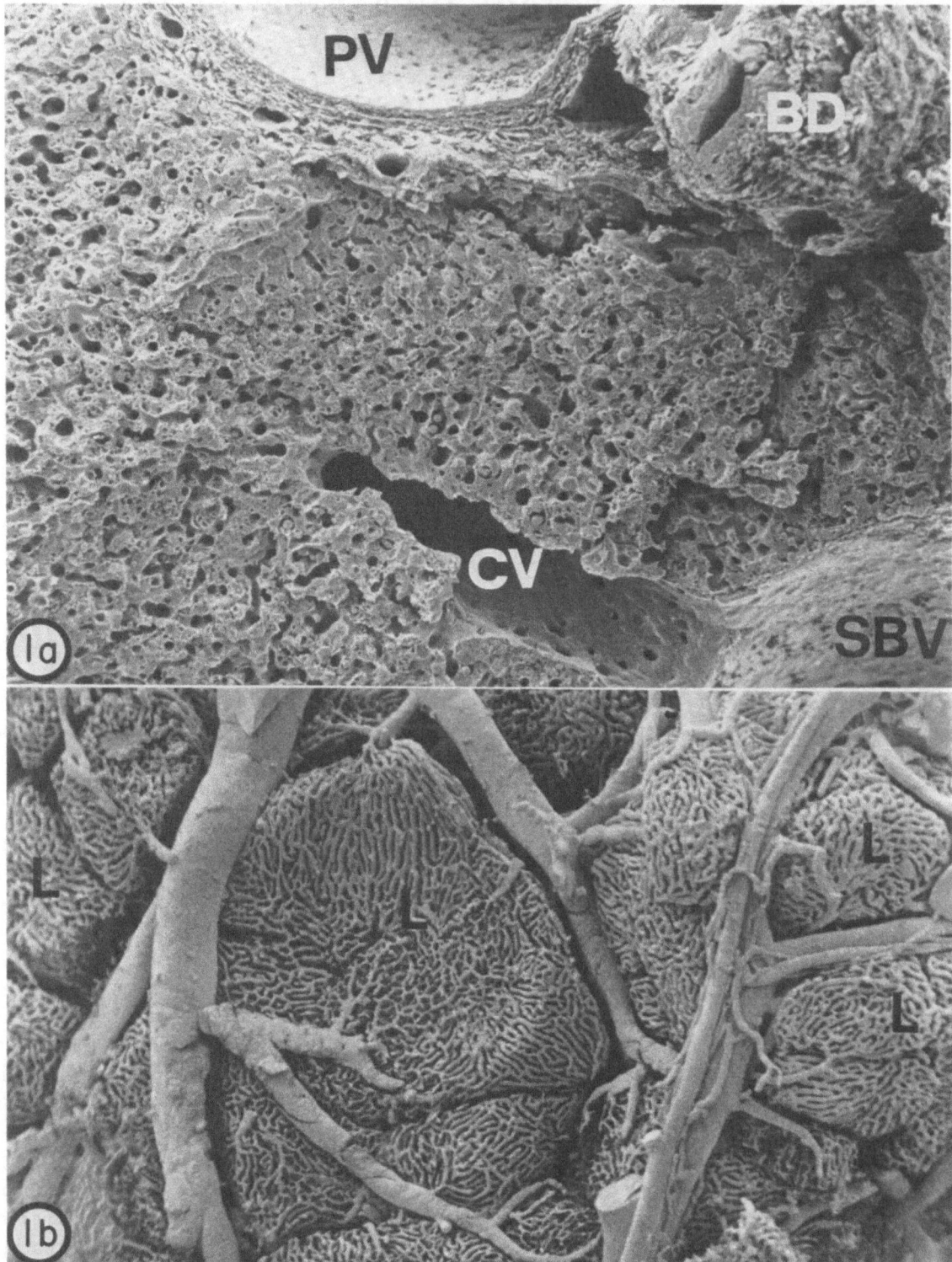

Figure 1. (*a*) Cat liver parenchyma showing hepatic laminae and sinusoids arranged around a central vein (CV). A portal area contains a branch of: portal vein (PV) and biliary duct (BD). SBV, sublobular vein; × 210. From Motta et al. (1978) *The liver. An atlas of SEM*. Courtesy of Igaku-Shoin, Tokyo/New York [7]. (*b*) Rat liver cirrhosis. The vascular casts clearly show the sinusoidal mass forming the (pseudo)lobules of Laennec (L). The areas of fibrotic invasion appear as dark zones within the lobules; × 180. Courtesy of Prof. T. Murakami and Igaku-Shoin, Tokyo.

liver in normal and pathological conditions [15] (see also chapter 6).

For example, typical "pseudolobules" of Laennec are revealed by vascular casts of cirrhotic liver that has been experimentally induced in the rat after treatment for half a year with a diet containing small amounts of CCl_4 [47]. The pseudolobules formed during the cirrhotic stage are apparent in the vascular casts after removal of the fibrotic liver parenchyma as irregularly rounded masses of dilated arterioles and sinusoids (Fig. 1b).

3. HEPATIC LAMINAE AND LIVER CELLS

The three-dimensional reconstruction of mammalian liver architecture reported in the classic histological studies by Elias 30 years ago [14] are readily verified by SEM. In fact, by SEM, the hepatic tissue consists of a continuous mass of polyhedral cells (hepatocytes) arranged in unicellular laminae (Fig. 1a).

The liver laminae are interconnected in a complex epithelial network (muralium) that encloses tunnels or spaces (lacunae) containing a meshwork of dilated capillaries (sinusoids) (Fig. 1a). Therefore, the perisinusoidal and perihepatocytic spaces form a labyrinth in which are contained circulating fluids the distribution of which in normal and pathological conditions can be easily evaluated by using SEM [6, 16].

One advantage of the SEM technique in the study of the liver is that when perfused liver fragments are dissociated with jeweler's forceps, or cut into thin slices with a razor blade, the hepatocytes often separate from one another along their common surfaces [8]. Other methods, such as fixing tissues in OsO_4 followed by soaking in a 1% solution of boric acid [17] or even reducing critical-point-dried liver specimens to a powderlike material by sandwiching them between two glass slides, also offer the possibility of obtaining fully isolated liver cells that can be then studied by using SEM (Fig. 2a).

As a consequence of such chemical and/or mechanical dissociation, hepatocytes tend to preserve their original shape and size, as when they were part of liver lobules. Therefore the surface heterogeneity displayed by isolated hepatocytes in SEM preparations, despite slight alterations produced dur-

ing preparation, essentially reflects the original position of single cells in hepatic tissue. This is likely the result of mechanical and functional factors [14].

SEM observations of single cells correlate well with the findings of quantitative stereological methods in which the structural heterogeneity of a population of liver cells is related to functional differences with respect to the topographical localization of the cells in the lobule [18].

Recently, the techniques of elutriation (counterflow centrifugation) developed by Wanson et al. [19, 20] have enabled the separation of hepatocytes into intact subpopulations of different sizes, which can then be easily studied by using SEM [21] (see chapter 5). Rat hepatocytes after isolation from pure fractions by elutriation and subsequent culture reveal important surface ultrastructural details. By these methods, in fact, different steps in cell dissociation can be distinguished and the reaggregation of hepatocytes into liver plates in vitro can be followed. Observations obtained from such cultured hepatocytes provide good reproducible images that correlate well with TEM and biochemical results [19, 20]. Similarly, SEM observations of isolated hepatocytes derived from liver tissues of known pathological and experimental conditions might offer considerable advantages in the analysis of the cell surface properties as related to absorption and/or secretion (see chapter 5).

Hepatocytes are polyhedral cells presenting a sinusoidal face that is exposed to the blood filtrate and an intercellular face that contains a portion of a bile channel (Fig. 2). The sinusoidal face is provided with numerous and short microvilli, pits, and occasional larger microprojections [6, 8, 16]. SEM enables a topographical evaluation of the distribution of such surface features in various experimental and pathological conditions [6, 7].

In normal situations, microvilli are often present on the hepatocytic sides where the subendothelial Disse space extends into intercellular spaces to form narrow recesses. These recesses are actually part of a continuous microlabyrinth of lacunae in which the hepatocytes project their rich microvillous surfaces. As a consequence of this, the total hepatocytic surface exposed to the blood filtrate circulating in the lacunar system of Disse is greatly enhanced. In this regard, it is interesting to note that when liver cells are isolated also the smooth sides

34

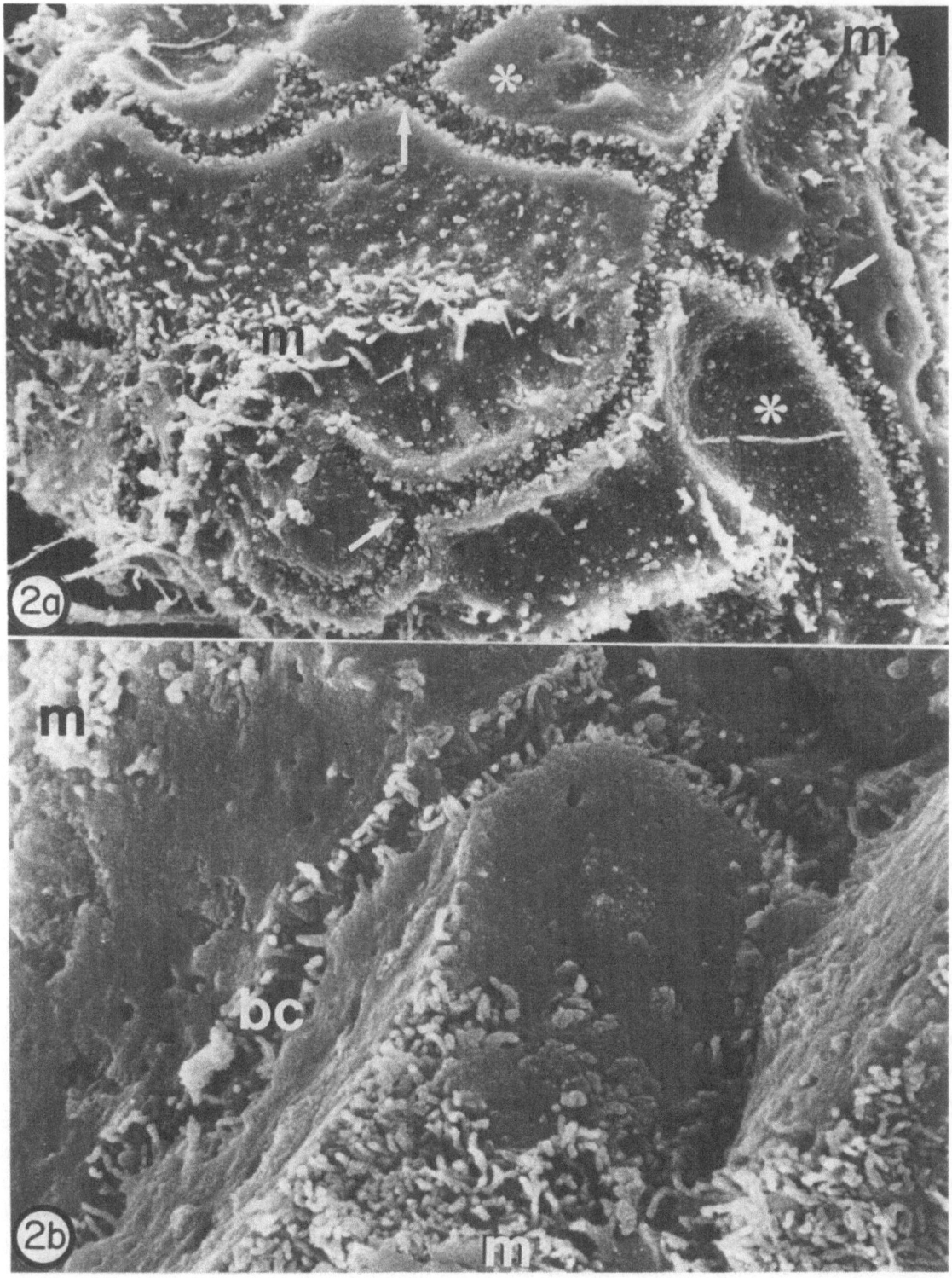

Figure 2. (*a*) Isolated liver cell showing smooth (asterisks) and microvillous (m) surfaces corresponding respectively to intercellular and tissue space facets. Half bile channels (arrows) are also evident. Rat; × 4000. (*b*) Bile channel (bc) on the smooth surface of a liver cell. The microvilli (m) populate the surface exposed to the blood filtratre (Disse space). Rat; ×8700.

that correspond to remnants of their intercellular faces are rapidly covered with microvilli while, by contrast, bile canaliculi totally disappear [21].

In cirrhotic liver, the portion of the hepatocyte surface covered by microvilli is greatly increased. The increased number of microvilli is paralleled by a corresponding reduction in the area occupied by the smooth-surfaced, narrow, intercellular spaces (Fig. 3a). Similarly, the microextensions occasionally noted in normal liver appear to increase according to the same increase noted in the connective tissue [22].

Collectively these results demonstrate that microvilli populating the hepatocytic surface are a temporary expression of a functional mechanism that is related to the free exposure of the cell surface to its environment.

The interhepatocytic surface is, as a rule, occupied in its center by a hemicanaliculus. Although only a single bile channel is present in the hepatocyte face, in other situations it may bifurcate into two or more ramifications on the same side of the cell. Some of these end blindly near the sinusoidal surfaces together with other short branches and/or lateral sacculations that may be present; thus the bile canaliculus is transformed into a tortuous channel. Although the tips of canalicular branches come close to the Disse space, a direct connection between these two channels is never observed [6, 8, 16] (Fig. 2).

Hemicanaliculi within the lobule measure about 0.1 μm in width, with the exception of those located in the portal ends of the liver plates [16, 23].

Microvilli obscure the interior of the narrow canaliculi, but appear to be clearly concentrated at the lateral margins in the larger channels [8, 24].

The interior wall of opened canaliculi often reveals small holes and pits [25]. Also bordered by microvilli are ramifications and lateral sacculations of the bile channels. Some of these, as seen in stereoscopic pair pictures, appear to arise from the subjacent cortical areas of the hepatocyte cytoplasm and can be interpreted as intracellular biliary branches [25].

The intercellular face of hepatocytes laterally bordering the bile canaliculus is rather smooth and contains only a few short microvilli, stubby protrusions, and numerous small pits (Fig. 2).

Although these smooth surfaces contain junctional complexes, as revealed by correlated freeze-etching and TEM preparations, their details cannot be revealed by using SEM alone. The numerous pits and holes in these areas indicate an intense traffic of fluids and other materials. The largest holes and protrusions most likely correspond to the stud processes described by TEM that are thought to have a role in cellular attachment [26, 27].

The smoothest part of the interhepatocytic surfaces is often a very narrow band running along the bile channel and measuring about 0.1 μm in width. These areas generally mark the intercellular spaces between adjacent hepatocytes and are the zones where the Disse spaces, with their recesses, come in closest contact, but not in open continuity, with the bile canaliculi. Such areas of minimal distance often appear in topographical SEM preparations [25] and, as indicated from reconstructions of serial thin sections [28], may serve as the sites of simple diffusion of substances having the same concentrations in the bile as in the blood [29].

Furthermore, these narrow zones may represent 'loci minoris resistentiae'. SEM studies of cholestatic liver obtained after choledocal ligation in the rat indicate open connections between Disse spaces and bile channels at the sites where such thin septa were previously present [7, 30].

Alterations of the liver cell facets bordering bile channels caused by different types of cholestasis are obviously suitable objects of SEM studies and freeze-etching preparations [31] (see also chapter 4).

The second day after ligation of the extrahepatic bile duct of adult rats, bile canaliculi appear more dilated, have lost their microvilli, and take a tortuous course presenting numerous and large smooth-surfaced saccular diverticula [32, 33]. Controversial results have been recently reported concerning the permeability of tight junctions after bile duct ligation in the rat [31–33]. Rat bile canaliculi, after infusion of various cholestatic agents (primarily bile acids) [34, 35], display comparable changes in bile channels when compared with those present after experimental ligation of the common bile duct. Variation in severity of ultrastructural changes produced by infusions of different chemicals probably results from the accumulation of bile salts in greater concentrations in hepatocytes near the portal triads [35]. Images showing very tortuous bile

36

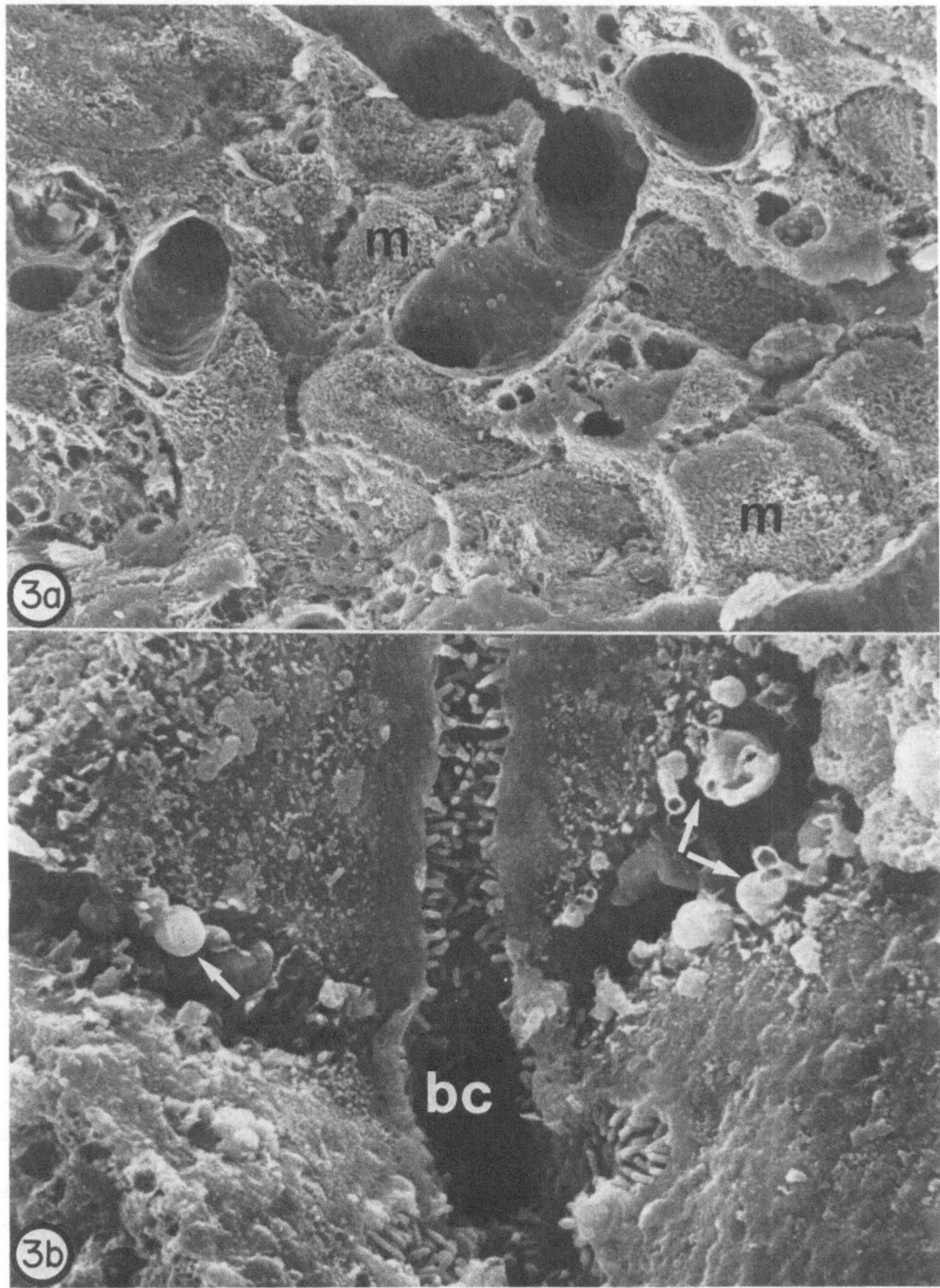

Figure 3 (*a*) Liver plates and sinusoids obtained from a patient diagnosed with primary biliary cirrhosis. The hepatocytic surfaces covered with microvilli (m) appear greatly increased; × 1350. (*b*) Biopsy sample of intrahepatic cholestasis. The bile channel (bc) is enlarged and amorphous material is present in the recesses of Disse (arrows) that are very close to the biliary wall. Human; × 5500.

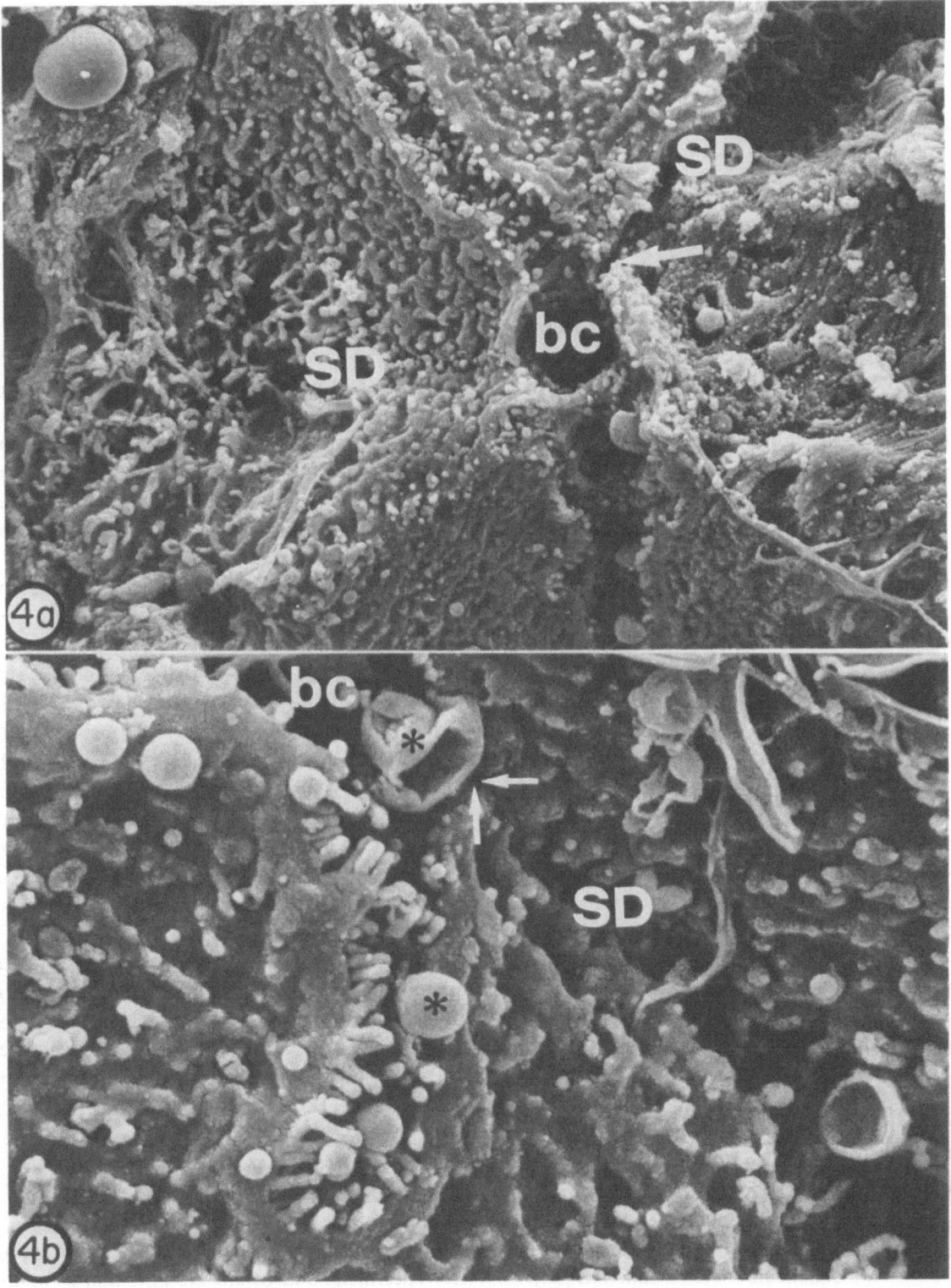

Figure 4a and b. The figures show hepatocytic surfaces populated by numerous irregular microvilli and microprojections on the facets provided with enlarged bile canaliculi (bc). These features together with possible free communication between the space of Disse (SD) and the wall of the bile channel (arrows) may, in this type of intrahepatic cholestasis, represent zones of regurgitation of the bile product (asterisk). Human, primary biliary cirrhosis; × 8500; × 14,000.

38

channels, with frequent lateral dilatations and loss of microvilli (Fig. 6a), may also be seen in laboratory mammals and in human obstructive jaundice, as well as in other nonobstructive intrahepatic cholestatic situations that arise in drug-induced hepatitis, viral hepatitis, pregnancy, and primary biliary cirrhosis. In many of these cases, SEM results indicate an increased accumulation of blebs and other irregular laminar extensions both within the lumen of the bile channels and also on their margins that are in association with the Disse space. Furthermore, the lumen of dilated bile channels may be occupied by large and free amorphous deposits that are also observed on the lateral surfaces of hepatocytes (Figs. 3 and 4) [36]. These surface features are probably an expression of both reabsorption of bile components through the wall of the biliary channel (transhepatocytic regurgitation) and/or through communication of the bile canaliculus with the Disse space. [30, 37].

Correlated TEM and SEM studies are a valuable approach to a systematic study of these morphodynamic aspects in pathology [30, 31, 33, 36, 38].

4. BILE DUCTS

Opened bile channels near portal zones are generally wider (1–2.5 μm) than those close to the central areas of the lobule (0.5–1 μm). The microvilli of the wider peripheral bile canaliculi are less numerous and often appear in association with intralobular ductules (of Hering), which are always lined by small cuboidal epithelial cells that are clearly different from hepatocytes.

The large peripheral bile channels are connected to the epithelial ducts of Hering through irregular diverticula of their wall (Fig. 5a). This intercalary tract is also termed the ampullar region or, more simply, *ampulla* and is lined by epithelial cells and hepatocytes, and corresponds to the canaliculoductular junction described in the TEM literature [23]. Finally, some bile canaliculi may open directly into the larger bile portal ducts without interposition of the canaliculoductular junction [23].

The luminal surface of ductular and duct tracts is covered by a number of short microvilli and single long cilia measuring about 0.2 μm in thickness and 5 μm in length [39]. In the wider bile ducts, the cilia

are more numerous and may be so long as to curve and twist, as in the process of crossing adjacent cilia within the ductal lumen (Fig. 5b). TEM examination shows that these cilia often possess a 9+2 microtubular pattern, and the possibility cannot be excluded that they have some functional motile or chemoreceptive role [6, 39]. Other features of the luminal surface of both intercalary tracts and bile ductules are numerous surface evaginations such as blebs, ruffles, and larger laminar extensions (Fig. 5). Such structures, together with masses of unknown material, are in the lumen of these regions and are probably an expression of sequestration (endocytosis) and/or secretion (exocytosis) of epithelial ductular cells [23]. Similar surface features in fact are observed in other epithelia where such activity occurs [40–42]. The above SEM findings suggest that the biliary ductules and ducts may have a role in an active process of reabsorption of biliary products [6].

In addition, the proliferation of bile ductules and preductules, canalicular dilatation, and the increased number of cilia present in cholestatic livers of rats subjected to ligation of the common bile ducts can all be easily followed by using SEM [7, 33, 38].

Generally, in primary biliary cirrhosis, the large (interlobular) bile ducts are altered by a remarkable fibrosis of their wall, with coupled intense lymphocyte infiltration. If observed by using correlated TEM and SEM, these ducts reveal a very thick basal lamina possessing various layers of collagen fibrils on the external surface, and a characteristic undulated and honeycomblike luminal surface, to which adhere epithelial cells [36]. The highly undulated lateral surfaces of these cells contain numerous lamellar projections and blebs that appear to be similar to structures present on epithelial cells that line the gallbladder during an intense process of material reabsorption (Fig. 6b).

5. VESSELS

The portal tract can be easily observed in fractured liver specimens and offers the potential of analyzing, in great detail, differences between hepatic arterial and venous vessels (ramifications of the hepatic artery and portal vein, respectively) (Fig. 1a). The luminal wall of hepatic arterial vessels is

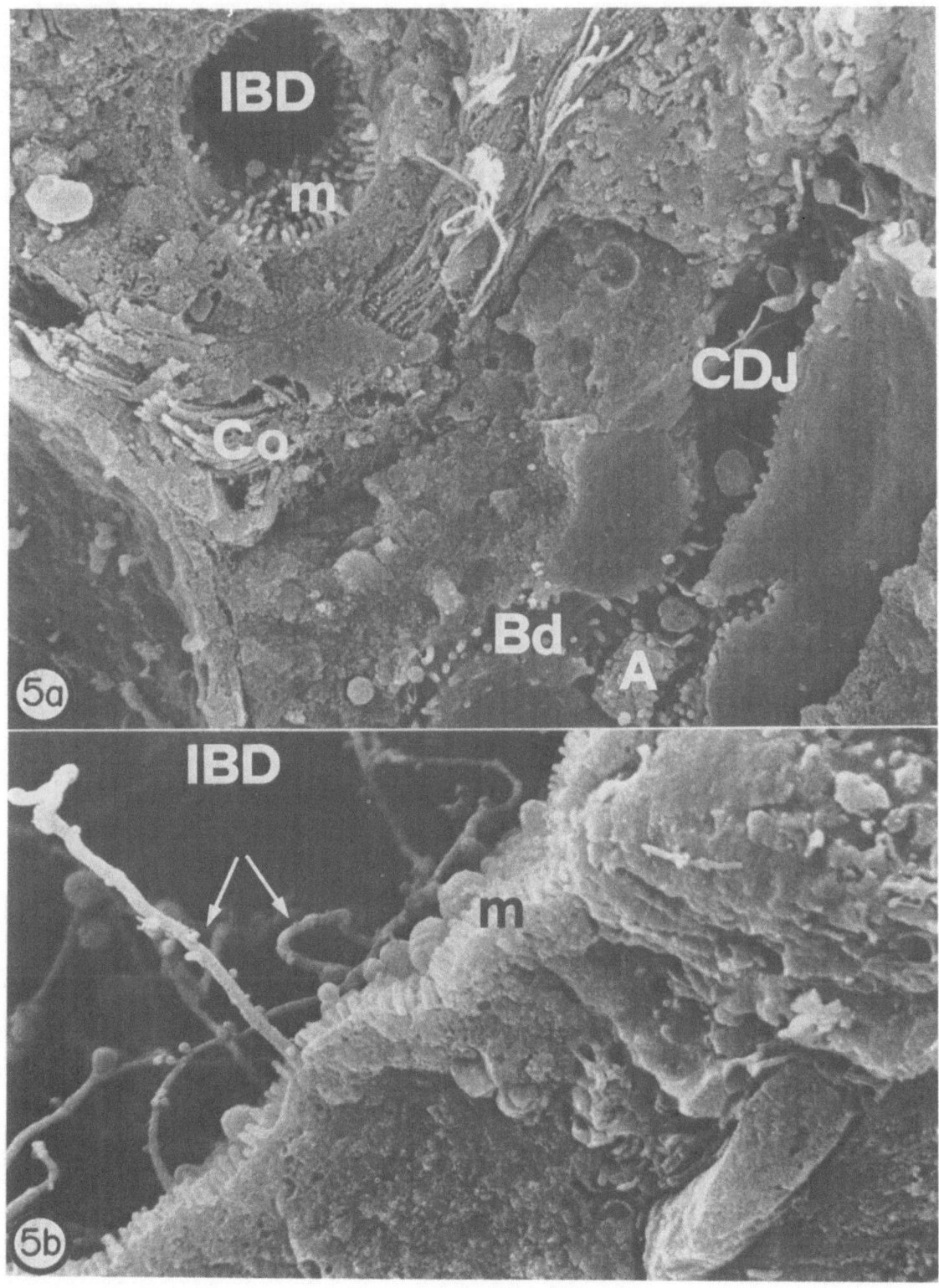

Figure 5a and b. Portal areas containing branches of canaliculoductular junction (CDJ) with the ampullar enlargement (A), bile ductule (Bd), and wide interlobular bile duct (IBD) showing numerous long cilia into the lumen (arrows). Co, collagen fibers; microvilli, blebs, and ruffles (m) populate the ductular lumen. Pig; ×1000; ×15,000.

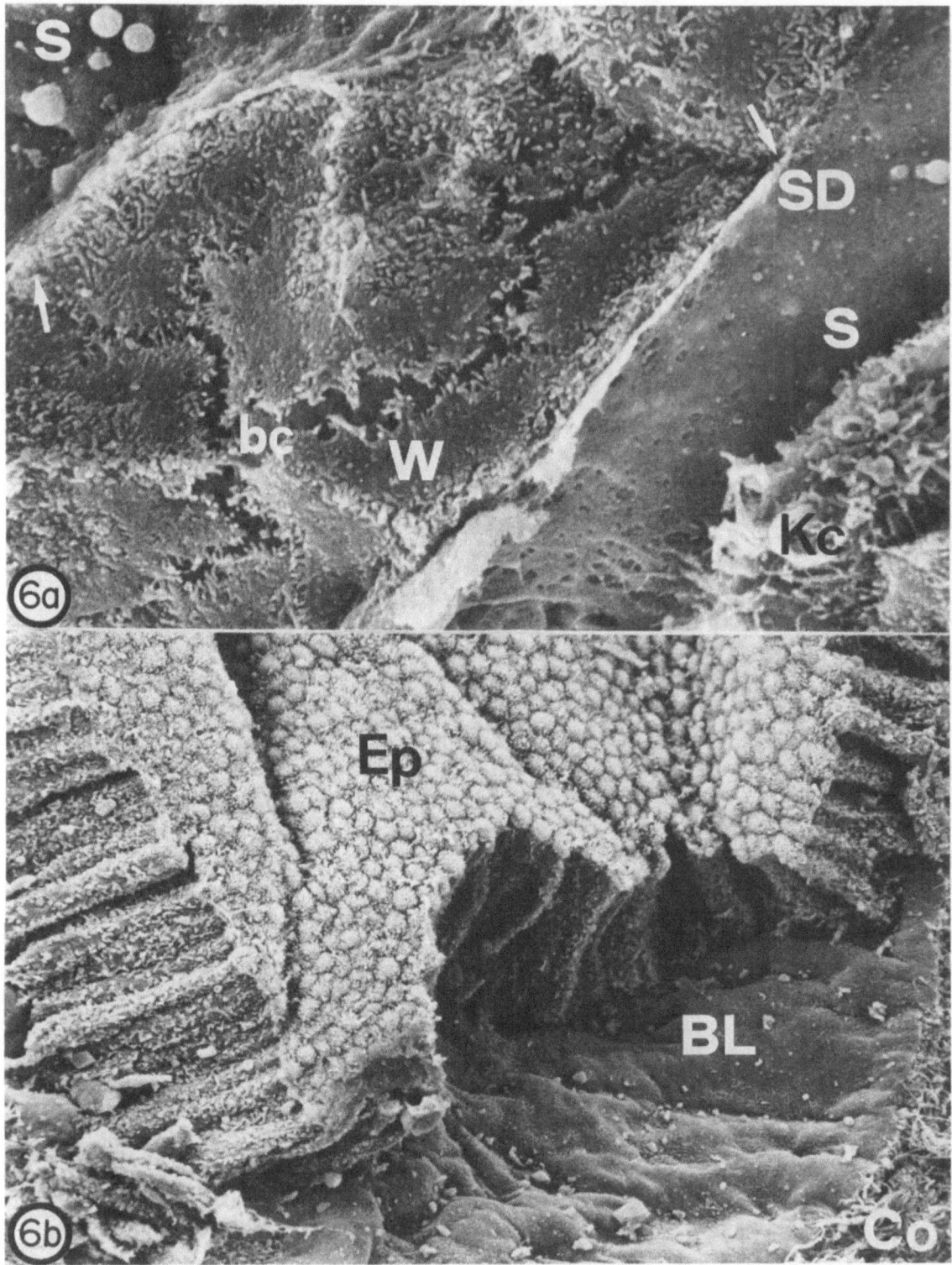

Figure 6. (*a*) Rat obstructive jaundice obtained seven days after ligation of the common duct. Bile canaliculi (BC) have a tortuous course and their marginal ridges show a 'wavy line' (W) provided with many diverticula. Apparent free communications between bile channels and spaces of Disse (SD) are noted (arrows). S, sinusoids; Kc, Kupffer cell; × 2600. From M. Nishi (1978) *Arch. Histol. Jpn.* 41:411 [30]. (*b*) Human primary biliary cirrhosis. Epithelial cells (Ep) covering the lumen of a large interlobular biliary duct. In this preparation the basal lamina (BL) surrounding the duct is very thickened and to it adhere numerous collagen fibers (Co); × 900.

frequently undulated and possesses longitudinal ridges that probably result from the contraction of the underlying muscular layer. The endothelial cells have a fusiform shape and are provided with few microvilli. In comparison with hepatic arteries, the luminal wall of the portal-vein ramifications shows a flattened and smooth endothelial coat. Microvilli are very rare and pits, together with small fenestrations, can be observed. A connective tissue rich in collagenous fibers surrounds these vessels and forms the support to all elements of the portal triad. The connective tissue of this area rapidly increases during liver fibrosis.

Liver sinusoids are special capillaries having a tortuous course. They form a radial and continuous network that connects the perilobular vessels with the central vein (Fig. 7a). As a consequence of this architecture, the wall of the central vein shows numerous small openings corresponding to the sinusoidal lumina (Fig. 7a). Under the SEM, the caliber of some of these openings appears so small that blood cells can be stopped. Not infrequently their sinusoidal lumen is also occupied by the bulging body of a Kupffer cell (Fig. 7c).

The endothelial wall of the central vein is very thin and has a few scattered microvilli, and flattened extensions provided with a number of small fenestrations similar to those of the sinusoids. Sinusoids are lined by very flattened endothelial cells showing scarce microvilli and isolated pits. Overlapping of thin endothelial extensions and zones of close cellular attachment can be observed when high-resolution SEM is employed [10]. The endothelial cell body, with the exception of the nuclear region bulging into the lumen, possesses very thin cytoplasmic expansions having two types of fenestrations. Some, very small (0.1–0.2 μm) are generally arranged in clusters ('sieve plates') while others are larger ($\sim$ 1 μm) and often subdivided by slender strands of cytoplasm [8, 24, 37, 43–47]. The small fenestrations are generally located intracellularly. The larger ones may be either intracellular or, more often, intercellular, as they actually occur between two cell margins [8–10].

A variety of causes probably infuences the size of endothelial fenestrations in normal as well in pathological conditions (hypoxia, cirrhosis, cholestasis, etc.). The larger gaps seem to arise by coalescence of the small ones [43, 48, 49]. As observed by using

SEM, Kupffer cells always display marked morphological differences from endothelial cells, and no transitional forms can be noted between either cell type in either adult or fetal liver [9, 44, 49–51]. In fact, Kupffer cells of different mammals and humans show an irregular and voluminous cell body provided with a variety of surface features such as blebs, microridges, holes, ruffles, lamellipodia, and filopodia (Fig. 7b) [7, 9, 10, 50, 52]. Three-dimensional analysis by SEM reveals that, as a rule, the Kupffer cells are located within the sinusoidal lumen and their cell body may lie on the luminal surface of the endothelial wall (Figs. 7 and 8).

In other situations, where large lamellipodia or long filopodia arise from the Kupffer cells, these projections clearly overlap thin endothelial extensions and contribute with these extensions to form a very delicate lining of the sinusoidal wall. These findings demonstrate that the overlapping of endothelial cells generally described in early TEM papers (for references see [37, 53]) can be, in several cases, due to Kupffer cell laminar extensions (lamellipodia). Junctional complexes are never found between Kupffer and endothelial cells. These two cell types are in close relationship, but do not attach to each other [7, 45]. On the basis of the above SEM results, it seems logical to suggest that Kupffer cells 'in vivo' are generally located within the sinusoidal lumen. When phagocytotic activity is particularly high (several physiopathological and experimental conditions), they may assume transitory interactions with the subjacent endothelial wall. These continuous and dynamic processes could generate the impression (when only sections by light microscopy and TEM are observed) that Kupffer and endothelial cells are a permanent component of the capillary wall [54, 55].

Furthermore, Kupffer cells are distributed not only in the sinusoids, but occasionally in the lumen of terminal hepatic and sublobular veins [52, 55]. In small vessels and capillaries, Kupffer cells bulge into the lumen such that their voluminous cell body and long cellular extensions thus reduce the caliber of the vessels and slow the blood flow, acting as a sort of sinusoidal sphincter [50, 52, 56].

In other cases the extensions of Kupffer cells (mainly filopodia and lamellipodia) are in proximity to endothelial fenestrations, or appear to

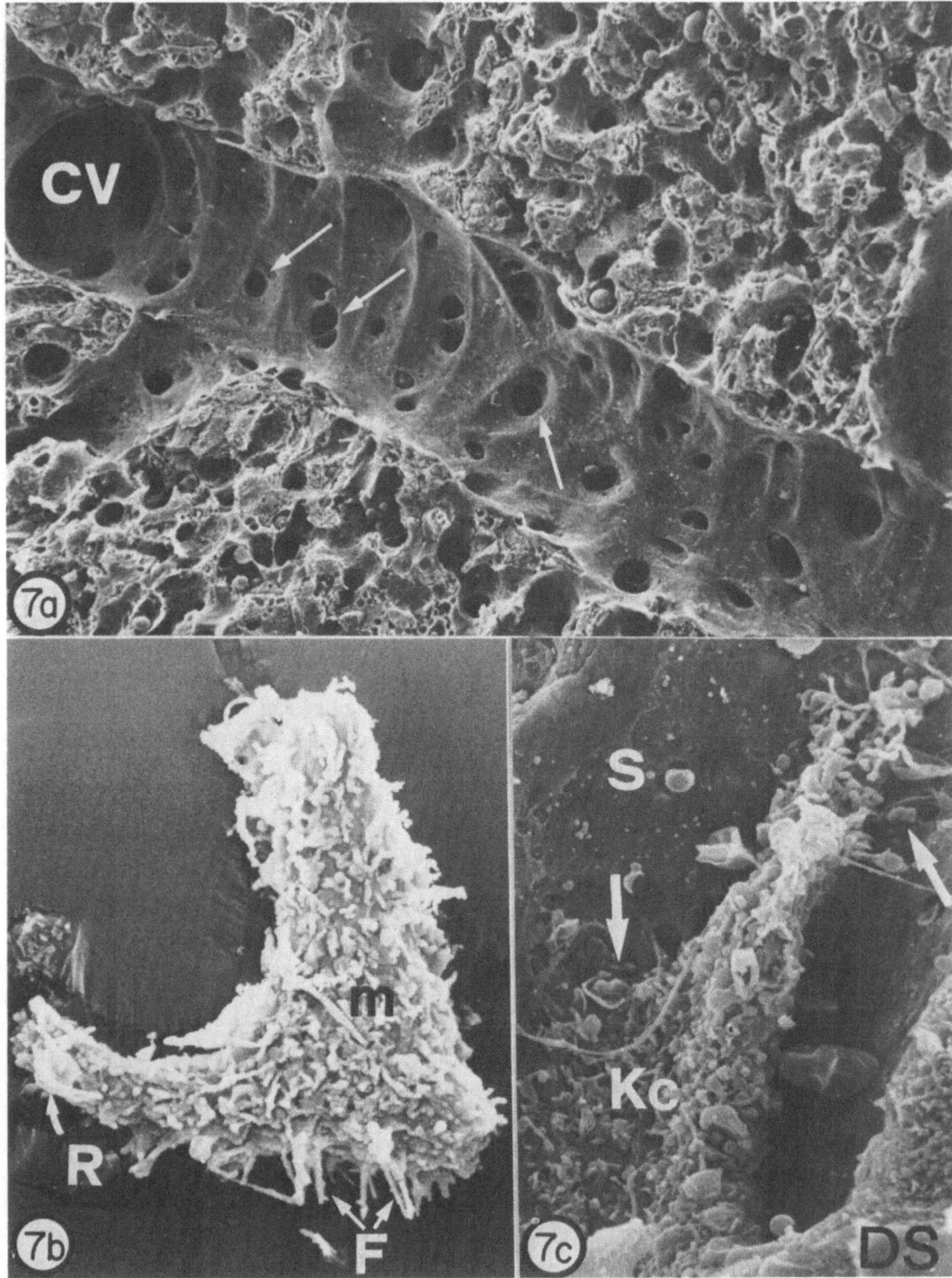

Figure 7. (*a*) Liver parenchyma showing a section of a central vein (CV) with numerous small openings corresponding to radiating lobular sinusoids (arrows). Cat; ×320. (*b*) An isolated Kupffer cell with numerous ruffles (R), blebs, microvilli (m), and filopodia (F) on its surface. (*c*) An activated Kupffer cell (Kc) within the lumen of a fenestrated liver sinusoid. Note the relationship between the surface features of the Kupffer cell (filopodia and lamellipodia) and the endothelial gaps (arrows). DS, Disse space. (*b*) Rat; ×6800. (*c*) Human, primary biliary cirrhosis; ×6200.

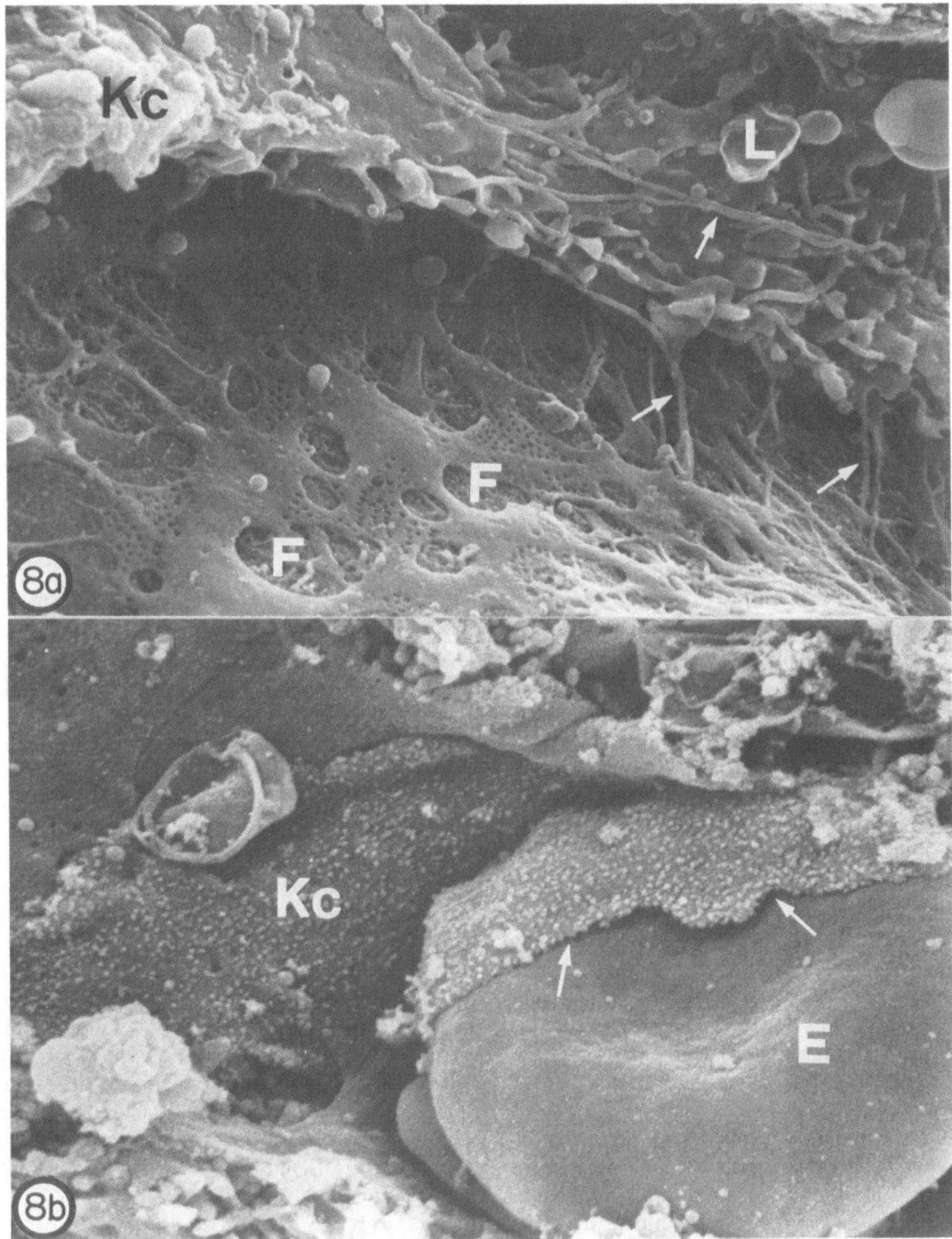

Figure 8. (*a*) This picture shows a highly fenestrated endothelium and an activated (phagocytosis) Kupffer cell (Kc) with numerous filopodia (arrows) and lamellar extensions (L) within the lumen of a sinusoid. Human; ×7500. (*b*) Kupffer cell (Kc) 5 min after portal infusion of glutaraldehyde-treated erythrocytes (E). The liplike extensions (arrows) of the Kupffer cell are covered with a number of granular precipitates, likely corresponding to cell coat substances. The phagocytosis of red cells by Kupffer cell extensions is shown in this figure. Rat; ×9500.

44

penetrate through them (Figs. 7 and 8). Although the possibility cannot be excluded that the appearance of larger endothelial gaps might be artifactual, the topographical relationship between Kupffer cell expansions and endothelial wall fenestrations, observable in the intact state only by SEM, should be considered when the delicate and perforated wall of the liver sinusoids is studied.

These observations suggest that the larger endothelial gaps (both intracellular and extracellular) always noted in liver sinusoids by different ultrastructural methods (TEM, freeze-etching, SEM) might depend upon a local activation of Kupffer cells (that actually are macrophages) [54, 55]. A similar dependence of large endothelial fenestrations upon the activation of Kupffer cells is also apparent in some SEM studies in which phagocytosis of Kupffer cells is experimentally induced in the rat by: (a) administration of drawing ink [57], or (b) introduction, via portal vein, of homologous red blood cells with chemically or immunologically modified surfaces (Fig. 8).

The results of these experiments demonstrate that erythrocytes are initially detected and then attached by one or more filopodia of Kupffer cells. The erythrocytes are subsequently attracted toward the cell body where they are finally engulfed by liplike projections of the Kupffer cells (Fig. 8). The capture and internalization of chemically treated erythrocytes occurs more vigorously and more rapidly than with antibody-coated cells [58].

In such experiments, the endothelial cells of the sinusoids are never involved in the process of phagocytosis [57–59]. Severe sinusoidal alterations are observed in SEM preparations of human liver pathology such as primary biliary cirrhosis and Banti syndrome, as well as in experimental conditions such as acute and chronic intoxication of the liver induced by various toxic chemicals (CCl_4 for example) [7] and estrogen treatment [60]. In some of these cases, the Kupffer cells may appear more active in phagocytosis. In these cases the endothelial wall is also provided with very large fenestrations, and displays wide interruptions along its surface (Figs. 7 and 8).

6. THE DISSE SPACE AND ITS CONTENTS

The Disse space, which is located between the hepatocytes and the cells lining the sinusoids, can be fully appreciated by using SEM techniques in adequately fixed and fractured preparations [8]. Under SEM, the Disse spaces form a continuous three-dimensional network of pericapillary and intercellular spaces in which sinusoids and liver cells are suspended. As seen topographically (mainly using stereo-views), the extensions of the Disse space are larger than was generally evident from TEM preparations alone. These ramifications extend out from adjacent hepatocytes and often form narrow intercellular channels connecting two or more adjacent pericapillary spaces. Because these recesses and channels are interrupted only where two hepatocytes are closely attached to form a bile canaliculus, they actually extend the subendothelial Disse spaces into a continuous labyrinthine system of intercellular spaces [61].

Into the Disse spaces are projected the hepatocyte microvilli. They contain a variable amount of fine collagen fibers there isolated or associated in bundles. In normal conditions, fat-storing cells (cells of Ito and Nemoto) and other pericytes (fibroblasts/fibrocytes) are occasionally encountered on the tissue side of the endothelium from where they extend their slender projections into the Disse recesses (Fig. 9).

The perisinusoidal fibers and/or nerve endings described in a number of recent TEM and histochemical studies [62–65] cannot be recognized by using only SEM methods [6, 66].

The Disse spaces have been observed in only a few experimental and pathological conditions, but the findings demonstrate that the alteration of this space can be of great diagnostic importance in a more exact topographical evaluation of its extensions and contents (collagen fibers and fibrocytes in cholestatis, fibrosis, cirrhosis; fat-storing cells and vitamin A effects, etc.) (Fig. 10) [7, 22, 30, 32, 36–38, 60].

7. THE LIVER SURFACE

The liver is provided with an investment of connective tissue that is rich in collagenous and elastic

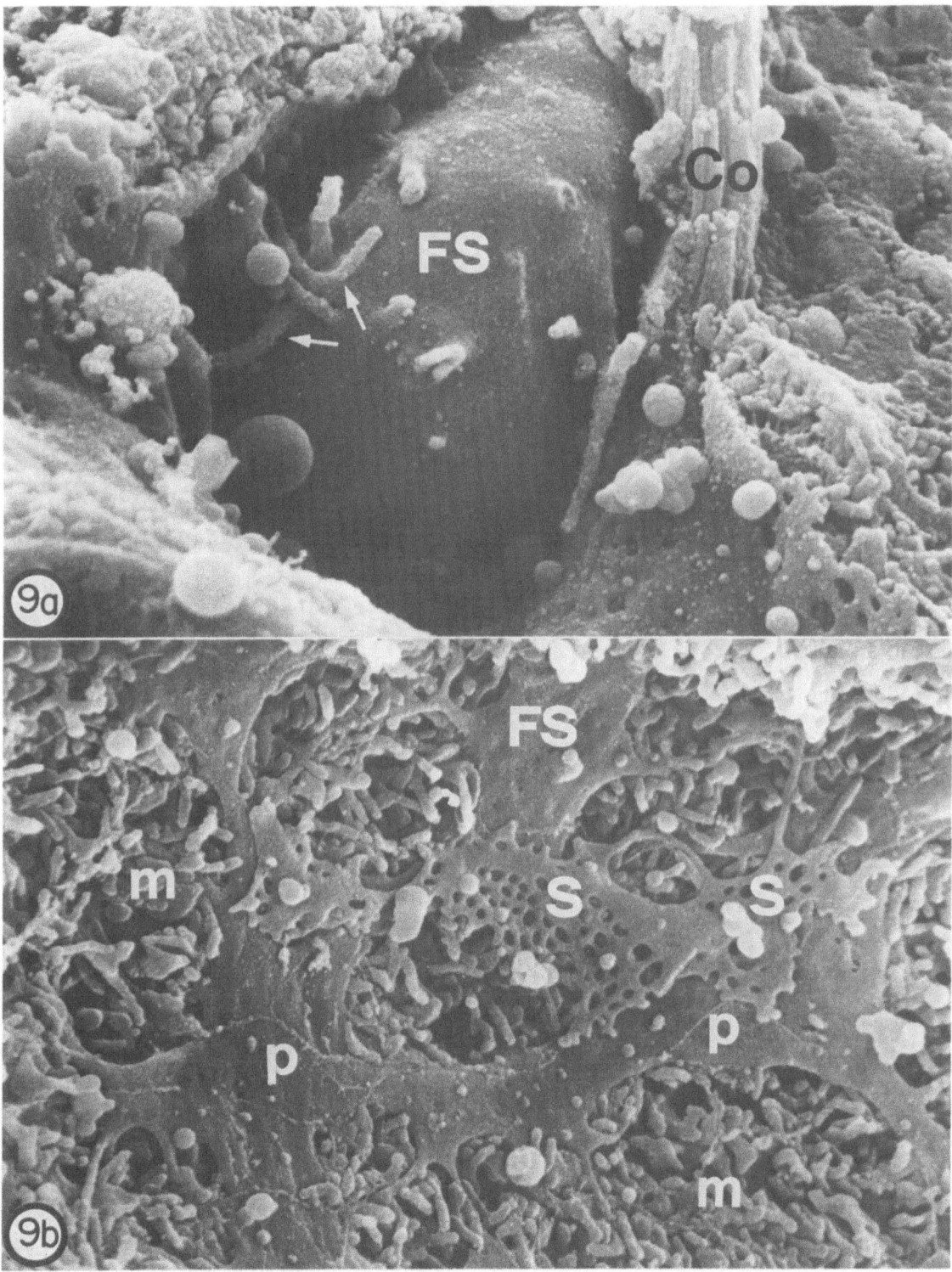

Figure 9. *(a)* Perisinusoidal space of Disse containing the cell body of a fat-storing cell (cell of Ito and Nemoto) (FS). Co, collagen fibers; microvilli and cellular extensions arising from the fat-storing cell (arrows). Rat; × 16,000. From Motta et al. (1978) *The liver. An atlas of SEM.* Courtesy of Igaku-Shoin Tokyo/New York [7]. *(b)* Probable subendothelial processes (p) of a large fat-storing cell (FS). The microvilli (m) belong to a subjacent hepatocyte; the fenestrated aspect of the sinusoidal endothelium is also evident (S). Rat; × 15,000.

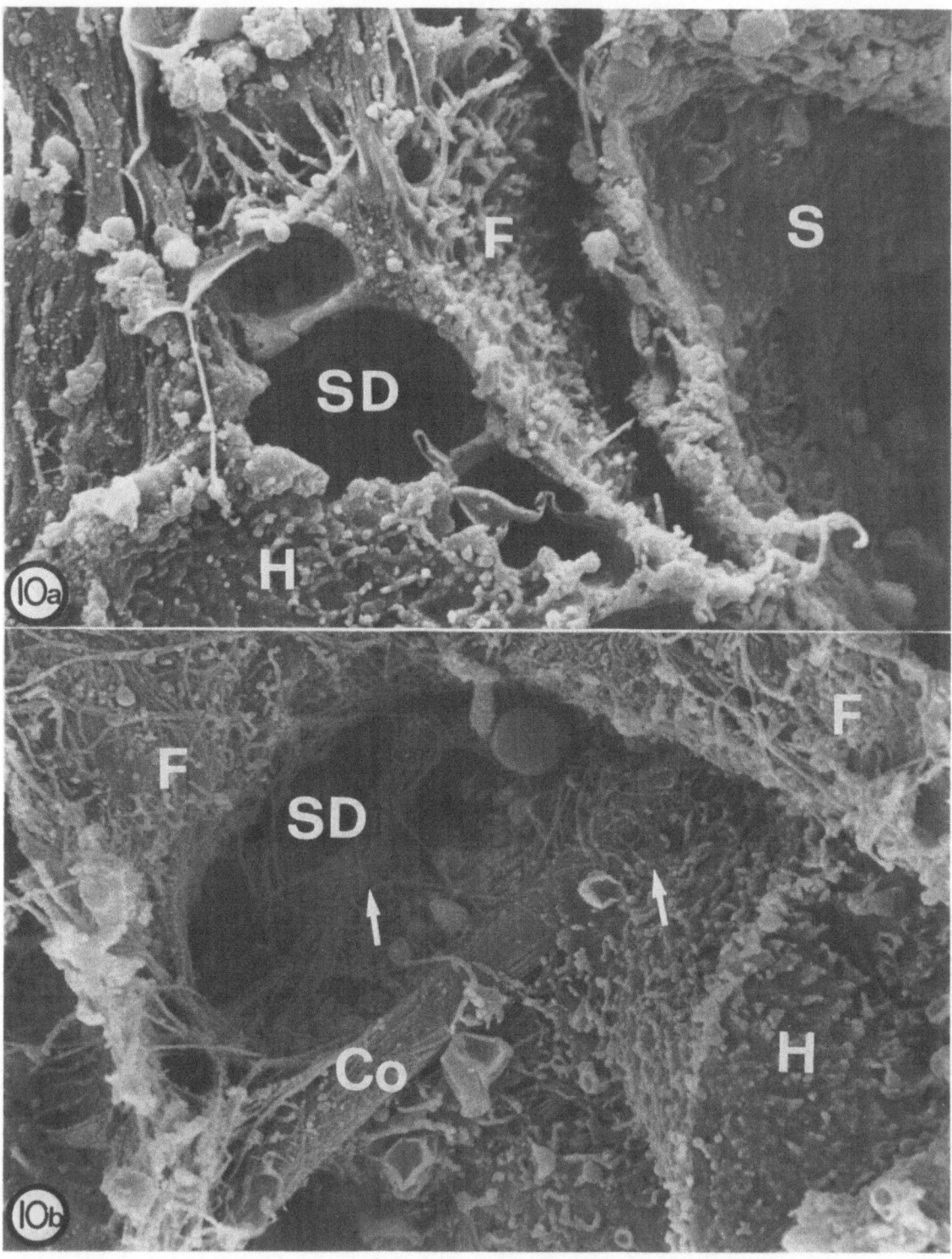

Figure 10a and b. The pictures show the space of Disse (SD) in a patient diagnosed with a primary biliary cirrhosis. Thick bundles of collagen fibers (Co) and irregularly shaped fibroblasts (F) are evident in these areas. The wall of the sinusoid is very thick (S) and the surface of the hepatocytes (H) is covered with numerous microvilli and irregular cell projections to which are attached collagen fibers (arrows). Human; ×8500; ×8200.

47

fibers and is covered by a continuous layer of serosal cells (Fig. 11). Serosa are flattened and/or cuboidal elements heavily populated by microvilli having a variable length. The microvilli surface is covered with fine strands of material highly colorable with rutenium red reacting material (glicocalix).

It has been suggested that mesothelial microvilli may function as a 'slippery cushion' capable of protecting the delicate serosa from surface friction

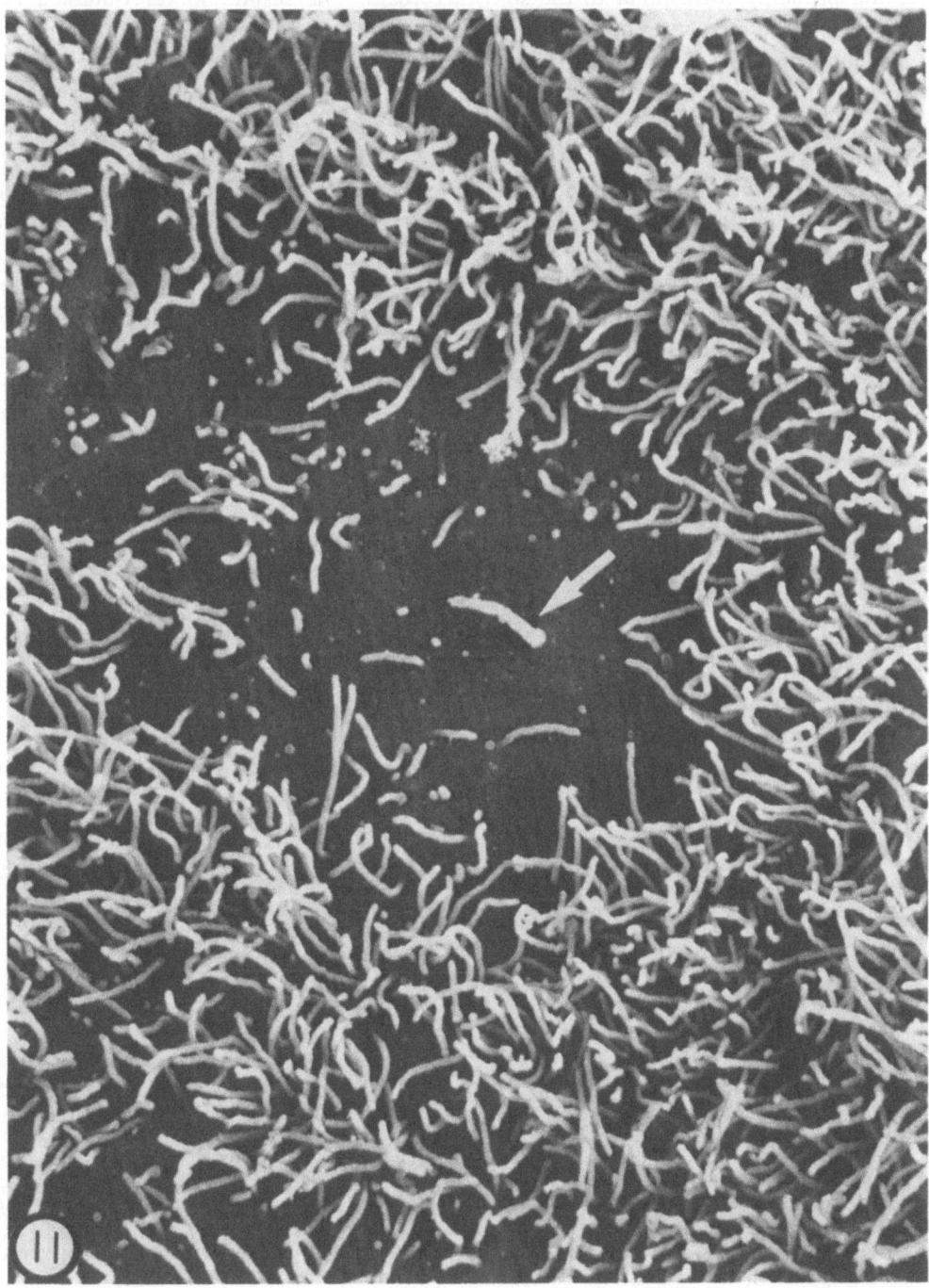

Figure 11. Capsular surface of liver. The serosal cells are covered with numerous microvilli and an isolated cilium (arrow). Cat; ×9500.

48

damage [67]. In other cases the serosal cells are devoid of microvilli and show rather smooth surfaces. Isolated cilia of various lengths, and numerous pinocytotic vesicles are on the free surface of these cells [68]. Furthermore, intercellular invaginations occasionally occur in these as well in other serosa layers, and probably correspond to the so-called stomata originally noted by von Recklinghausen [69] and more recently carefully described by using correlated SEM and TEM [68, 70].

The numerous pinocytotic vesicles on the serosal surface are related to a high exchange of fluids between the liver parenchyma and the peritoneal cavity in normal conditions. In fact, as it is known, the tissue spaces beneath the serosa contain fluids arising from the labyrinthine system of Disse spaces, which can be considered to be transformed lymphatic lacunae. The free flow of plasma substances from the fenestrated sinusoids to the Disse spaces, and from there to the area subjacent to the serosal layer, explains the importance of the hepatic capsule as source of ascites during liver cirrhosis.

In cirrhotic rats with ascites, the mesothelial cells covering the liver are thickened and show numerous vacuoles and intercellular fluid-filled dilatations [37]. These findings demonstrate a probable increase in intrahepatic hydrostatic pressure of the lymph and provide reason for increased ascitic fluid transudates on the liver surfaces [37]. Scanning SEM has not been used to study the altered liver surface during cirrhosis and it seems to be an appropriate approach to investigate dynamics of ascites fluids.

8. CONCLUDING REMARKS

The utility of scanning electron-microscopic techniques in the visualization of 'real' three-dimensional microanatomy of the liver is clearly indicated by the numerous articles published within the last six years. The results so far obtained have been directed primarily toward a definition of a normal morphology. Furthermore, the parallel improvement of chemical and mechanical dissociation techniques that expose the internal surfaces of liver parenchyma are invaluable in elucidating the exact topography of hepatic components. The development of such techniques, together with the progressive development of higher-resolution instruments, prove that the SEM may be an important tool in clarifying dynamic alterations in liver morphology in response to altered physiopathological conditions. These processes may be useful in the rapid evaluation of human liver biopsies [7, 10]. This latter approach may prove particularly useful, as indicated by the impact of SEM on gastrointestinal research [71].

Comparisons of results from various concurrent TEM and SEM techniques enable an understanding of the synthesis of organ structure and function in three dimensions with much greater speed and certainty [71]. This is simply to say that SEM is closer than other microscopic techniques to reproducing, as a frame out of a cinema, the spatial and temporal status of a dynamic living object.

Acknowledgments. We gratefully acknowledge the expert assistance offered by Dr. J. Van Blerkom during the preparation of this manuscript. We would also like to thank Mr. K. Adachi and Mr. G. F. Franchitto for the photographic work and Mrs. A. Andreani for typing this chapter. This work was supported by CNR grant CT 80.00521.04.

REFERENCES

1. Fujita T, Tokunaga J, Inoue H (1971) Atlas of scanning electron microscopy in medicine. Tokyo: Igaku-Shoin
2. Motta PM, Andrews PM, Porter KR (1977) Microanatomy of cell and tissue surfaces. Philadelphia: Lea and Febiger
3. Hayat MA (1978) Introduction to biological scanning electron microscopy. Baltimore: University Park
4. Kessel RG, Kardon RH (1979) Tissues and organs: a text–atlas of scanning electron microscopy. San Francisco: WH Freeman
5. Fujita T, Tanaka K, Tokunaga J (1981) SEM atlas of cells and tissues. Tokyo: Igaku-Shoin
6. Motta P (1977) The three-dimensional fine structure of the liver as revealed by scanning electron microscopy. Int Rev Cytol [Suppl 6]: 347–399
7. Motta P, Muto M, Fujita T (1978) The liver. An atlas of scanning electron microscopy. Tokyo: Igaku-Shoin
8. Motta PM, Porter KR (1974) Structure of rat liver sinusoids and associated spaces as revealed by scanning electron microscopy. Cell Tissue Res 148: 111–125
9. Muto M (1975) A scanning electron microscopic study on endothelial cells and Kupffer cells in rat liver sinusoids. Arch Histol Jpn 37:369–386
10. Muto M, Nishi M, Fujita T (1977) Scanning electron microscopy of human liver sinusoids. Arch Histol Jpn 40: 137–151

11. Kiernan F (1833) The anatomy and physiology of the liver. Philos Trans Roy Soc London 123: 711–770
12. Mall FP (1906) A study of the structural unit of the liver. Am J Anat 5: 227–308
13. Rappaport AM, Borony ZJ, Lougheed WM, Lotto WN (1954) Subdivision of hexagonal liver lobules into a structural and functional unit: role in hepatic physiology and pathology. Anat Rec 119: 11–34
14. Elias H, Sherrick JC (1969) Morphology of the liver. New York: Academic
15. Murakami T, Itoshima T, Shimada Y (1974) Peribiliary portal system in the monkey liver as evidenced by the injection replica scanning electron microscope method. Arch Histol Jpn 37: 245–260
16. Grisham JW., Nopanitaya W, Compagno J, Nagel AEH (1975) Scanning electron microscopy of normal rat liver. The surface structure of its cells and tissues components. Am J Anat 144: 295–322
17. Vial JD, Porter KR (1975) Scanning microscopy of dissociated tissue cells. J Cell Biol 67: 345–360
18. Loud AV (1968) A quantitative stereological description of the ultrastructure of normal rat liver parenchymal cells. J Cell Biol 37: 27–46
19. Wanson JC, Drochmans P, May C, Penasse W, Popouski A (1975) Isolation of centrolobular and perilobular hepatocytes after phenobarbital treatment. J Cell Biol 66: 23–41
20. Wanson JC, Bernaert D, Mày C (1979) Morphology and functional properties of isolated and cultured hepatocytes. In: Popper H, Schaffner F (eds) Progress in liver disease, vol 6. New York: Grune and Stratton, pp 1–22
21. Penasse W, Bernaert D, Mosselmans R, Wanson JC, Drochmans P (1979) Scanning electron microscopy of adult rat hepatocytes in situ after isolation of pure fractions by elutriation and after culture. Biol Cell 34:175–186
22. Nopanitaya W, Grisham JW, Carson JL, Dotson MM (1976) Surface features of cirrhotic liver. Virchows Arch Pathol 273:97–108
23. Marinozzi G, Muto M, Correr S, Motta PM (1977) Scanning electron microscope observations of intrahepatic biliary tree. I. Canaliculo-ductular junction. Bile ducts and ducts. J Submicrosc Cytol 9:127–143
24. Brooks SEH, Haggis GH (1973) Scanning electron microscopy of rat's liver. Application of freeze-fracture and freeze-drying techniques. Lab Invest 29:60–64
25. Motta PM, Fumagalli G (1975) Structure of rat bile canaliculi as revealed by scanning electron microscopy. Anat Rec 182:499–514
26. Bruni C, Porter KR (1965) The fine structure of the parenchymal cell of the normal rat liver. I. General observations. Am J Pathol 46:691–755
27. Tandler B, Hoppel CL (1974) Subsurface cisterns in mouse hepatocytes. Anat Rec 179:173–284
28. Matter W, Orci L, Rouiller C (1969) A study on the permeability barrier between Disse's space and the bile canaliculus. J Ultrastruct Res [Suppl 2]:1–71
29. Brauer RW (1963) Liver circulation and function. Physiol Rev 43:115–213
30. Nishi M (1978) Scanning electron microscope study on the mechanism of obstructive jaundice in rats. Arch Histol Jpn 41:411–426
31. Metz J, Aoki A, Merlo M, Forssmann WG (1977) Morphological alterations and functional changes of interhepatocellular junctions induced by bile duct ligation. Cell Tissue Res 182:299–310
32. Compagno J, Grisham JW (1974) Scanning electron microscopy of extrahepatic biliary obstruction. Arch Pathol 97:348–351
33. Brooks SEH, Reynolds P, Audretsch JJ, Haggis G (1975) Scanning electron microscopy of proliferating bile ductules. Lab Invest 33:311–315
34. Layden TJ, Schwarz J, Boyer JL (1975) Scanning electron microscopy of the rat liver. Studies of the effect of taurolithocholate and other models of cholestasis. Gastroenterology 69:724–738
35. Miyai K, Richardson AL, Mayr W, Javitt ND (1977) Subcellular pathology of rat liver in cholestasis and choleresis induced by bile salts. I. Effects of lithocholic 3β-hydroxy-5-cholenoic, cholic and dehydrocholic acids. Lab Invest 36:249–258
36. Nishi M, Kawamura T, Kamimura T, Murayama H, Sasaki H, Ichida F (1976) Scanning and transmission electron microscopic observation of primary biliary cirrhosis. J Clin Electron Microsc 9:5–6
37. Tanikawa K (1979) Ultrastructural aspects of the liver and its disorders, 2nd edn. Tokyo: Igaku-Shoin
38. Carpino F, Gaudio E, Marinozzi G, Melis M, Motta PM (1981) A scanning and transmission electron microscopic study of experimental extrahepatic cholestasis in the rat. J Submicrosc Cytol (in press)
39. Motta PM, Fumagalli G (1974) Scanning electron microscopy demonstration of cilia in rat intrahepatic bile duct. Z Anat Entwicklungsgesch 145:223–226
40. Enders AC, Nelson DM (1973) Pinocytotic activity of the uterus of the rat. Am J Anat 138:277–300
41. Motta PM, Andrews PM (1976) Scanning electron microscopy of the endometrium during the secretory phase. J Anat 122:315–322
42. Barberini F, Sartori S, Van Blerkom J, Motta PM (1978) Changes in the surface morphology of the rabbit endometrium related to the estrous and progestational stages of the reproductive cycle. A scanning and transmission electron microscopic study. Cell Tissue Res 190:207–222
43. Nopanitaya W, Grisham JW (1975) Scanning electron microscopy of mouse intrahepatic structures. Exp Mol Pathol 23:441–458
44. Itoshima T, Kobayashi T, Shimada Y, Murakami T (1974) Fenestrated endothelium of the liver sinusoids of the guinea pig as revealed by scanning electron microscopy. Arch Histol Jpn 37:15–24
45. Wisse E, Knook DL (1979) The investigation of sinusoidal cells: a new approach to the study of liver function. In: Popper H, Schaffner F (eds) Progress in liver diseases, vol 6. New York: Grune and Stratton, pp 153–171
46. Ishimura K, Okamoto H, Fujita H (1978) Freeze-etching images of capillary endothelial pores in the liver. Thyroid and adrenal of the mouse. Arch Histol Jpn 41:187–193
47. Montesano R, Nicolescu P (1978) Fenestrations in endothelium of rat liver sinudoids revisited by freeze-fracture. Anat Rec 190:861–870
48. Frenzel H, Kremer B, Mucker H (1977) The liver sinusoids under various pathological conditions. A TEM and SEM study of rat liver after respiratory hypoxia, telecobalt-irradiation and endotoxin application. In: Wisse E, Knook DL (eds) Kupffer cells and other liver sinusoidal cells. Amsterdam: Elsevier/North-Holland, pp 213–222
49. Motta PM (1977) Kupffer cells as revealed by scanning electron microscopy. In: Wisse E, Knook DL (eds) Kupffer cells and other liver sinusoidal cells. Amsterdam: Elsevier/North-Holland, pp 93–102
50. Motta PM (1975) A scanning electron microscopic study of

the rat liver sinusoid. Endothelial and Kupffer cells. Cell Tissue Res 164:371–385

51. Motta PM, Makabe S (1980) Foetal and adult liver sinusoids and Kupffer cells as revealed by scanning electron microscopy. In: Liehr H, Grun M (eds) The reticulo-endothelial system and the pathogenesis of liver disease. Amsterdam: Elsevier/North-Holland, pp 11–16

52. Vonnahme FJ (1977) A scanning electron microscopic study of Kupffer cells in the monkey liver. In: Wisse E, Knook DL (eds) Kupffer cells and other liver sinusoidal cells. Amsterdam: Elsevier/North-Holland, pp 103–108

53. David H (1964) Submikroskopische Ortho- und Pathomorphologie der Leber. Berlin: Akademie-Verlag

54. Motta PM (1978) A three-dimensional microscopic study of Kupffer cells [Abstr]. J Cell Biol 79:40

55. Motta PM (1979) The location of Kupffer cells in the liver of different mammals. A three dimensional analysis by scanning electron microscopy. Verh Anat Ges 73:827–830

56. McCuskey RS (1966) A dynamic and static study of hepatic arterioles and hepatic sphincters. Am J Anat 119:455–478

57. Satodate R, Sasou S, Oikawa K, Hatekeyama N, Katsura S (1977) Scanning electron microscopical studies on the Kupffer cell in phagocytotic activity. In: Wisse E, Knook DL (eds) Kupffer cells and other liver sinusoidal cells. Amsterdam: Elsevier/North-Holland, pp 121–129

58. Muto M, Fujita T (1977) Phagocytotic activities of the Kupffer cell: a scanning electron microscope study. In: Wisse E, Knook DL (eds) Kupffer cells and other liver sinusoidal cells. Amsterdam: Elsevier/North-Holland, pp 109–119

59. Munthe-Kaas AC, Kaplan G, Seljelid R (1977) On the mechanism of internalization of opsonized particles by rat Kupffer cells in vitro. Exp Cell Res 103:201–212

60. Tanikawa K (1979) Liver pathology. In: Trump BF, Jones RT (eds) Diagnostic electron microscopy, vol 2. New York: John Wiley and Sons, pp 15–46

61. Motta PM, Porter KR (1974) Rat liver cells and associated spaces of Disse as revealed by scanning electron microscopy. In: Saunders JV, Goodchild DJ (eds) Proceedings 8th International Congress of Electron Microscopy, vol 2. Canberra: Australian Academy of Sciences, pp 410–411

62. Yamada E (1965) Some observations on the nerve terminals on the liver parenchymal cell of the mouse as revealed by electron microscopy. Okajimas Folia Anat Jpn 40:663–677

63. Forssmann WG, Ito S (1977) Hepatocyte innervation in primates. J Cell Biol 74:299–313

64. Mazzanti L, Del Tacca M, Breschi MC (1977) Histochemical studies of noradrenergic innervation of the liver in untreated and dannomycin-pretreated guinea pigs. Histochemistry 53:17–24

65. Ungvary G, Donath T (1969) On the monoaminergic innervation of the liver. Acta Anat (Basel) 72:446–459

66. Skaaring P, Bierring F (1976) On the intrisic innervation of normal rat liver. Histochemical and scanning electron microscopical studies. Cell Tissue Res 171:141–155

67. Andrews PM, Porter KR (1973) The ultrastructural morphology and possible functional significance of mesothelial microvilli. Anat Rec 177:409–426

68. Barberini F, Carpino F, Renda T, Motta PM (1977) Etude au microscope électronique à balayage du péritoine du rat. Anat Anz 142:486–496

69. Von Recklinghausen. F.T. (1865) Zur Fettresorption. Virchows Arch Pathol Anat 26:172–208

70. Leak LV, Rahil K (1978) Permeability of the diaphragmatic mesothelium: the ultrastructural basis for 'stomata'. Am J Anat 151:557–594

71. Toner PG, Carr KE (1979) The digestive system. In: Hodges GM, Hallowes RC (eds) Biomedical research applications of scanning electron microscopy, vol 1. New York: Academic, pp 203–272

4. FREEZE-FRACTURE OF HEPATIC FINE STRUCTURE UNDER NORMAL AND EXPERIMENTAL CONDITIONS

J. METZ

1. INTRODUCTION

The freeze-fracture method is a special preparatory procedure that is utilized in ultrastructural studies and has been applied to biological and medical investigations for more than twenty years. The historical development as well as theoretical aspects of the method have been reviewed in several previous publications [1–3]. Since its inception, the method has been widely used and continuously improved. A particularly impressive current development is quick freezing whereby tissue can be solidified without perceptible structural changes, allowing electron-microscopic specimen analysis close to or resembling that of the 'in vivo conditions' [4].

The liver was one of the first organs on which ultrastructural investigations were carried out by using the freeze-fracture method [5]. In practice, tissue is chemically fixed by using routine techniques of electron microscopy [6, 7]. Prior to cryofixation, antifreeze agents are applied and the tissue is rapidly brought to liquid nitrogen temperature. In a vacuum apparatus, internal faces of the frozen tissue are exposed to temperatures between $-90°$ C and $-115°$ C either by means of a microtome (freeze-cleaving) or a fracture device (freeze-fracturing). A replica of the exposed surface is made by an evaporation of platinum–carbon. In standard shadow-cast replicas, a three-dimensional image is obtained by directing the platinum shadowing at an angle of 45°. For transmission electron microscopy, the replica is removed from the fractured specimen. The resolution by using this method is in the range of 25 Å.

In combination with standard thin section and negative staining methods, freeze-fracturing offers additional advantages not only in exposing cellular membranes, and their geometry, but also providing further information concerning their associated processes. Structural details of membranous components, such as intramembranous protein particles, can be analyzed as well. In the last few years the study of intercellular connections has captured the attention of numerous investigators, which was particularly facilitated by the development of this method.

Misinterpretations stemming from the development of the freeze-fracture method primarily concerned the fracture levels in membranes, which were also evident in liver tissue [5, 8, 9] and have since been corrected [10, 11]. According to these data, fracture levels, which run along a membrane, usually follow the central hydrophobic plane of the lipid bilayer. Thus, the inner faces of membranes are exposed in the freeze-fracture procedure. According to the nomenclature that was established in 1975 [12], the part of the bilayer which is adjacent to the cytoplasm is called the P-face, while the E-face is the part directed to the extracellular space.

In the following review, major emphasis will be given to the presentation of membrane architecture and membrane-associated processes of the liver parenchyma, which has mainly been investigated with the freeze-fracture method.

2. LIVER PARENCHYMA

The typical arrangement of liver tissue is captured in a three-dimensional view upon observation by freeze-fracture replicas. The ultrastructure of cellular elements, intercellular structures, and compartments can be clearly differentiated. Furthermore, the principal cell types that are present within the parenchyma, such as hepatocytes, endothelial

52

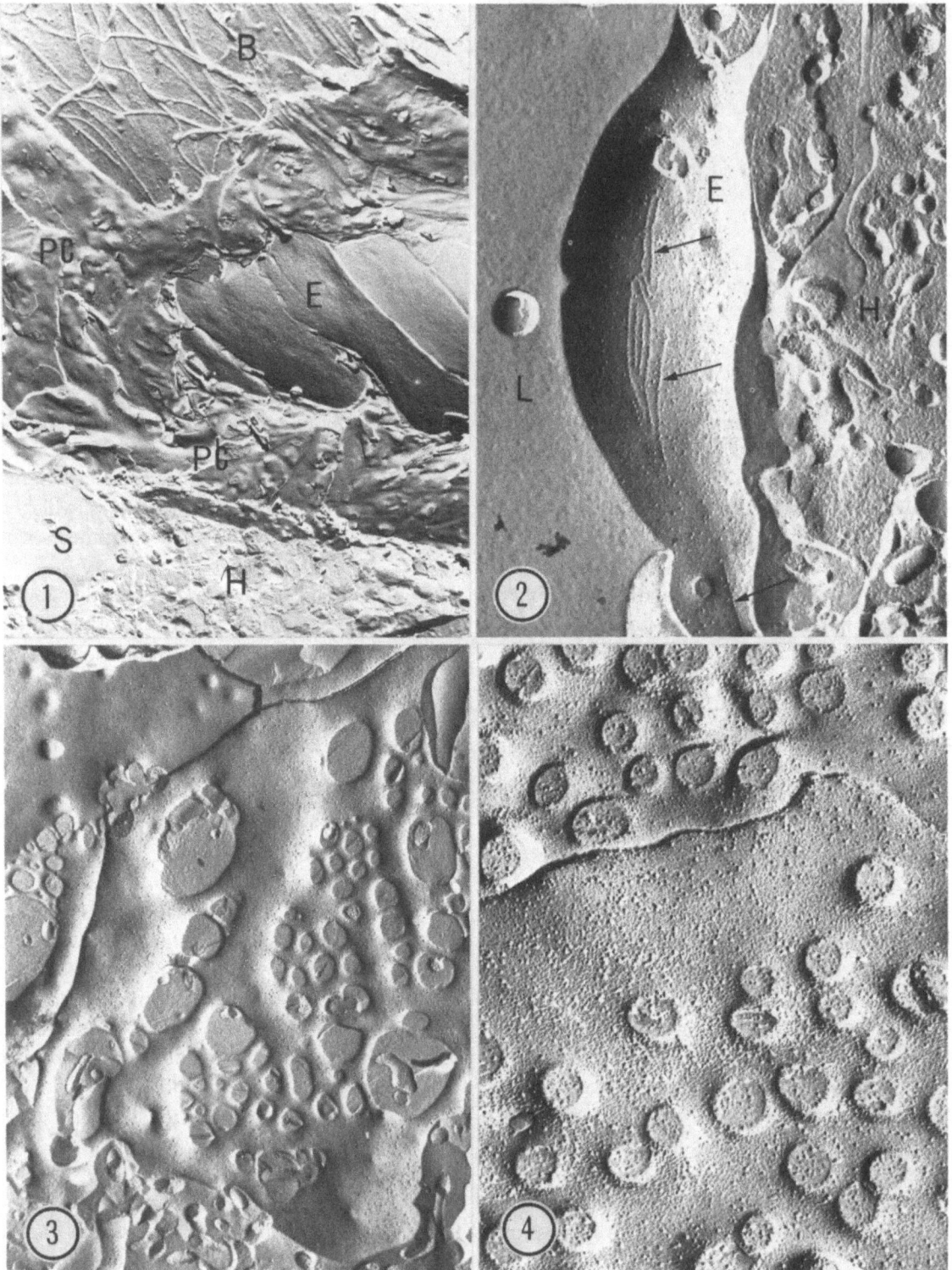

Figure 1. Rat liver. The wall of an interlobular branch of the portal vein is fractured stepwise: Endothelial cells (E) with pinocytotic activity, a basal lamina (B), and pericytes (PC) are identified. A sinusoid (S) runs in the direction of the parenchyma. H, hepatocytes; ×5200.

Figure 2. Rat liver. Endothelial cell (E) fractured along the interendothelial membrane region. Particulate tight junctional strands (arrows) are discontinuously arranged on the P-face, of the endothelial membrane. H, hepatocyte; L, lumen; ×37,000.

cells, and Kupffer cells, can be readily recognized in the replicas from characteristic morphological features. Cells within the liver are fractured either crosswise, revealing cytoplasm and cell organelles, or intramembranously, exposing faces of the plasmalemma at variable degrees. In addition, cross-sectional fractures reveal information concerning the membranes of cell organelles, such as the endoplasmic reticulum or the Golgi apparatus. Problems do arise, however, in identifying cell organelles that possess similar forms and sizes and whose inner structure is not adequately exposed. These structures include microbodies, lysosomes, and vacuoles.

2.1. Liver sinusoid

The sinusoids originate from interlobular branches of the portal vein (Fig. 1) and constitute a rich intralobular vascular network that converges from the lobular periphery in the direction of the central veins. The walls of the sinusoids consist primarily of flat endothelial cells (Fig. 2). Kupffer cells, fat-storing cells, and pit cells are not as numerous. Endothelial cells are located in the strategically important area between the blood and the hepatocytes. Their inner surfaces delineate the blood space, while the outer surfaces border on the perisinusoid Disse space, into which countless microvillous processes of the hepatocytes project (Figs. 3 and 4).

In most mammals, endothelial cells form a continuous wall that displays numerous openings. Narrow clefts between processes of neighboring endothelial cells are irregularly closed by a few or single strands (Fig. 2) that are considered as macular types of tight junctions. Often no more than single junctional particles provide punctate contacts between both membranes [13]. The intercellular connections seem to possess only minor importance with respect to a permeability barrier for blood plasma substances. Numerous fenestrations are typically seen in endothelial cells (Fig. 3), although there is as yet no exact information available on their number, size, geometry, or location [69]. The fenestrations vary in size, but it appears that blood cells down to the level of thrombocytes are restricted from passage, as well as chylomicrons, which appear unable to proceed readily into the perisinusoidal space [14]. Serotonin apparently has a constrictive effect on the diameter of the fenestrations [14], while high perfusion pressure [15] results in their enlargement.

The Kupffer cells can easily be differentiated from the endothelial cells by their irregular surface structure. Long cellular processes frequently reach through the fenestrations into the perisinusoidal space. Numerous membrane-enclosed vesicles, which are mainly lysosomes, are present within these cells.

2.2. Hepatocyte

2.2.1. Cytoplasm. Special attention is drawn to a few characteristics of individual cell organelles that in comparison with other methods are seen to better advantage in freeze-fracture replicas [16].

Within the large, polyhedral hepatocytes, one or two round nuclei are generally centrally located. Characteristic pores between the outer and inner membranes are distributed randomly over the nuclear surface (Fig. 7). Freeze-fracture results indicate that the pore system comprises about 8% of the total nuclear surface [17], while sectioned material give smaller values [18]. The outer membrane of the nuclear envelope is smooth, whereas the inner membrane shows numerous associated particles. Mitochondria exhibit relatively smooth external membrane (E-) faces, while their inner (P-) faces are occupied by numerous particles (Figs. 5 and 6). The interior arrangement of crosswise-fractured mitochondria is clearly distinguishable only in deeply etched specimens. Cisternae of rough endoplasmic reticulum are slightly curved and appear as parallel lamellae that often exhibit typical fenestrations (Figs. 5 and 6). Anastomosing tubular and caveolar

Figure 3. Rat liver. P-face of endothelial cells facing the perisinusoidal side. Numerous fenestrations interrupt the cellular continuity. In the interspaces are located fractured microvillous structures of hepatocytes; ×30,000.
Figure 4. Rat liver. P-faces of the perisinusoidal membrane area of hepatocytes exhibit numerous transversely fractured microvillous structures; ×64,000.

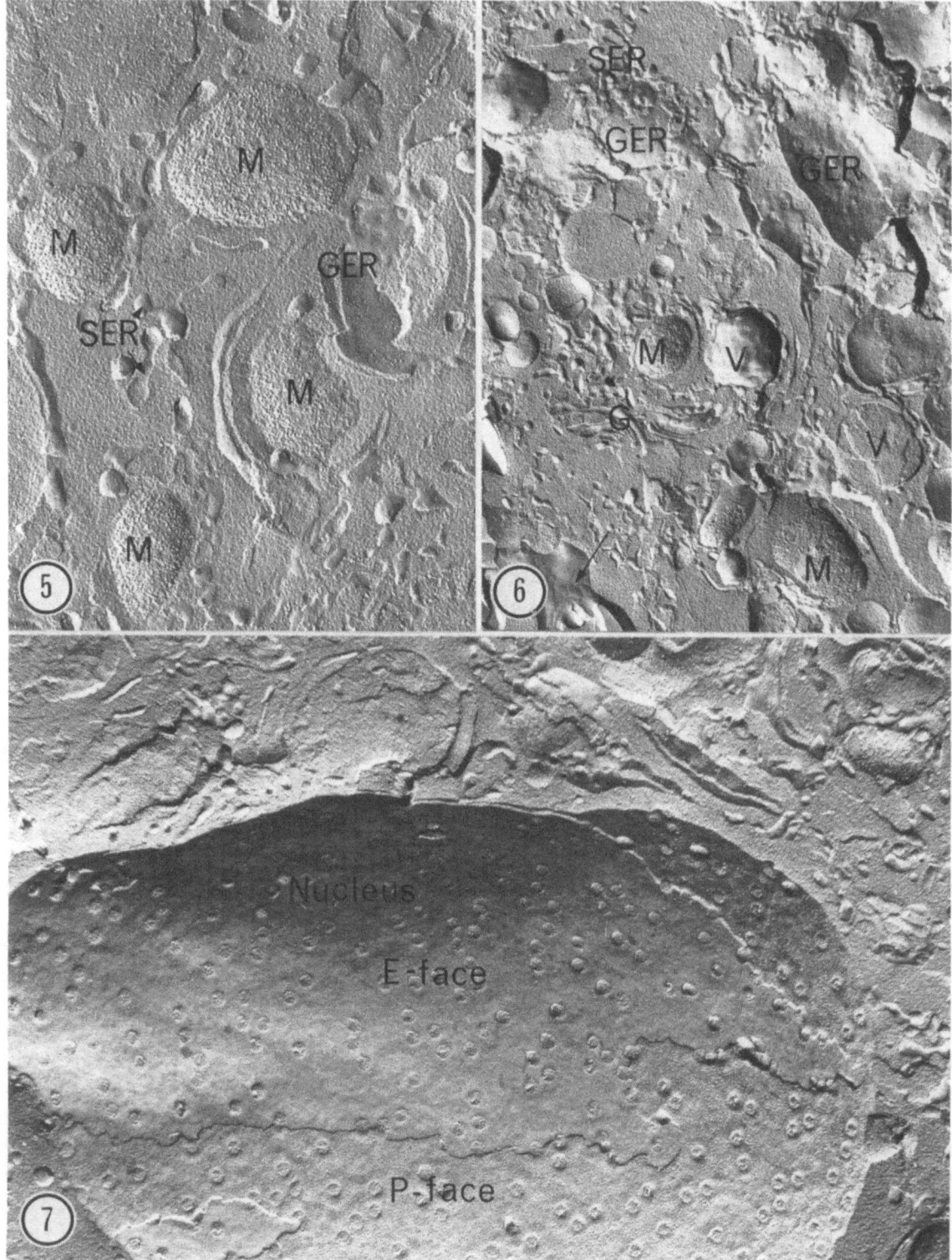

Figure 5. Rat liver. Within the transversely exposed hepatocytic cytoplasm mitochondria (M), cisternae of the granular endoplasmic reticulum (GER), and smooth endoplasmic reticulum (SER) are situated. The inner (P-)face of the mitochondrial membrane is scattered by many particles; × 38,000.

Figure 6. Rat liver. A Golgi region (G) near the bile canalicular area (arrow), mitochondria (M), smooth (SER) and granular endoplasmic reticulum (GER), and vesicular structures (V) are localized with the hepatocytic cytoplasm; × 23,000.

structures are prominent in smooth endoplasmic reticulum, building an irregular, intricate network. The Golgi complex is found in the area of the bile canaliculi and consists of closely packed, parallel, membranous lamellar structures that exhibit lateral enlargements (Fig. 6). Faces of their membranes possess numerous vesicles that probably are undergoing transfer. Numerous corpuscular structures in the range of 0.2–2.0 μm, which are distributed throughout the cytoplasm of the hepatocytes, represent lysosomes, fat droplets, or vacuoles.

2.2.2. Plasmalemma. Differences in the surface structure and the selective arrangement of specialized membrane connections indicate a functional polarization of the hepatocytes. Depending on the arrangement and location of the hepatocytes in the lobule, at least three principal membrane areas (domains) on the cell surface can be differentiated: (1) membrane surfaces that are in interhepatocytic contact (lateral hepatocyte membrane) (Figs. 8, 9, 11, and·12); (2) membrane surfaces that limit the bile canaliculi (bile canalicular hepatocyte membrane) (Fig. 12); and (3) membrane surfaces that border the perisinusoidal Disse space (basal or perisinusoidal hepatocyte membrane) (Fig. 4). These membrane areas exist on most hepatocytes. In addition, there are special membrane areas that are found in only a limited number of cells, for example those areas that contact portal connective tissue (Fig. 1).

2.2.2.1. Lateral hepatocyte membrane. The plasmalemma of adjacent hepatocytes exhibits infrequent interdigitations. Large, bulky microvilli are present on the juxtasinusoidal (basolateral) transitions of the cell surface. Various types of membrane specializations are observed in mediolateral and juxtabiliary areas. Extensive species variations exist in the structure of gap junctions (nexus) and desmosomes (maculae adherentes). Tight junctions are situated on the demarcation of the bile canaliculi.

Numerous membrane-associated particles occur on the P-face of the hepatocyte membrane (Figs. 8, 9, and 13). They range in size from 60 to 120 Å and are randomly distributed. Fewer particles are generally found on the E-face (Fig. 12). Experimental evidence indicates that the particles are protein components of membrane, while the smooth areas between the particles represent lipid molecules. The unequal relation of the particles suggests membrane asymmetry, but as yet there is no information as to the location of specific membrane proteins.

2.2.2.1.1. Gap junction (nexus, macula communicans). Unlike the randomly distributed particles seen on the P- and E-faces of the hepatocyte membrane, particle aggregations are found only on the P-face of interhepatocytic membranes [10, 19] (Figs. 8, 9, 12, and 13). Situated between the juxtabiliary and the juxtasinusoidal regions, these structures have been found in all animal species examined, including the human [17]. Particle aggregations are irregularly formed macular arrays that are not associated preferentially with depressions or protrusions of the membrane. The course of the fracture plane occasionally runs across the intercellular space from one cell to the next (Figs. 8 and 10); areas of pits on the E-face correspond to the intramembranous particles on the P-face of the membrane (Fig. 10). A particulate-free area that is found around the particle aggregations in other organs is relatively narrow or absent in hepatocyte membranes. Particle aggregations situated within juxtabiliary membrane regions are often closely associated with tight junctional strands. Clusters of a few particles, seen as small particle aggregations, are usually integrated between the anastomosing and intersecting strands (Fig. 13). There is general agreement that large particle aggregations on the lateral hepatocyte membranes correspond to the gap junctions that are observed in ultrathin sections [9, 20] (Fig. 11).

The formation of gap junctions between cells was investigated in embryonic tissue (Fig. 9) [17, 21] and in cell cultures [22]. According to these studies, 'large' precursor particles appear within formation plaques on the plasmalemma. They assemble in progressively enlarging polygonal arrangements of

Figure 7. Rat liver. A nucleus of a hepatocyte exhibits numerous pores, the inner (P-) and outer (E-) membrane faces of the nuclear envelope; ×29,000.

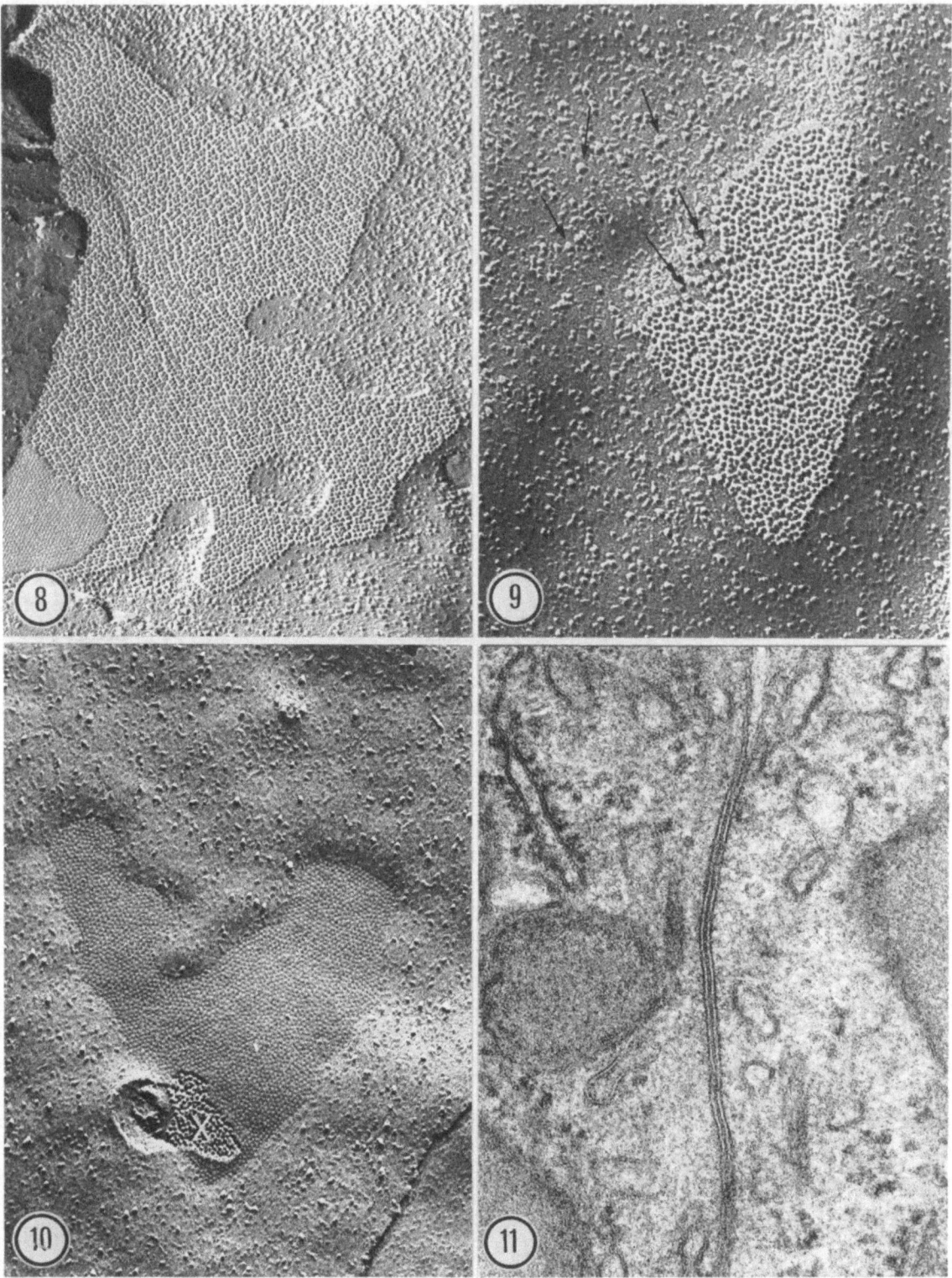

Figure 8. Rat liver. Particle aggregation on the P-face and pits on the E-face of the lateral hepatocyte membrane; ×80,000.
Figure 9. Fetal human liver. Developing particle aggregation on the P-face of the lateral hepatocyte membrane. 'Large' precursor particles (arrows) of the junction are intermingled within the randomly distributed particles and assemble (double arrow) toward the aggregation; ×80,000.

junctional particles, which seem to be smaller than the precursor particles. Similar results are obtained as will be reported later, in hepatectomized [23] or cholestatic animals [24], where disappearance and reconstitution of gap junctions were studied.

The number and size of the particle aggregations vary extensively among species. In preliminary studies of a 22-week-old human fetus, less than 0.5% of the total hepatocyte membrane surface was occupied by these structures [17]. They showed no specific localization on the lateral hepatocyte membrane when observed in the juxtabiliary as well as juxtasinusoidal regions. In *Tupaia belangeri*, rabbits, and guinea pigs, similar amounts are present [17]. Particle aggregations within the tight junctional strands are rarely seen in these species. In rats and mice, however, significantly more particle aggregations occupy the lateral hepatocyte membrane [23, 24]. These are frequently much larger (from 0.7 to 1.0 μm^2) and account for about 1.5% of the total hepatocyte membrane or 2.9%–3.6% of the lateral membrane area [23, 24]. Particle aggregations that range in size 0.002–0.02 μm^2 are integrated into or are frequently associated with the tight junctional strands. The species differences in the structure of particle aggregations are possibly due, at least in part, to differences in the innervation of the hepatocytes [17]. Remarkably, the liver parenchymal cells of species with little innervation [25], such as the rat or mouse, have more particle aggregations than humans, *Tupaia belangeri* and guinea pigs, which are highly innervated [25, 26], but contain only a few particle aggregations.

Among different specimens analyzed in the electron microscope, there is considerable variation in the lattice constant and the center-to-center distance between the particles. Evidence suggests that these parameters can vary depending on the preparative procedure. In the mouse liver, which is fixed with aldehydes, most junctional particles are irregularly packed with average center-to-center spacing of about 9–10 nm [9]. On the P-face the particle arrangement is usually disordered, but on the E-face the lattice of pits often exhibits long-range regularity similar to the hexagonal patterns seen with Lanthanum [20] and in negative stain [27–29]. Small areas of fairly regularly arranged hexagonal packings of particles exhibit an average particle spacing of 9.2–9.5 nm [29, 30]. On the other hand, following extended glutaraldehyde fixation, tight packing (8.5 nm) of junctional particles is observed. When tissues are quick frozen with no chemical fixation or cryoprotective agents, interparticular distances of 10 nm and more are measured [31]. In cases where chemical fixation is inadequate, annulate forms occur [32]. Structural changes of the particle aggregations are also seen after specific uncoupling procedures [30, 33]. In hypoxic liver, the junctional particles form regular hexagonal packings in which the average center-to-center particle spacing is about 8.5 nm. Similar changes are seen in specimens treated with 2,4 dinitrophenol (DNP). In liver perfused with hypertonic disaccharide solutions, most junctions dissociate [34]. The separate junctional membranes then contain particles which are also regularly arranged and tightly packed.

X-ray diffraction and electron-microscopic analyses on isolated gap junctions show constant patterns with the interparticular distance varying between 80 and 90 Å [35–37]. Furthermore, biochemical studies indicate that gap junctions are comprised of units called connexons that are hexagonally arranged in the pair of connected cell membranes [35]. Connexons span double membranes like hollow cylinders with a length of about 75 Å, an outer diameter of 60 Å, and an inner diameter of 20 Å [36, 37]. Apparently, these are protein-lined hydrophilic channels that transverse adjacent cell membranes [28, 29, 36, 37].

Gap junctions are specialized membrane regions of intercellular contact that can serve as the pathway for cell-to-cell communication [28, 38–40]. Experimentally, communication can be defined as the intercellular transfer of ions, metabolites, or both. Thus, communicating cells may be referred to

Figure 10. Rat liver. Macular array of pits on the E-face of the lateral hepatocyte membrane. In a small area (X), corresponding particles on the P-face of the adjacent cell are exposed: × 80,000.
Figure 11. Fetal human liver. Gap junction between two hepatocytes; × 76,000.

58

as electrotonically or metabolically coupled. Although the intercellular passage of porcion yellow between hepatocytes has been demonstrated [17, 41], it is not possible to predict on the basis of routine freeze-fracture studies to which degree all particle aggregations are coupled, since gap junctions uncouple during aldehyde fixation [42].

2.2.2.1.2. Tight junction (zonula occludens). The tight junctional complex represents a specialized area in the juxtabiliary region of the hepatocyte membrane and modifies the intercellular space before broadening into the bile canaliculus. Generally found on two sides of the bile canaliculus, the tight junction forms a continuous zone of intimate contact between the membranes of neighboring liver cells. No apparent structural differences are seen between species, at least those studied in humans (Fig. 12), *Tupaia belangeri*, guinea pigs, rats (Fig. 13) and mice. In freeze-fracture replicas, the junctional structure is regularly confined to narrow belt-like arrays and usually consists of 3–5 continuous strands on the P-face of the membrane. The lumen is lined by an uninterrupted strand, in which anastomoses extend laterally to other parallelly arranged strands. Aggregations of particles are occasionally seen where the strands intersect. Often grooves or pits corresponding either to the strands or to the particle aggregations can be identified on the E-face of the membrane (Fig. 12). On the blind originations of the bile canaliculi, strands are more numerous and perpendicularly arranged with longer extensions reaching the lateral hepatocyte membrane. Similarly, at points where three hepatocytes abut, the tight junctional meshwork is also modified (Fig. 13). On the P-face, horizontally arranged strands extend at various levels from a thick, perpendicularly running strand and connect in a ladder-like fashion to other vertical elements.

Varying conditions of fixation lead to characteristic modifications in the arrangements of particles on both the E-face and the P-face of the membrane [43, 44]. Glutaraldehyde appears to crosslink and polymerize tight junctional substructures effecting a lateral binding of junctional protein particles which give rise to the formation of strands, as well as a fixation of the strands to the protein-rich inner cytoplasmic side of the membrane. In chemically unfixed or lightly fixed tissue, the junctional

particles are found predominantly on the E-face of the membrane. However, following long fixation, strands appear mainly on the P-face.

Particle aggregations that are intercalated between strands are regarded as gap junctions [19, 23]. Data indicate that these structures can arise in the juxtabiliary region under experimental conditions [23, 24, 32]. They are also considered as part of a pool of unorganized structural subunits of tight junctional strands [24, 45, 46]. Difficulty in identification arises where these junctional structures are mixed.

The formation of the tight junctions is similar to that in other organs. In embryonic liver, tight junctions appear around the newly developing bile canaliculi [21]. The junctional structures grow by aligning particles within the presumptive pericanalicular region of the plasmalemma. After subsequent fusion into beaded ridges, they in turn become confluent and transform into smooth unbroken lines. Multiple chains often are arranged in discontinuous networks and are characteristically associated with small clusters of tightly packed particles that probably represent developing or mature gap junctions.

In cultured explants of fetal liver, tight junctios develop both in the bile canalicular region and in the processes of cells at the free surface [47]. Individual particles and rows of particles appear in preexistent lines of the lipid matrix and these eventually develop into continuous strands that are normally seen in glutaraldehyde-fixed tissue. Together with observations made under other experimental conditions (Fig. 15) [17, 23, 48], it may be concluded that the capability of the hepatocyte membrane in establishing junctional specializations is not restricted to the pericanalicular region.

In cell cultures of isolated adult rat hepatocytes, a broad range of tight junction-like structures appears in typical locations near the bile canaliculi [49]. These differ, however, from the corresponding in vivo structures in that they have an atypical length. Only a few particulate proximal strands are transformed into ridges that build the definite tight junctional barrier around the bile canaliculi, while the remaining, more peripheral regions or particles probably regress or serve as precursors of other types of junctions.

Functionally, tight junctions around the bile

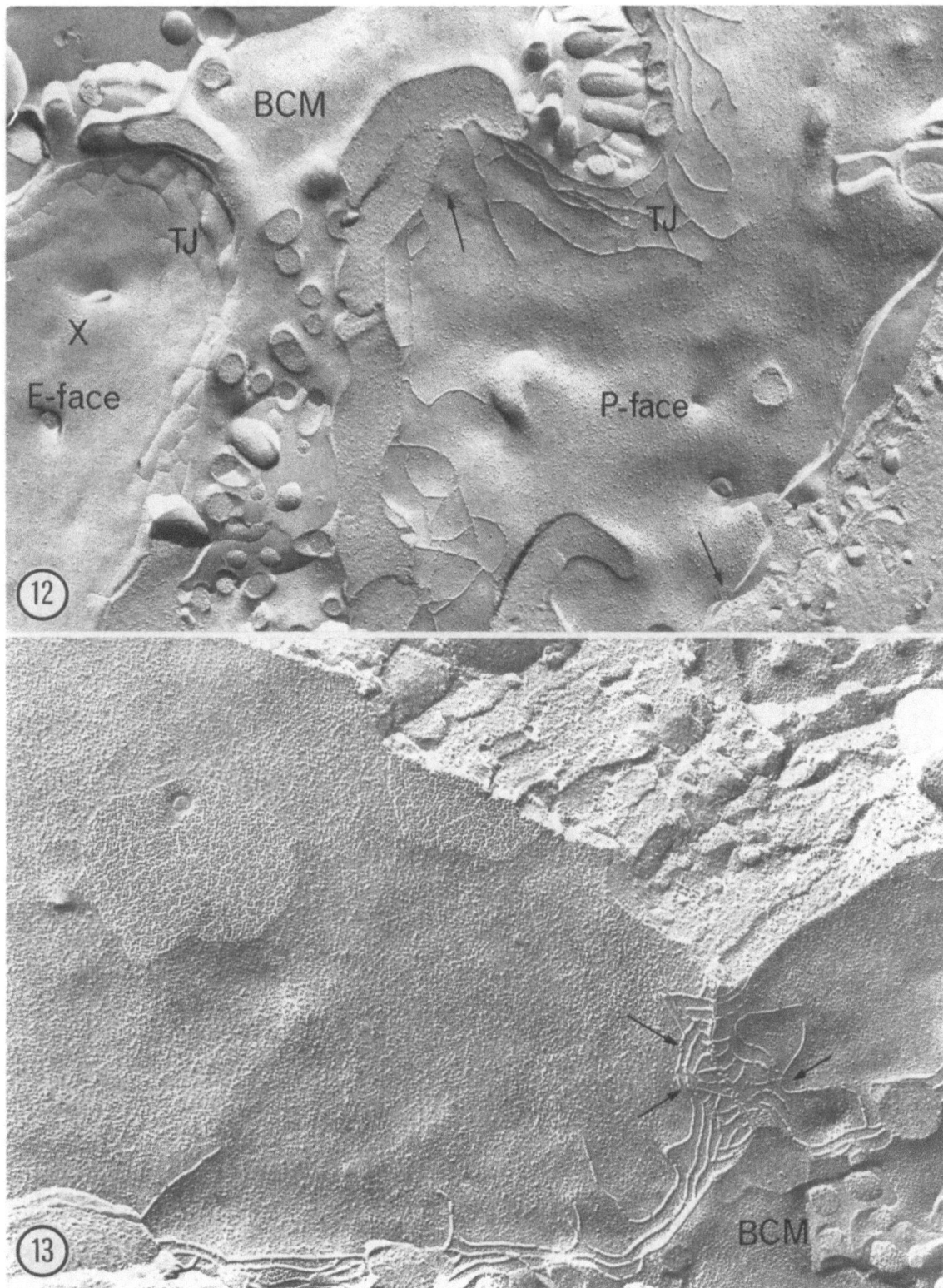

Figure 12. Fetal human liver. Bile canalicular membrane (BCM) with microvilli are seen as well as tight junctions at the E-face and the P-face of the juxtabiliary area of a hepatocyte. The tight junctional structures (TJ) exhibit grooves on the E-face and strands on the P-face. Desmosomes (X) and small particle aggregations (arrows) are observed as well; ×35,000.

Figure 13. Rat liver. Bile canalicular membrane (BCM) and accompanying tight junctional strands with the formation of a triple junction (arrows) are exposed on the P-face of a hepatocyte membrane. Small particle aggregations are intermixed within the meshwork of strands. Large particle aggregations are situated on the lateral membrane area; ×45,000.

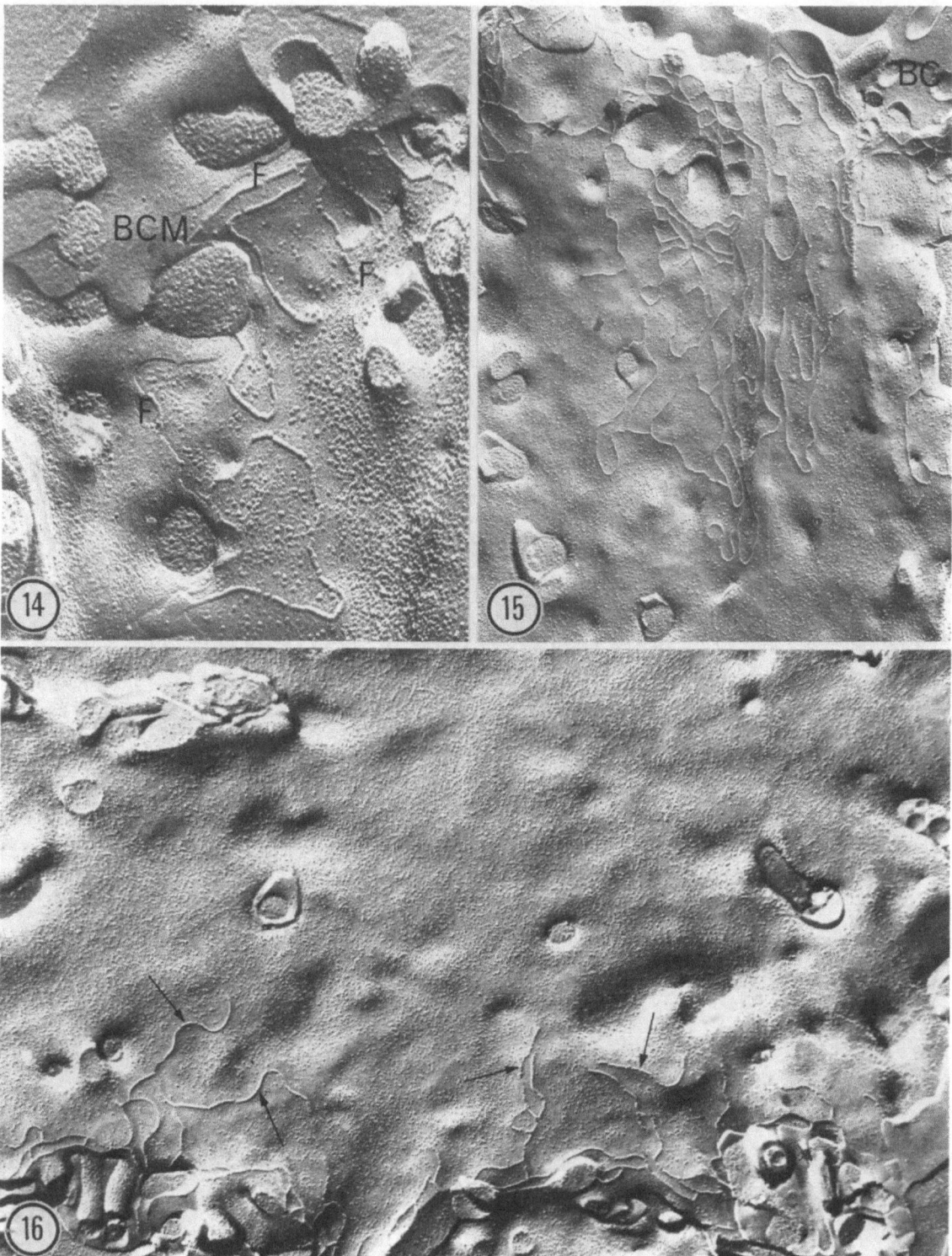

Figure 14. Rat liver after bile duct ligation. The bile canalicular membrane (BCM) is lined by 1–2 irregularly arranged and discontinuous strands. Fragments (F) of strands exhibit a particular substructure on the P-face; ×80,000.

Figure 15. Rat liver after bile duct ligation. Proliferation of tight junctional strands on the P-face of the lateral hepatocyte membrane. BC, bile canaliculus; ×34,000.

Figure 16. Rat liver after bile duct ligation. The lateral hepatocyte membrane area is free of gap junctions. The number of strands is reduced and single extended strands (arrows) migrate toward the lateral area. Membrane-associated particles are less numerous in the close vicinity of the strands; ×35,000.

canaliculi appear to build a permeability barrier between the biliary and interhepatocytic compartments, restricting paracellular transfer. This was shown in studies where electron-dense tracers were applied via the blood circulation [46, 50, 51]. Functional conclusions based solely on the freeze-fracture image of the tight junctional arrangement can be made only with reservation, since the nature of intercellular sealing is still unsolved.

2.2.2.1.3. Desmosome (macula adherens). Desmosomes are found in variable amounts at the lateral hepatocytic membrane of several species. In humans, they are frequently found located predominantly in the proximal regions of the bile canaliculi. The freeze-fracture image exhibits numerous granules and short segments of filaments on the E- and P-faces (Fig. 12).

In isolated adult rat hepatocytes, hemidesmosomes develop within 4 h of incubation and induce the differentiation of symmetric structures in neighboring, intimately associated cells [49].

2.2.2.2. Bile canaliculus. The canaliculi are small bile spaces that arise as blind branches between hepatocytes and continue into larger canalicular structures. They have a diameter of 0.5–1.5 μm and are often located centrally between neighboring parenchyma cells. Microvilli and larger protrusions project from the wall into the lumen (Figs. 12 and 13). The membrane of the bile canaliculi is smooth. Vacuoles (0.1–1.0μm in size) are sometimes seen in the lumen. Occasionally only a small distance exists between the Disse space and the bile canaliculus, though always separated by tight junctions.

2.2.2.3. Perisinusoidal (basal) hepatocyte membrane. Hepatocyte membranes that extend toward the perisinusoidal space exhibit numerous microvillous and irregularly shaped cytoplasmic protrusions (Fig. 4). Collagen bundles and nerve fibers are located within the perisinusoidal space. The nerve fibers, which are parasympathetic and sympathetic, often end in small swellings on the hepatocyte cell membrane.

3. LIVER CELLS UNDER EXPERIMENTAL AND PATHOLOGICAL CONDITIONS

3.1. Cholestasis

Many studies examining the pathological changes occurring within the liver during cholestasis have been carried out. These have been performed either by obstructing the bile duct system (extrahepatic cholestasis) or by administering drugs (intrahepatic cholestasis). Freeze-fracture has been utilized by only a few authors to delineate membrane alterations [24, 46, 52, 53] that occur following these procedures.

3.1.1. Extrahepatic cholestasis. Obstructive syndromes of the bile duct system involve changes of the bile canaliculi and cholestasis with regurgitation of bile constituents into the blood (e.g. [54]). Freeze-fracture studies initially indicated that congested bile reaches the blood space directly via altered tight junctions between hepatocytes [46]. Additional confirmation was obtained by tracer experiments and biochemical analyses [46]. Freeze-fracture reveals gradual changes in the geometry of tight junctional structures that occur in the vicinity of the bile canaliculi of rats shortly after ligation of the common bile duct. The number of strands occasionally becomes reduced and their continuity appears interrupted. Although the strands exhibit a particulate substructure, particle aggregations are seldom associated with the zonula occludens. With progressing cholestasis, the number of strands and anastomosing branches in tight junctions concomitantly decrease. There are increasing interruptions in formerly intact strands on the P-face (Fig. 14) that are accompanied by a disappearance of the grooves on the E-face of the membrane. These alterations probably represent changes that occur when tight junctions become leaky and then contribute to a breakdown of the bile–blood barrier. Electron-dense tracers support this idea [46]. Under the supposition of continuous bile secretion into the canaliculi after ligation of the common duct, elevated intracanalicular pressure could well promote plastic deformation of walls of the bile compartment involving alterations of the integrity of the zonula occludens. The amount of regurgitation should depend primarily on the extent of blockage in bile flow within the canaliculi. Changes in junctional structures apparently occur before the integrity of the plasmalemma is compromised, which is in agreement with other experimental approaches [55–57]. Contrary to these early changes, an increase in junctional depth has been reported after one to three weeks [53]. However, freeze-fracture and tracer studies were carried out on a small number of immersion-fixed specimens in which intracanalicular pressure was reduced before and during the experiment.

Besides changes of the tight junctional meshwork and arrangement within the juxtabiliary region, proliferation of tight junctional structures on the lateral hepatocyte membrane is rarely observed after bile duct ligation (Fig. 15). Similar processes have been found in fetal liver explants [47], in regenerating liver [23], or after phalloidin application [48].

Changes in gap junctions occur at the same time that the hepatocytic membrane is altered during experimental cholestasis [46]; 48 h after ligation of the common bile duct, gap junctions are reduced from control values of 3.6% of the lateral hepatocyte membrane area to less than 0.02% (Fig. 16). Removal of the gap junctions from the cell surface, for example, by an uptake into lysosomes [58] or the formation of annulate gap junctions [59], could be ruled out. The junctional particles are apparently not merely dispersed, since isolated larger particles are not seen between the smaller randomly distributed membrane particles. It is conceivable that the junctional particles are dispersed into smaller subunits that probably mix with the other intramembranous particles. Biochemical and biophysical experiments indeed reveal substructures of gap junctions on control hepatocytes [35, 37], lending support to this hypothesis. The disappearance of gap junctions could contribute to imbalances in metabolic activity within the liver, a possibility that requires additional investigation.

When ligatures are released and the common bile duct successfully rechannels, membrane as well as junctional structures of the biliary tree reestablish their original configurations within 72–90 h [24].

Reformation of tight junctions begins immediately (Fig. 17). Small clusters of particles within the intersections of strands appear to contribute to their reconstitution (Fig. 18). The strands become

continuous, increase in number, and irregularities in their structure disappear. Although bilirubin values return to normal within 24 h after rechanneling, the geometry of the tight junctions is similar to that in control animals only after 72–96 h.

The first stages of gap junction reformation are characterized by aggregations of single particles, which progessively assemble into clusters and groups (Figs. 18 and 19). Since these structures appear within the tight junctional meshwork, in the juxtabiliary region as well as in the area of the lateral hepatocyte membrane, it is probable that reformation occurs at more than one site [24]. Gap junctions appear in excess at least temporarily in the juxtacanalicular area, suggesting that they form predominantly in this region. After 72–96 h, however, the distribution and appearance of gap junctions on the hepatocytes is again similar to controls.

It is clear from this experimental model that freeze-fracture can potentially provide significant information concerning the behavior of intercellular junctions and this may contribute to a better understanding of human pathology.

3.1.2. Intrahepatic cholestasis. Intrahepatic cholestasis can be induced by certain drugs and chemicals [60]. Some pathogenetic mechanisms of these agents may be similar to those involved in extrahepatic cholestasis that results from obstruction of the bile system.

3.1.2.1. Bile salts. After parenteral administration of litocholates into rats, ultrastructural changes in the bile canaliculi and in the pericanalicular regions result, which are probably due to high concentrations of these substances [61]. Freeze-fracture studies reveal a transformation of the wall of the bile canaliculi, especially of the microvilli. A clear variation in the distribution and concentration of the intramembranous particles is also present in the altered areas of the canalicular membrane. It is concluded that bile substances pass into the interhepatocytic space as a result of increased membrane permeability [61]. It should be noted, however, that the structure of the zonulae occludentes was not analyzed in these studies.

3.1.2.2. ANIT. Cholestasis and hyperbilirubinemia can be produced in rats by a single dose of

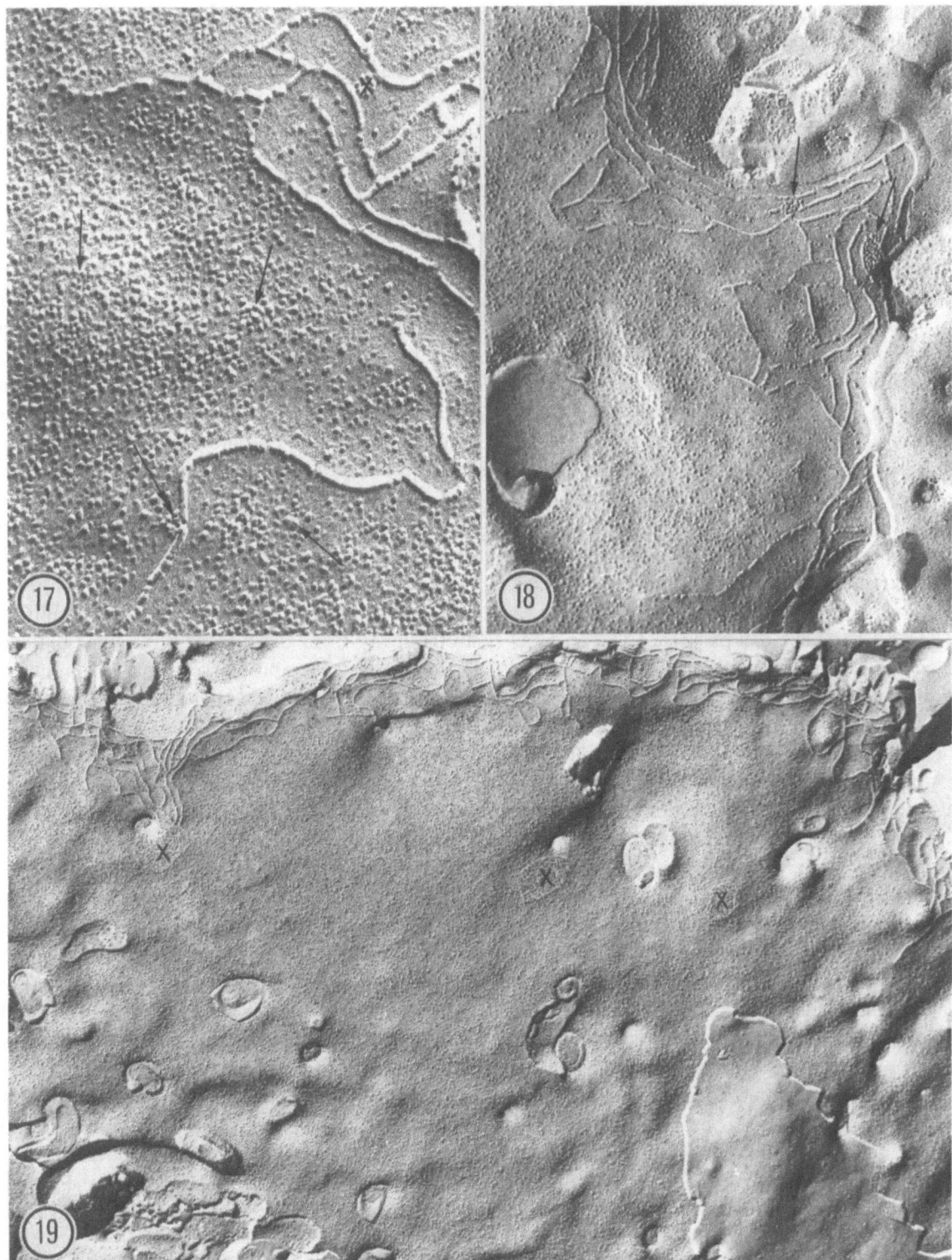

Figure 17. Rat liver 45 min after ligature release. A cluster of particles is visible within the meshwork of tight junctional strands (x) and one is attached to a single strand (double arrow). Small groups of particles are also seen apart from the strands (arrow); ×95,000.

Figure 18. Rat liver 4 h after ligature release. The tight junctions are disarranged. Particle aggregations (arrows) are integrated within the network on the P-face of the membrane; ×65,000.

Figure 19. Rat liver 24 h after ligature release. Intermediate-sized particle aggregations (x) are localized either in apposition to the strands or apart on the lateral hepatocyte membrane; ×28,000.

α-naphthylisothiocyanate (ANIT) [60]. In these animals, tight junctional strands are altered within 12–24 h after oral application of the drug (250 mg/kg body weight) [62]. Progressive changes occur in the arrangement and geometry of the strands. The strands frequently become discontinuous and less numerous. Increased permeability of the tight junctions is suggested by biochemical assays. Although the structural changes in the tight junctions seen in freeze-fracture are similar to those found in obstructive cholestasis, the gap junctions on the lateral side of the hepatocytes are not affected. It appears then that changes in tight junctions and gap junctions are not necessarily coupled and they occur independently, varying with the type of primary liver damage.

3.2. Hepatectomy

Partial hepatectomy has been employed to examine the plasmalemma in hepatocyte regeneration [23, 32].

An almost complete disappearcnce of gap junctions occurs in the remaining liver tissue within 24–36 h after resection. The tight junctions also exhibit changes in their geometry and localization on the plasmalemma. Although the continuity of the zonulae occludentes along the bile canaliculi is preserved, many strands of the zonula occludens disappear from their pericanalicular locations. Frequently, macular types assume complex configurations on large membrane areas. After 36 h, the gap junctions reappear in the form of small particle aggregations that are chiefly associated with the tight junctional strands. These are localized either in the pericanalicular region or within macular tight junction formations on the lateral hepatocyte membrane. Within 44 h after partial hepatectomy, morphometric analysis shows the number of gap junctions to be similar to that in control animals. The cycle of the disappearance and reappearance of the gap junctions in regenerating liver was found to be quite reproducible in various rat strains. It is thought that connexons disperse within the membrane and intermediary forms are seen, as that which is seen in obstructive cholestasis [24, 46]. Phenoxybenzamine, a substance that reduces the cAMP concentration in the liver of partially hepatectomized rats, promotes gap junc-

tional appearance in much higher numbers than in normal livers [32, 63]. This phenomenon occurs within the first 28 postoperative hours. Although the number of gap junctions is increased, the proportion of the perisinusoidal membrane that is occupied by gap junctions remains reduced.

3.3. Hepatocyte necrosis

3.3.1. Phalloidin. Parenteral administration of phalloidin to laboratory animals results in a characteristic hemorrhagic dystrophy of the liver that leads to death within hours [64]. Previous biochemical and ultrastructural studies indicate that phalloidin primarily affects the plasma membrane of the hepatocytes and interferes with actin-like proteins beneath the inner membrane [65]. After long-term administration of relatively small doses of phalloidin to rats, extensive development of tight junctions is induced, which has been verified in freeze-fracture studies [48]. The junctional strands lose their parallel orientation to the canaliculi and stretch away from the lumen in irregular patterns that cover large membrane areas apart from the bile canaliculi. It is probable that these changes result from both a proliferation and a reorganization of the junctional elements [48].

3.3.2. Carbon tetrachloride. A single dose of carbon tetrachloride causes hepatocyte necrosis and is followed within 3–4 days by a proliferation of tight junctions in the rat liver [66]. Proliferation occurs through a *de novo* formation of junctional elements, by inclusion of intramembranous particles, and by reorganization of preexisting junctional ridges. Two different types of strands are seen on the lateral side of the hepatocyte plasmalemma. The first exhibits an almost equal distribution of particles arranged in rows. The linear chains are derived from discrete growth centers on the lateral surface. Such strands have also been described in other developmental systems. They are regarded as a stage in the process of de novo formation of junctional strands. The second type consists of short 'ridges' that likely represent strands derived from fragmented zonulae occludentes that have migrated laterally. Intermediate stages which run together and form large macular tight junctions on the lateral face possibly exist. Five days later these structures are no longer

65

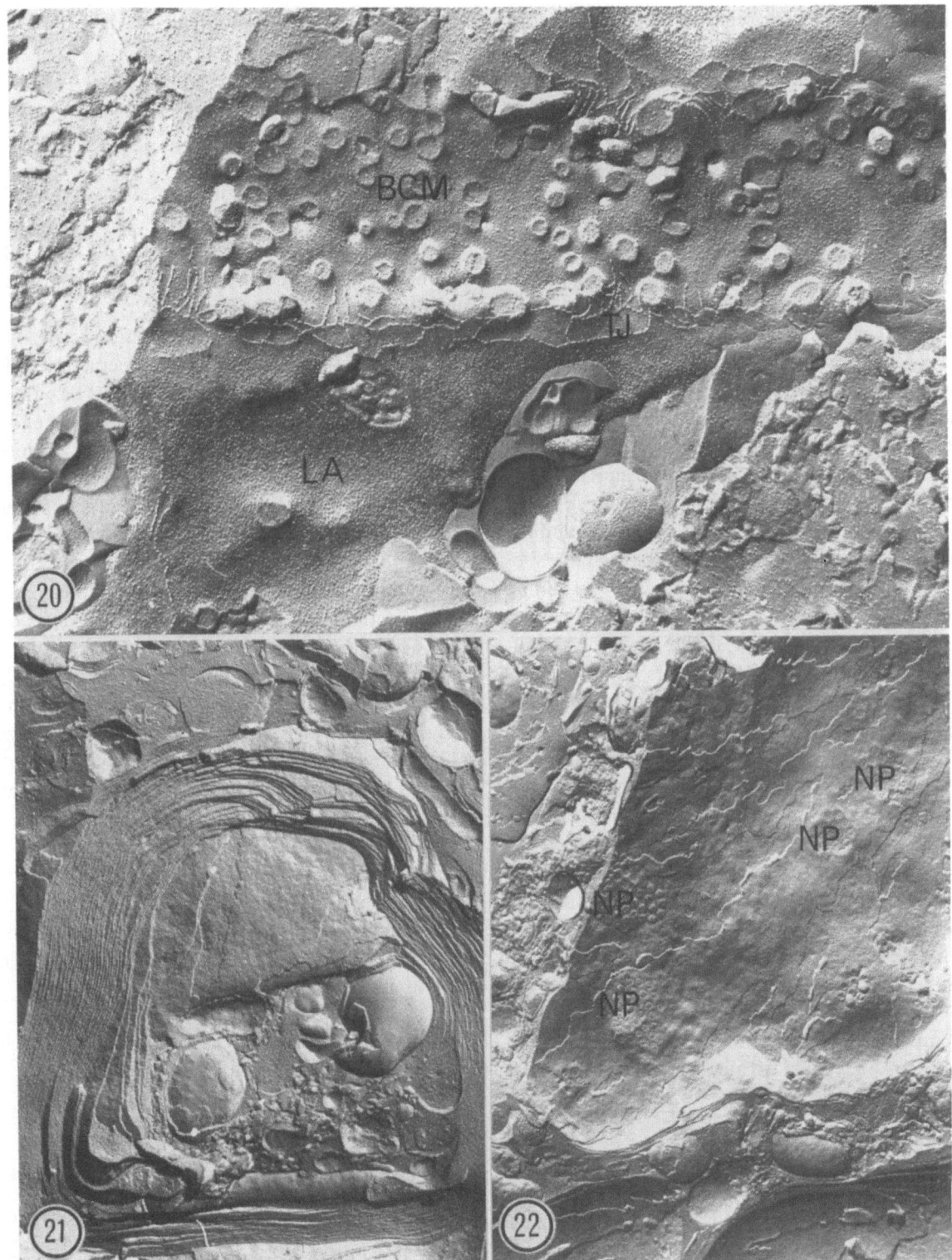

Figure 20. Rat liver after galactosamine treatment. The tight junctional strands (TJ) are disarranged, reveal a particulate structure, and are occasionally dislocated toward the lateral hepatocyte area (LA) or toward the bile canalicular membrane (BCM); ×34,000.
Figure 21. Rat liver after galactosamine treatment. Lamellar formation within the cytoplasm of hepatocyte consists of multiple membranous layers and contains cytoplasm and organelles; ×14,000.
Figure 22. Rat liver after galactosamine treatment. The nucleus of an hepatocyte exhibits local assemblies of nuclear pores (NP); ×13,000.

found, and are therefore regarded as transitory [66].

3.3.3. Galactosamine. After the administration of the amino sugar D-galactosamine, to rats, a dose-dependent development of diffuse hepatocellular injury with focal necrosis and an inflammatory infiltration of the periportal regions occur [67]. Secondary lesions resulting from an inhibition of uracil-nucleotide-dependent synthesis of macromolecules occur and structural disturbances of cell organelles, particularly nucleoli, endoplasmic reticulum, and plasmalemma are evident [68].

At 24 h after administration of 500 mg/kg of galactosamine, freeze-fracture replicas reveal large areas of the liver parenchyma that contain gap junctions and zonulae occludentes [17]. Focally, the number of gap junctions is reduced and the tight junctional meshwork becomes disarranged (Fig. 20). The number of strands is often reduced and the continuity interrupted, revealing a particulate substructure of the strands. Perpendicularly running strands appear in a direction toward the lateral hepatocyte membrane and also toward the canalicular membrane area. After application of 1500 mg/kg, however, severely necrotic areas with disintegration of parenchymal cell groups are observed. Gap junctions and zonulae occludentes diminish and are often absent from their typical location within the hepatocyte membrane. Separated and dislocated fragments of zonulae occludentes are seen on the lateral hepatocyte membrane. Lamellar structures that consist of whirled membranes are particularly conspicuous in the cytoplasm of parenchymal cells in freeze-fracture replicas (Fig. 21). Cisternae of the rough endoplasmic reticulum are frequently continuous with the lamellar structures. The nuclear pores are diminished in number and frequently aggregated within groups on the nuclear

envelope (Fig. 22), suggesting a large disturbance of the nuclear metabolism.

4. CONCLUSION

The freeze-fracture method is used to analyze the ultrastructure of the liver under normal and experimental conditions. This procedure is especially advantageous for the investigation of membranes and their associated processes.

In crossfractures through the interior of liver cells, principal information is obtained from fractures along membranes of cell organelles, i.e., about nuclear pores, fenestrations of the granular endoplasmic reticulum, or membrane structure of mitochondria. Different areas of the plasmalemma of liver cells are characterized, e.g., the perisinusoidal, lateral, or bile canalicular hepatocyte membrane regions. Among the various intercellular junctions species variations particularly concern the nexus, while the tight junctions exhibit a relatively constant arrangement around the bile canaliculi.

The individual membrane areas and especially the intercellular connections are significantly changed under experimental conditions. Altered freeze-fracture images constitute the morphological substrate of functional consequences that occur within intracellular as well as intercellular compartments. Future aspects of the freeze-fracture method are to be considered in correlation with other morphological and functional analytical methods in order to contribute to further information on the normal functioning liver as well as on the pathogenesis of hepatic diseases.

Acknowledgments. The author is indebted to Mr. R. Eichler for excellent technical assistance and to Mrs. A. Miehle for preparing the manuscript.

REFERENCES

1. Benedetti EL, Favard P (eds) (1973) Freeze-etching techniques and applications. Paris: Société Francaise de Microscopie Electronique
2. Koehler JK (ed) (1973) Advanced techniques in biological electron microscopy. Berlin: Springer
3. Rash JE, Hudson CS (eds) (1979) Freeze fracture: methods, artefacts and interpretations. New York: Raven
4. Heuser JE, Reese TS, Dennis MJ, Yan Y, Yan L, Evans L (1979) Synaptic vesicle exocytosis captured by quick freezing and correlated with quantal transmitter release. J Cell Biol 81:275–300
5. Kreutziger G (1968) Freeze-etching of intercellular junctions of mouse liver. Proc Electron Microsc Soc Am, pp 234–235
6. Karnovsky MJ (1965) A formaldehyde-glruraldehyde fixative of high osmolality for use in electron microscopy. J Cell Biol 27:137
7. Forssmann WG, Ito S, Weihe E, Aoki A, Dym M, Fawcett DW (1977) An improved perfusion fixation method for the testis. Anat Rec 188:307–314
8. Spycher MA (1970) Intercellular adhesions. An electron

microscope study on freeze-etched rat hepatocytes. Z Zell-forsch 111:64–74

9. Goodenough DR, Revel JP (1970) A fine structural analysis of intercellular junctions in the mouse liver. J Cell Biol 45:272–290

10. Chalcroft JP, Bullivant S (1970) An interpretation of liver cell membrane and junction structure based on observation of freeze-fracture replicas of both sides of the fracture. J Cell Biol 47:49–60

11. Pinto da Silva P, Branton D (1970) Membrane splitting in freeze-etching. J Cell Biol 45:598–605

12. Branton D, Bullivant S, Gilula NB, Karnovsky MJ, Moor H, Mühlethaler K, Northcote DH, Packer L, Satir B, Satir P, Speth V, Stachelin LA, Steere RL, Weinstein RS (1975) Freeze-etching nomenclature. Science 190:54–56

13. Yee AG, Revel JP (1975) Endothelial cell junctions. J Cell Biol 66:200–204

14. Wisse E, Knook DL (1979) The investigation of sinusoidal cells, a new approach to the study of liver function. In: Popper H, Schaffner F (eds) Progress in liver diseases, vol 6. New York: Grune and Stratton, pp 151–171

15. Meairs S, Nimmrich H, Weihe E, Metz J, Forssmann WG (1979) Scanning electron microscopy for the study of vascular endothelia [Abstr]. In: 5th European Anatomical Congress, Prague, 1979, p 451

16. Orci L, Matter A, Rouiller C (1971) A comparative study of freeze-etch replicas and thin sections of rat liver. J Ultrastruct Res 35:1–19

17. Metz J (1979) Unpublished results

18. Barnes BG, Davis JM (1959) The structure of nuclear pores in mammalian tissues. J Ultrastruct Res 3:131–146

19. Friend D, Gilula N (1972) Variations in tight and gap junctions in mammalian tissues. J Cell Biol 53:757–776

20. Revel J, Karnovsky J (1967) Hexagonal array of subunits in intercellular junctions of the mouse heart and liver. J Cell Biol 33:7–12

21. Montesano R, Friend DS, Perrelet A, Orci L (1975) In vivo assembly of tight junctions in fetal rat liver. J Cell Biol 57:310–319

22. Johnson R, Hammer M, Sheridan J, Revel J (1974) Gap junction formation between reaggregated Novikoff hepatoma cells. Proc Natl Acad Sci USA 71:4536–4540

23. Yee AG, Revel J-P (1978) Loss and reappearance of gap junctions in regenerating liver. J Cell Biol 78:554–564

24. Metz J, Bressler D (1979) Reformation of gap and tight junctions in regenerating liver after cholestasis. Cell Tissue Res 199:257–270

25. Metz W, Forssmann WG (1980) Innervation of the liver in guinea pig and rat. Anat Embryol 160:239–252

26. Forssmann WG, Ito S (1977) Hepatocyte innervation in primates. J Cell Biol 74:299–313

27. Benedetti EL, Emmelot R (1965) Electron microscopic observations on negatively stained plasma membranes isolated from rat liver. J Cell Biol 26:299–305

28. Payton BW, Bennet MVL, Pappas GD (1969) Permeability and structure of junctional membranes at an electronic synapse. Science 166: 1641–1643

29. McNutt NS, Weinstein RS (1970) The ultrastructure of the nexus: a correlated thin-section and freeze-cleave study. J Cell Biol 47:666–687

30. Peracchia C (1977) Gap junctions. Structural changes after uncoupling procedures. J Cell Biol 72:628–641

31. Raviola G, Raviola E (1978) Intercellular junctions in the ciliary epithelium. Invest Ophthalmol Vis Sci 17:958–981

32. Yancey SB, Easter D, Revel J-P (1979) Cytological changes in gap junctions during liver regeneration. J Ultrastruct Res 67:229–242

33. Peracchia C, Dulhunty AF (1976) Low resistance junctions in cray fish: structural changes with functional uncoupling. J Cell Biol 70:419–439

34. Goodenough DA, Gilula NB (1974) The splitting of hepatocyte gap junctions and zonulae occludentes with hypertonic disaccharides. J Cell Biol 61:575–590

35. Goodenough DA (1975) Methods for the isolation and structural characterization of hepatocyte gap junctions. In: Korn ED (ed) Methods in membrane biology, vol 3. New York: Plenum, pp 51–80

36. Caspar D, Goodenough D, Makowski L, Phillips W (1977) Gap junction structures: I. Correlated electron microscopy and X-ray diffraction. J Cell Biol 69:605–628

37. Makowski L, Caspar D, Phillips W, Goodenough D (1977) Gap junction structures: II. Analysis of the X-ray diffraction data. J Cell Biol 74:629–645

38. Dewey MM, Barr L (1962) Intercellular connections between smooth muscle cells: the nexus. Science 137:670–672

39. Dreifuss JJ, Giradier L, Forssmann WG (1966) Etude de la propagation de l'excitation dans le ventricule du rat au moyen de solutions hypertoniques. Pfluegers Arch 292:15–33

40. Gilula N, Reeves O, Steinbach A (1972) Metabolic coupling, ionic coupling and cell contacts. Nature (London) 235: 262–265

41. Revel J (1979) Personal communication

42. Bennett MVL (1973) Function of electronic junctions in embryonic and adult tissues. Fed Proc 32:65–75

43. Bullivant S (1978) The structure of tight junctions. In: Sturgess JM (ed) Electron microscopy. Canada: Imperial, pp 659–672

44. Van Deurs B, Luft JH (1979) Effects of glutaraldehyde fixation on the structure of tight junctions. A quantitative freeze-fracture analysis. J Ultrastruct Res 68:160–172

45. Elias P, Friend D (1976) Vitamin A induced mucous metaplasia: an in vitro system for modulating tight and gap junction differentiation. J Cell Biol 68:173–188

46. Metz J, Aoki A, Merlo M, Forssmann WG (1977) Morphological alterations and functional changes of interhepatocellular junctions induced by bile duct ligation. Cell Tissue Res 182:299–310

47. Montesano R, Mira-Moser F, Stefan Y, Perrelet A, Orci L (1978) Tight junctions in fetal rat liver explants grown in vitro. J Ultrastruct Res 64:182–190

48. Montesano R, Gabbiani G, Perrelet A, Orci L (1976) In vivo induction of tight junction. Proliferation in rat liver. J Cell Biol 68:793–798

49. Wanson J-C, Drochmans P, Mosselmans R, Ronveaux M-F (1977) Adult rat hepatocytes in primary monolayer culture. Ultrastructural characteristics of intercellular contacts and cell membrane differentiations. J Cell Biol 74:858–877

50. Forssmann WG, Matter A, Rouiller Ch, Westphal U (1966) Le problème des communications entre l'espace de Dissé et les canalicules biliaires [Abstr]. Acta Anat (Basel) 65:614

51. Matter A, Orci L, Rouiller C (1969) A study on the permeability barriers between Disse space and the bile canaliculus. J Ultrastruct Res [Suppl] 11

52. De Vos R, Desmet VJ (1978) Morphologic changes of the junctional complex of the hepatocytes in rat liver after bile duct ligation. Br J Exp Pathol 59:220–227

53. Koga A, Todo S (1978) Morphological and functional changes in the tight junctions of the bile canaliculi induced by bile duct ligation. Cell Tissue Res 195:267–276

54. De Vos R, De Wolf-Peeters C, Desmet V, Bianchi L, Rohr

HP (1975) Significance of liver canalicular changes after experimental bile duct ligation. Exp Mol Pathol 23:12–34

55. Wade JD, Karnovsky MJ (1974) Fracture faces of osmotically disrupted zonulae occludentes. J Cell Biol 62:344–350

56. Metz J, Forssmann WG, Ito S (1977) Exocrine pancreas under experimental conditions: III. Membrane and cell junctions in isolated acinar cells. Cell Tissue Res 177:459–474

57. Metz J, Merlo M, Billich H, Forssmann WG (1978) Exocrine pancreas under experimental conditions: IV. Alterations of intercellular junctions between acinar cells following pancreatic duct ligation. Cell Tissue Res 186:227–240

58. Staehelin A (1974) Structure and function of intercellular junctions. Int Rev Cytol 39:191–283

59. Merk F, Albright J, Botticelli C (1973) The fine structure of granulosa cell nexuses in rat ovarian follicles. Anat Rec 175:107–125

60. Plaa GL, Priestly BG (1977) Intrahepatic cholestasis induced by drugs and chemicals. Pharmacol Rev 28:207–273

61. Miyai K, Mayr WW, Richardson AL (1975) Acute cholestasis induced by lithocholic acid in the rat. Lab invest 32:527–535

62. Krell H, Höke H, Pfaff E, Metz J (1979) Development of intrahepatic cholestasis induced by α-naphthylisothiocyanate: increased permeability of tight junctions [Abstr]. Falk Symp no. 27, S. 36

63. Yancey SB, Easter D, Revel DP (1978) Cytological changes in gap junctions during liver regeneration. J Cell Biol 79:230a

64. Wieland Th, Wieland O (1972) The toxic peptides of Amanita species. Microbiol Toxicol 8:249–254

65. Govindan VM, Rober G, Wieland Th, Agostini B (1973) Binding of phallotoxin to protein filaments of plasma membrane of liver cell. Hoppe Seylers Z Physiol Chem 354: 1159–1161·

66. Robenek H, Themann H, Ott K (1979) Carbon tetrachloride induced proliferation of tight junctions in the rat liver as revealed by freeze-fracturing. Eur J Cell Biol 20:62–70

67. Decker K, Keppler D (1974) Galactosamine hepatitis: key role of the nucleotide deficiency period in the pathogenesis of cell injury and cell death. Rev Physiol Biochem Pharmacol 71:77–106

68. El Mofty SK, Scrutton MC, Serroni A, Nicolini C, Farber JL (1975) Early reversible plasma membrane injury in galactosamine-induced liver cell death. Am J Pathol 79: 579–595

69. Montesano R, Nicolescu P (1978) Fenestrations in endothelium of rat liver sinusoids revisited by freeze-fracture. Anat Rec 190:861–870

5. MORPHOFUNCTIONAL FEATURES OF CULTURED LIVER CELLS

J.-C. Wanson†, D. Bernaert, R. Mosselmans, and W. Penasse

1. INTRODUCTION

Freshly prepared suspensions of well-preserved hepatocytes are currently obtained in high yields by using collagenase perfusion [1–3]. The isolated liver parenchymal cells have been established in primary monolayer cultures in an attempt to maintain during time the phenotypic expression of several specific metabolic functions occurring in normal hepatocytes in vivo [4–10]. Morphofunctional properties of adult rat hepatocytes in short-term primary cultures depend on the nutrient and hormonal microenvironment. Addition of various hormones such as insulin [8, 11], corticosteroids [9, 12], triiodothyronine [13], or glucagon [14], alone or in combination [15], stimulates individual enzymatic inductions. Moreover, the use of collagen or collagen gels [16] improves the hormonal regulation of enzymatic activities and enhances the survival period of hepatocytes in culture. In this respect, a prolonged survival of well-differentiated hepatocytes was obtained by using symbiotic cultures of sinusoidal cells and hepatocytes, extracted separately from rat livers by appropriated enzymatic techniques [17, 18].

This chapter illustrates ultrastructural properties of short-term primary hepatic cultures under the transmission and scanning electron microscopes. Adult rat hepatocytes in culture form trabeculae provided with specific cell membrane differentiations [10, 19], and reconstitute heterogeneous cell surfaces [20]. The cytochemical analysis of glucose-6-phosphatase and its biochemical quantification reveals a homogeneous intracellular distribution of the enzyme in culture, which slowly decreases with time. Moreover, albumin synthesis and secretion confirms the integrity of adult rat hepatocytes in culture [21] and their ability to constitute, for at least two to three days, an interesting experimental model for the study of specific metabolic functions. Finally, the symbiotic culture that enhances the survival period of liver parenchymal cells in culture forms an attractive model whose ultrastructural characteristics will be described.

2. ADULT RAT PARENCHYMAL CELLS IN CULTURE

2.1. Isolation and culture conditions

Adult rat hepatocytes were isolated, under sterile conditions, by continuous recirculating perfusion of the liver in situ in the presence of 0.1% collagenase (200 IU/mg) and 0.1% hyaluronidase (460 IU/mg) [3, 19, 22]. This treatment results in a collapsed organ, which contains single hepatocytic cell plates embedded in a partially digested connective tissue framework. After disruption of the Glisson capsule, hepatocytic cell plates are liberated into the suspension by gentle dissociation with a spatula and later separated into single cells by rolling the cell suspension in a siliconized flask, using a rotary evaporator. The hepatocytic cell population is then filtrated on Perlon (polyamide PA 6) of 63-μm pore size and washed by a 1-g sedimentation for 10 min at room temperature. Filtration enables purification of the liver parenchymal cell suspension by retaining large cell aggregates on the filter, while sedimentation eliminates subcellular debris, damaged hepatocytes, and nonparenchymal cells in the supernatant. Finally, the isolated hepatocytes resuspended in an enriched Dulbecco medium are incubated for 30–60 min at room temperature in a gyratory shaker. During this preincubation, hepatocytes become round and acquire homogeneous cell surfaces covered with uniformly distributed microvilli [20, 23].

Isolated hepatocytes (3×10^6 cells suspended in 3 ml medium) were plated in 60-mm plastic Petri dishes, in the presence of Dulbecco medium supplemented with 4 mM glutamine, 5–20 mM glucose, 17% fetal calf serum, and antibiotics. Petri dishes were incubated under air and CO_2 (in a ratio of 95:5) at 37°C. The medium was renewed each day.

2.2. Development of hepatic cell cords, provided with newly formed cell membrane differentiations

This section summarizes some of our ultrastructural data obtained during the last few years in the field of hepatocytic cultures. The ultrastructural and biochemical aspects of the behavior of isolated liver parenchymal cells were analyzed at different steps in culture [10, 11, 19, 24]. Hepatocytes reaggregate in cell cords and flatten in a bidimensional monolayer within 24 h. As illustrated in Figure 1, reconstituted cell trabeculae (T) are spread on the bottom of the Petri dishes. Free cell surfaces are covered with numerous thin microvilli (Fig. 1, mv), while interhepatocytic faces are intimately associated and develop specific cell membrane specializations, such as bile canaliculi, tight junctions and desmosomes. As illustrated in Figure 2, numerous newly formed bile channels are regularly encountered in a string of beads, after 24 h culture. Successive villous bile canalicular spaces are distinguished (Fig. 2, BC), separated from each other by densely stained tight junction-like structures (Fig. 2, ti). Hemidesmosomes (Fig. 2, HD), already detectable after 4 h culture, are the precursors of mature desmosomes. Finally, paraplasmatic smooth cisternae (Fig. 2, pp), totally absent in isolated cells, reappear symmetrically in both adjacent cytoplasms. Inside the cells, a Golgi biliary polarity is restored. Numerous Golgi complexes (Fig. 2, GO), composed of smooth cisternae, micro- and macrovesicles, regain their classic peripheral cytoplasmic localization by migrating in the vicinity of the bile canaliculi. Their role in rehandling and secretion of bile products is still being debated.

2.3. Cell surface characteristics as revealed by SEM

Hepatocytes in culture were fixed overnight in 2.5% cacodylate-buffered glutaraldehyde at room temperature. After brief washings, pieces of the Petri dishes were dehydrated in a graded series of alcohols and critical-point dried in a Sorvall apparatus by using CO_2. Specimens coated with a 20-nm-thick layer of gold were examined in a Jeol JSM 35 scanning electron microscope at 35 kV.

Figure 3 illustrates the high degree of flattening of 24-h-cultured hepatocytes. Polyhedral cells spread on the bottom of the dishes and are recovered by spherical, damaged hepatocytes. We furthermore notice, in this micrograph, the presence of a network of filamentous structures, which could correspond to secretory proteins (Fig. 3, fi). The liver parenchymal cells established in cell cords are separated from each other by large fractures (Fig. 3, arrows). These artifactual fractures that occur between adjacent hepatocytes result from the critical-point-drying procedure and enable the visualization of the interhepatocytic cell surfaces. At higher magnification, as shown in Figure 4, the cell surface properties of free (Fig. 4, FS) and interhepatocytic faces (Fig. 4, IHS) are well differentiated, which confirms the recovery by cultured hepatocytes of a specific cell surface heterogeneity. The free surfaces display numerous microvilli (Fig. 4, mv) while interhepatocytic areas offer villous bile canalicular regions (Fig. 4, BC) separated by smooth surfaces (Fig. 4, asterisk). In conclusion, the artifact of shrinkage due to retraction of the biological material, during the preparation for SEM, reveals interhepatocytic faces that display similar characteristics to those observed in situ [20, 25].

3. CYTOCHEMICAL DISTRIBUTION OF G-6-PASE IN MONOLAYER CULTURES

The cytochemical localization of G-6-Pase was analyzed in parenchymal cell cultures. Monolayers of adult rat hepatocytes were fixed for 1 min in 2.5% cacodylate-buffered glutaraldehyde, briefly washed and quickly frozen in liquid nitrogen in order to allow a homogeneous penetration of the substrate. The cells were then incubated in Wachstein-Meisel medium, slightly modified according to Hugon [26], at 37°C for 30 min. Hepatocytes were later rinsed, postfixed, dehydrated, and embedded in Epon. Parallelly, biochemical determinations were carried

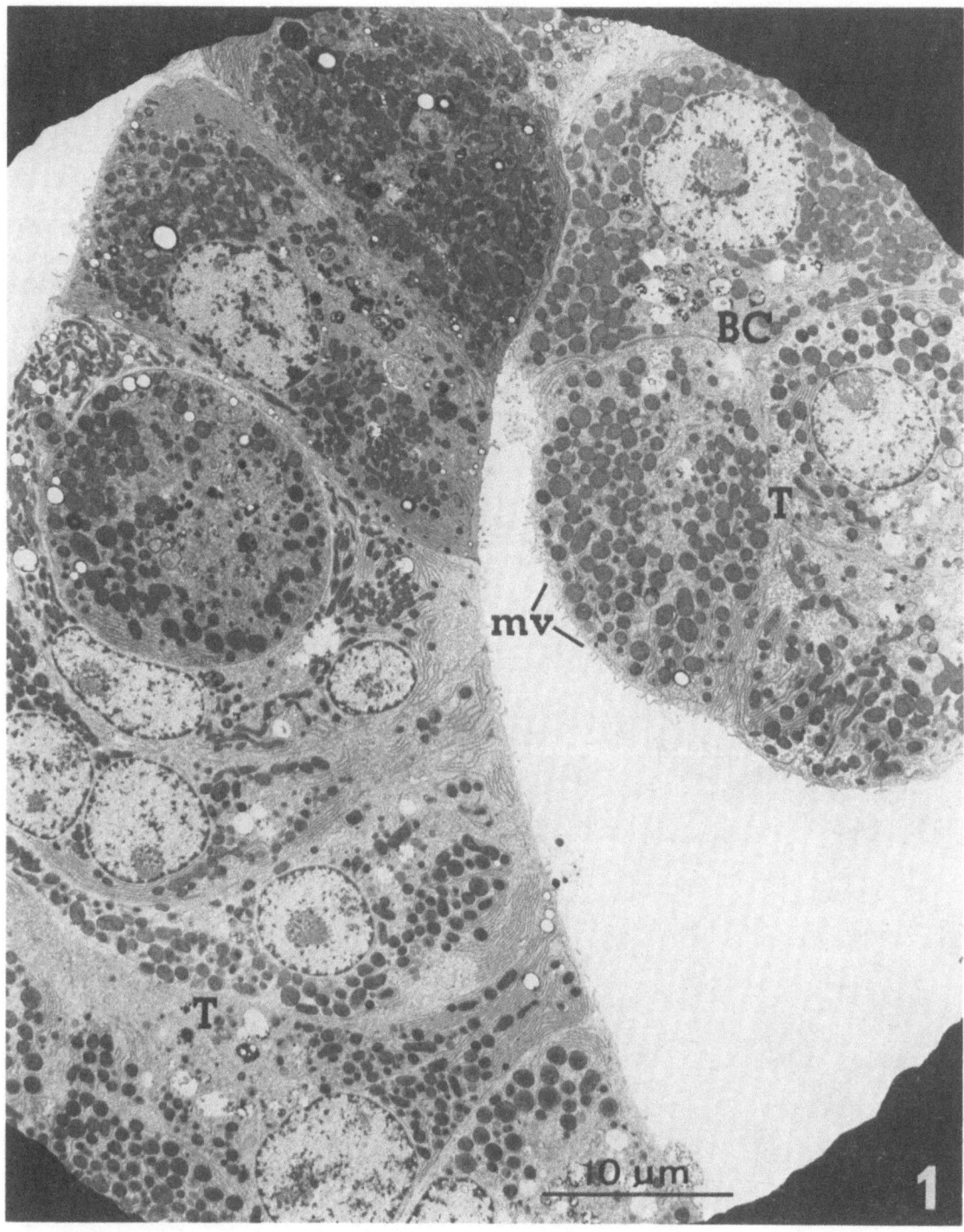

Figure 1. Hepatocytes cultured for 24 h, sectioned in a plane parallel to the bottom of the Petri dish. Cell trabeculae (T) are reconstituted, provided with newly formed bile canaliculi (BC). Microvilli (mv) are detected on the free cell surfaces.

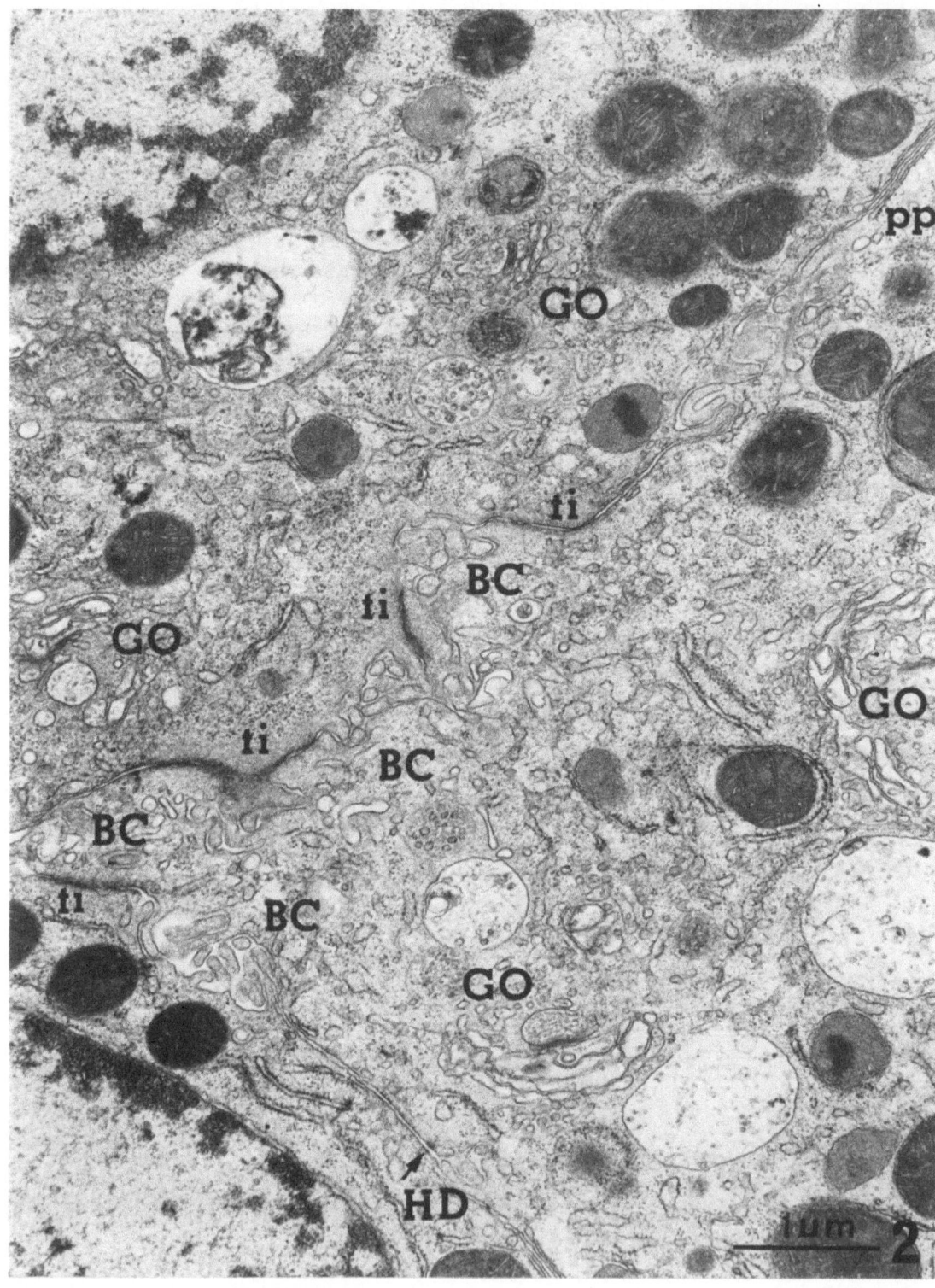

Figure 2. High-magnification view of 24-h-cultured hepatocytes. Golgi complexes (GO) are polarized toward newly formed villous bile canaliculi (BC), endowed with tight junctions (ti). HD, hemidesmosome; pp, paraplasmatic cisternae.

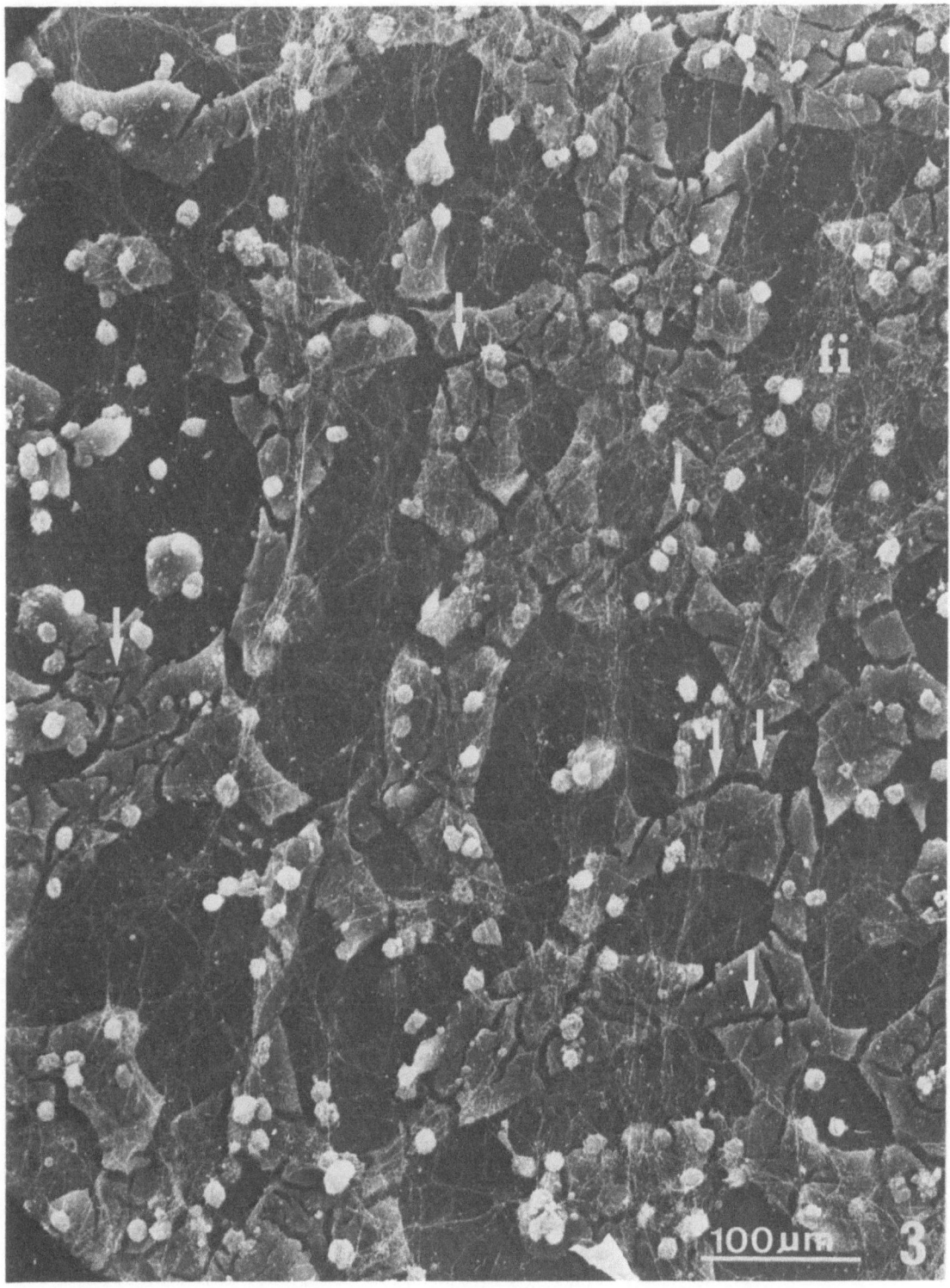

Figure 3. 24-h-cultured hepatocytes. Cells offer a high degree of flattening and present granular damaged round cells on their upper surface. Arrows point to artifactual fractures inbetween adjacent hepatocytes. A network of filamentous structures (fi) is frequently encountered.

74

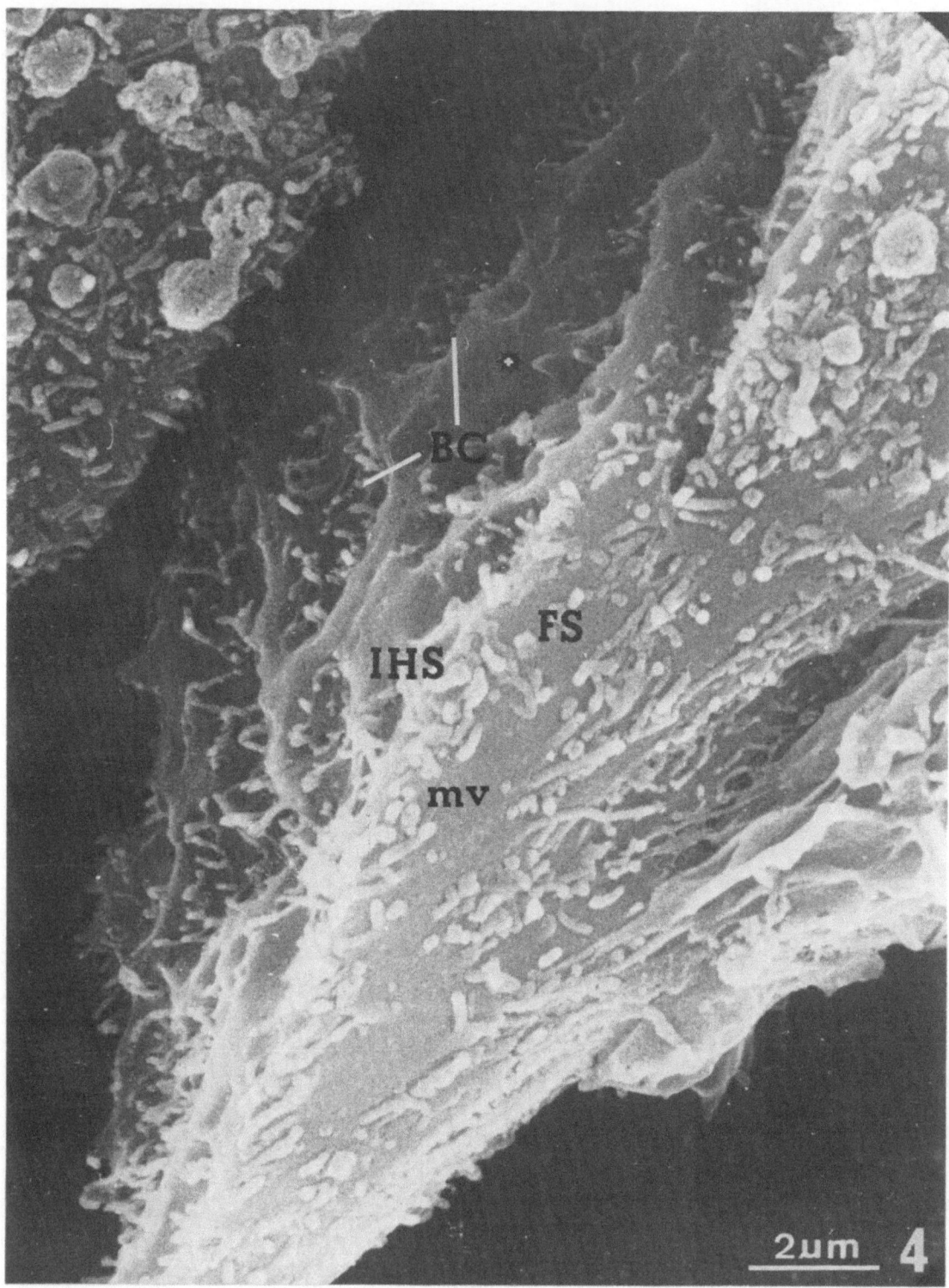

Figure 4. High-magnification view of hepatocytic surfaces of 24-h-cultured parenchymal cells. Free cell surfaces (FS) exhibit numerous microvilli (mv) while interhepatocytic faces (IHS) show newly formed villous bile canaliculi (BC), separated by smooth areas (asterisk).

out after 24, 48, and 72 h culture, according to a method previously described [23].

After 24 h culture, adult rat hepatocytes reveal a homogeneous distribution of G-6-Pase. Figure 5 illustrates a low-magnification view of positively reacting parenchymal cells, intimately reassociated in cell cords. Heavy lead-phosphate deposits are regularly observed within the cisternae of the smooth (SER) and rough (RER) endoplasmic reticulum and in the nuclear envelope (NE). No lead precipitates are encountered on the plasma membrane. At higher magnification (Fig. 6), the enzymatic localization is clearly detected in the smooth and rough ER (Fig. 6, SER and RER). In the peripheral cytoplasm, the smooth ER frequently constitutes a well-developed network of anastomosed tubules, closely connected to the rough ER. The latter is composed either of stacks of numerous parallel-running cisternae or of single cisternal units intimately related to mitochondria. G-6-Pase appears uniformly distributed in these two different topographical arrangements of the RER.

After 48 h culture, hepatocytes are more flattened and present thin cytoplasmic extensions. They still display a positive, but less intense, G-6-Pase cytochemical reaction, as illustrated in Figure 7. Lead-phosphate precipitates offer a regular and continuous distribution in the previously described cell organelles, i.e., SER, RER, and nuclear envelope (NE). Hepatocytes exhibit specific membrane differentiations, such as bile canaliculi (Fig. 7, BC) that are maintained for several days in culture. Moreover, we notice an increased amount of cytolysosomes (Fig. 7, CYL) containing cell debris at different stages of degradation. As confirmed by our biochemical data, the G-6-Pase specific activity decreases progressively in culture. In isolated parenchymal cells, the enzymatic activity reaches the mean value of 116.9 ± 4.3 nmol P/min/mg proteins. After 24 h and 48 h culture, the G-6-Pase activity represents, respectively, about 70% and 50% of the values of the original isolated cell population. The partial loss of enzymatic activity could be attributed either to the high glucose concentration present in the incubation medium or to an important lysosomal degradation rate, which can be suspected by the increased number of cytolysosomes in cultured cells, as revealed by our electron micrographs.

4. SYMBIOTIC CULTURES OF SINUSOIDAL CELLS AND HEPATOCYTES

4.1. Behavior and ultrastructure of parenchymal and nonparenchymal cells in culture

The experimental model of cocultures between parenchymal and nonparenchymal cells was introduced three years ago, thanks to a fruitful collaboration established between the group of Dick Knook in Rijswijk (The Netherlands) and our group in Brussels. Our aim was to reconstitute in vitro, through the association of both cell types, a situation close to that existing in situ. Adult rat hepatocytes were isolated by collagenase perfusion and sinusoidal cells were extracted from the liver parenchyma by pronase digestion [27]. Cocultivation was started by adding 3×10^6 hepatocytes per 60-mm Falcon Petri dish to 10^7 sinusoidal cells, previously cultured for 24 h in Dulbecco medium supplemented with 17% fetal calf serum.

The ultrastructural properties of isolated and cocultured cells, their behavior, and viability have been described in detail in previous publications [17, 18, 28–30]. Briefly, transmission electron-microscopic studies of the cocultured cell populations have shown the potentialities of both cell types to recover and to maintain specific cell properties for several days in culture. *Hepatocytes* reassociate in cell cords and recover their cell surface specializations. Inside the cell, Golgi complexes and lysosomes are polarized toward newly formed bile canaliculi after 24 h culture. Hepatocytes remain well differentiated for more than one week in coculture, i.e., they still retain large areas of smooth endoplasmic reticulum, glycogen particles of the α- and β-types, localized inbetween the network of anastomosed tubules, numerous peroxysomes, and stacks of rough endoplasmic cisternae. *Endothelial cells and Kupffer cells* in culture develop ultrastructural features that make them clearly recognizable, and exhibit specific functional properties such as endocytosis and phagocytosis. The isolated round-shaped endothelial cells, which remain unattached in single cultures, present a higher degree of cell spreading on the bottom of the collagen-coated Petri dishes after the addition of hepatocytes. They flatten in close relation with the parenchymal cells and progressively lose their

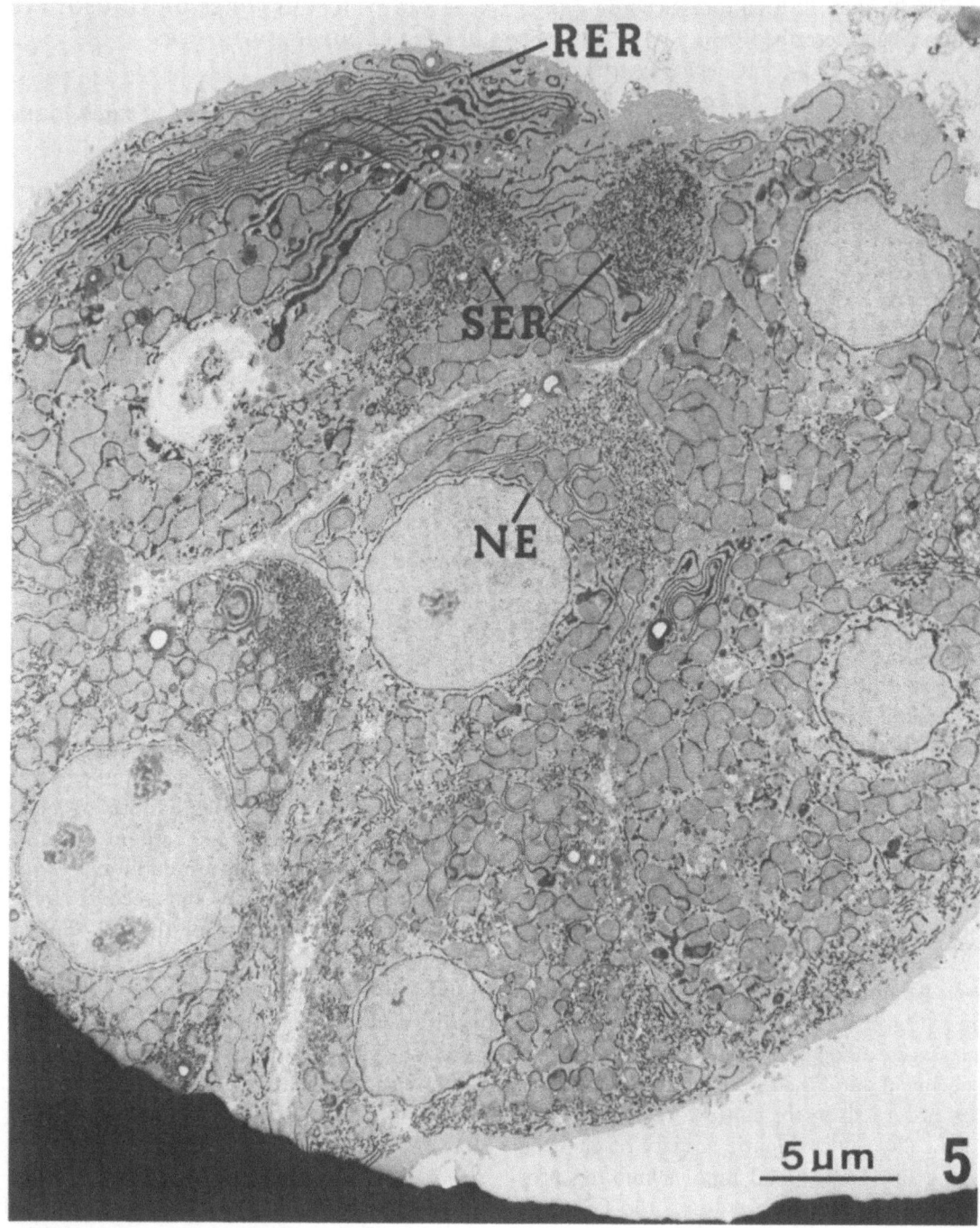

Figure 5. 24-h-cultured hepatocytes incubated for 30 min in the modified Wachstein-Meisel medium for the detection of G-6-Pase. The reaction product is homogeneously distributed in the lumen of the smooth (SER) and rough (RER) endoplasmic reticulum and in the nuclear envelope (NE).

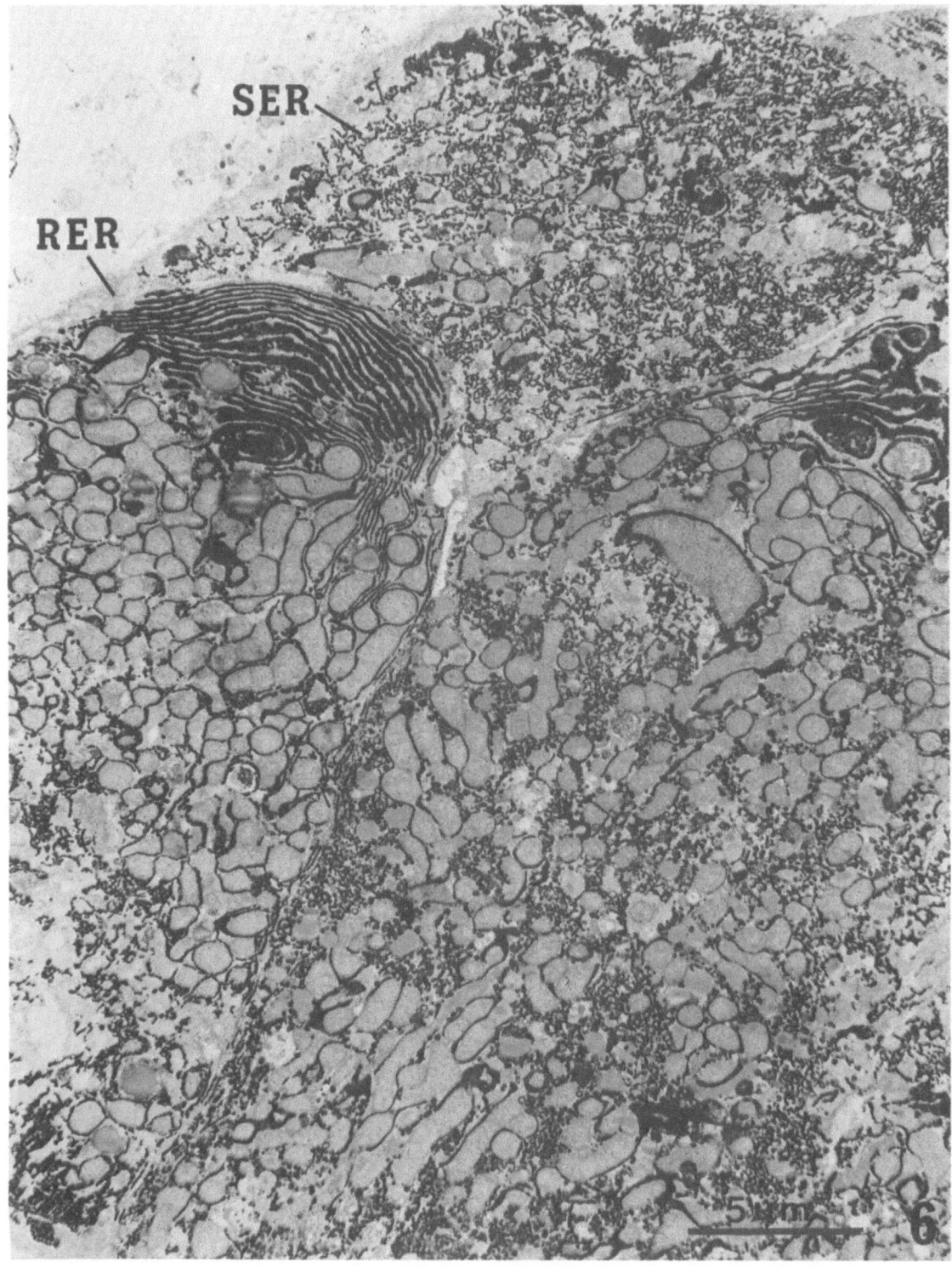

Figure 6. High-magnification view of 24-h-cultured hepatocytes incubated 30 min for G-6-Pase activity. An intense cytochemical reaction is present in the smooth (SER) and rough (RER) endoplasmic reticulum.

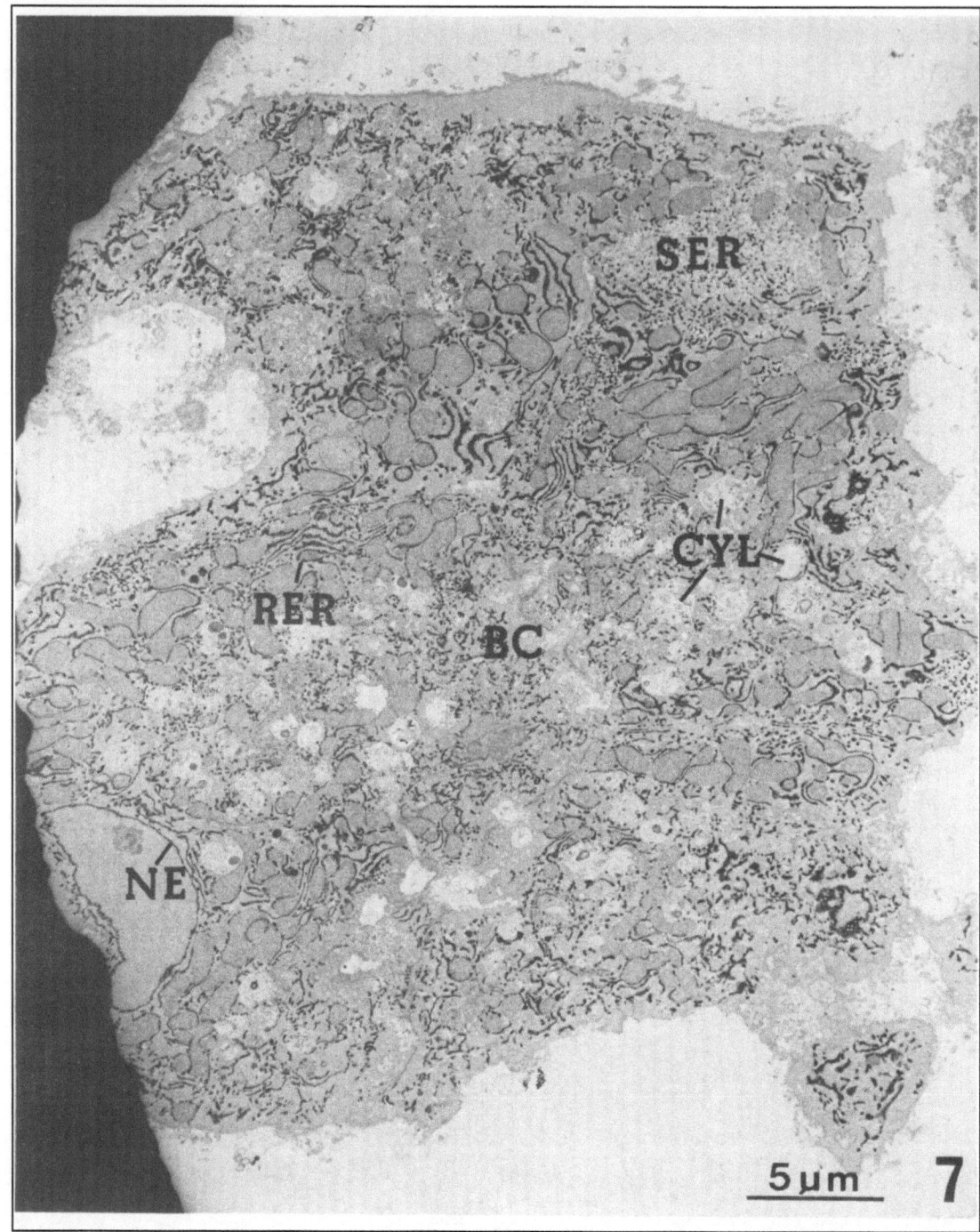

Figure 7. Cytochemical distribution of G-6-Pase activity in 48-h-cultured hepatocytes. A homogeneous but decreased enzymatic activity is observed. SER, smooth ER; RER, rough ER; NE, nuclear envelope; CYL, cytolysosomes; BC, bile canaliculi.

fenestrae. Endothelial cells display numerous micro- and macropinocytic vacuoles, giving evidence of intense endocytic activity. Kupffer cells, on the other hand, rapidly adhere to and spread on the plastic in a few hours. They offer numerous digestive vacuoles containing fat globules, glycogen particles, and membranes of various organelles at different stages of degradation. Phagocytosis of foreign material was clearly demonstrated by the uptake in culture of latex particles, 0.8 μm in diameter, or the engulfing of damaged hepatocytes or red blood cells. Kupffer cells in culture recover specific cell membrane differentiations, such as microvilli, bristle-coated micropinocytic vacuoles, and wormlike structures [30, 31]. These latter structures, visualized after 24 h culture, correspond to invaginations of the cell surface, containing a dense midline of fuzzy-coat material. Finally, few *pit cells* and few *fat-storing cells* were detected by transmission electron microscopy in our preparations. The coculture enables an important improvement of the survival period of hepatocytes in culture. This prolonged survival seems to be related either to the high phagocytic activity of Kupffer cells or to the intercellular cooperation that would exist between both cell types.

4.2. Cell surface properties of sinusoidal cells and hepatocytes in single and cocultures

Single and symbiotic cultures of sinusoidal cells and hepatocytes were prepared for scanning electron microscopy (SEM) as previously described in section 2.2. This technique offers the advantage of enabling the estimation of the proportion of the different sinusoidal cell types collected after isolation, and the analysis their behavior in culture. Starting from a population of isolated spherical cells, it is interesting to recognize, in single and cocultures, the various sinusoidal cells through specific and reproducible cell surface characteristics.

Three sinusoidal cell types, at least, were distinguished by using SEM after 24 h culture: (a) *Kupffer cells*, which represent the majority of cells, attach to the bottom of the dishes. They develop, as illustrated in Figure 8a and b, cytoplasmic extensions varying in number and size and in degree of flattening (K). Despite their variety in shape and

form, Kupffer cells still remain recognizable by the presence of ruffles and lamellipodia covering their free surfaces. (b) *Fat-storing cells* (Ito cells) are regularly detected after 24 h culture. They appear as oblong and fusiform cells, which offer a cell body dressed with numerous thin, closely apposed microvilli (Fig. 8a, FSC). These spindle-shaped cells frequently have smooth, elongated cytoplasmic extensions that end in goose-foot structures (Fig. 8a, arrows). These cells, examined under the transmission electron microscope, are particularly rich in fat droplets. Their fibroblastic behavior in culture and their lack of uptake of latex particles constitute additional arguments in favor of the definitive diagnosis of fat-storing cell [31, 32]. (c) *Endothelial cells* are less frequent in single cultures. They remain round shaped and adhere to the collagen-coated dishes by short cytoplasmic extensions (Fig. 8b, E).

In cocultures, the three sinusoidal cell types are regularly encountered and display the same morphological features. Endothelial cells and fat-storing cells appear intimately related to hepatocytes. Figure 9 illustrates, under the scanning electron microscope, the cell surface properties of sinusoidal cells cultured for 48 h, associated with hepatocytes incubated for 24 h. Liver parenchymal cells reform cell cords (Fig. 9, H) and exhibit villous free surfaces, clearly distinguished in this micrograph (Fig. 9, mv). Sinusoidal cells, in particular endothelial cells (Fig. 9, E) and Kupffer cells (Fig. 9, K), establish loose contacts with hepatocytes. Kupffer cells are responsible for the high degree of cleanliness observed in cocultures.

In conclusion, endothelial cells, Kupffer cells, and fat-storing cells exhibit, in single cultures and cocultures, specific and different cell surface properties and behavior that enable an accurate differential diagnosis of each cell type.

5. CONCLUSIONS AND PERSPECTIVES

It appears from our actual ultrastructural and biochemical data that the 24- to 48-h hepatocytic cultures constitute an appropriate experimental model that is close to the situation in situ. We would like to stress the advantages of our experimental models in the future development of various

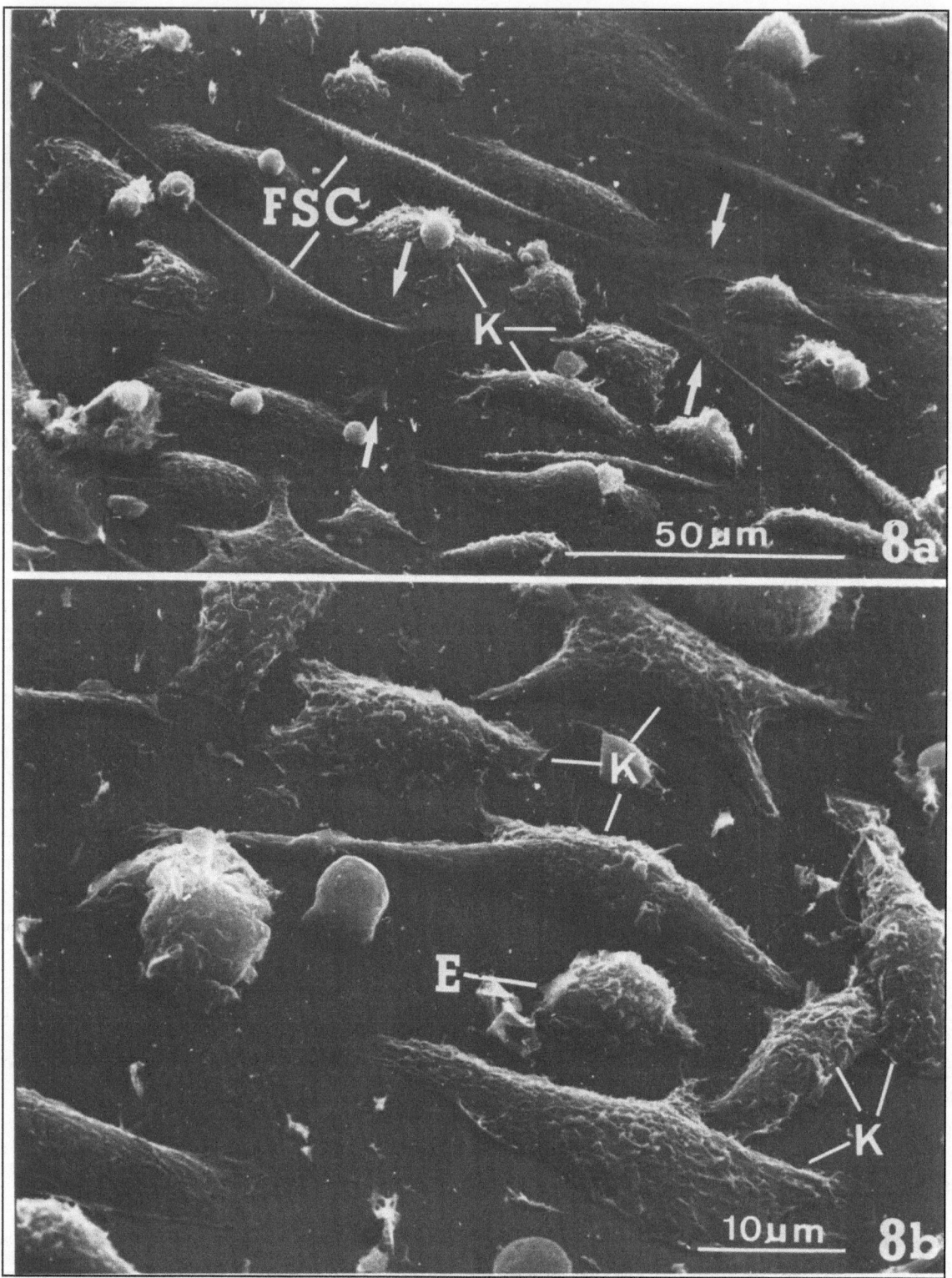

Figure 8a and b. Single cultures of 24-h-cultured sinusoidal cells. Kupffer cells (K), dressed with ruffles and lamellipodia, adhere to the collagen-coated dishes and form numerous cytoplasmic extensions. Fat-storing cells (FSC) appear as spindle-shaped cells. Their cell body is covered with numerous thin, closely apposed microvilli while their peripheral cytoplasmic extensions appear smooth and end in goose-foot structures (arrows). Endothelial cells (E) remain round-shaped and are poorly adhering cells.

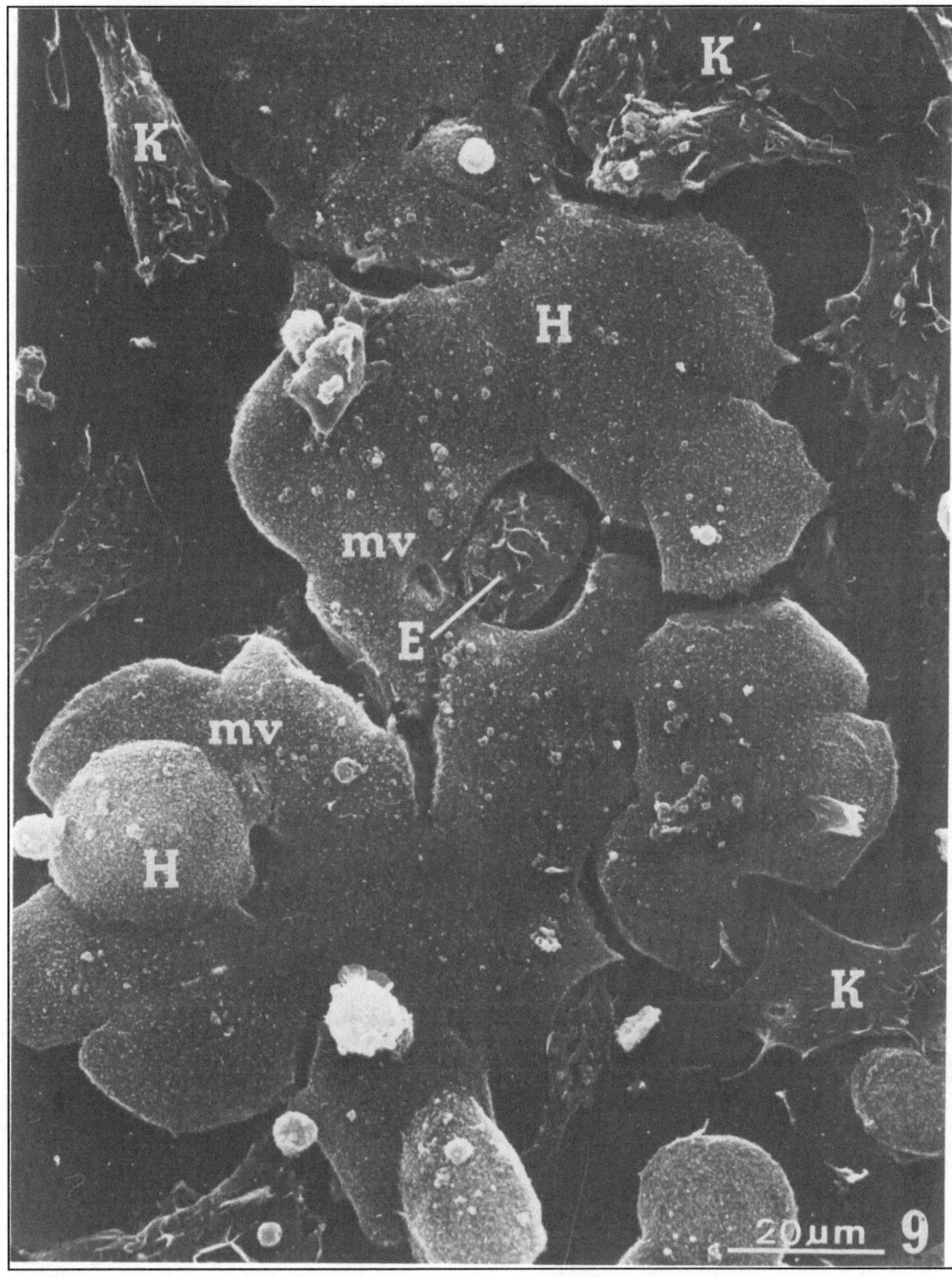

Figure 9. Cocultures of 24-h-cultured hepatocytes and 48-h-cultured sinusoidal cells. Hepatocytes reform cell cords and exhibit villous free surfaces (mv). Endothelial cells (E) and Kupffer cells (K) establish loose cell contacts with hepatocytes (H).

types of metabolic studies. Physiological processes such as endocytosis and exocytosis, the fate of plasma membranes, i.e., retrieval and intracellular redistribution, can be successfully analyzed in vitro. Preliminary cinetic studies of fixation and internalization of cationized ferritin were performed in vitro under the conditions proposed by Farquhar [33]. Fusions between coated vesicles and Golgi-condensing vacuoles were frequently observed, which suggests that plasma liver parenchymal cell membranes interiorized by endocytosis may recycle back to the cell surface without transit through the lysosomal compartment [34].

Turnover of specific plasma membrane enzymatic activities, i.e., 5'nucleotidase (5'NT), Mg^{++} dependent ATPase, or adenylate cyclase, can be followed in situ. The first important problem consists in defining the relative proportion of enzymes bound to the cell surface and localized inside the cell. In the particular case of 5'NT, our recent cytochemical results show that the enzyme is homogeneously distributed on the cell surface of isolated and cultured hepatocytes, and is detected inside the cells, in micropinocytic-coated vesicles and in cytolysosomes, at different stages of development [35]. Finally, the presence of galactose and fucose receptors was demonstrated on adult rat hepatocytes established in primary monolayer cultures [36, 37]. These highly specific receptors play an important role in the hepatic clearance of galac-

tose and fucose terminating glycoproteins. Glycosylated derivatives of bovine serum albumin (BSA), i.e., N-acetyl-lactosamine-BSA and fucose-BSA, were specifically incorporated by hepatocytes in culture. Single cultures and cocultures could be used in the future to test the relative distribution of carbohydrate receptors on parenchymal and non-parenchymal cells.

Our experimental models of isolation and culture of adult rat parenchymal cells have been successfully used to analyze the morphological and biochemical alterations of hepatocytes during the carcinogenic transformation induced by chemicals, i.e., N-nitrosomorpholine [38, 39] and diethylnitrosamine [40, 41]. Specific ultrastructural modifications occur during hepatocarcinogenesis at the level of preneoplastic and hyperplastic foci, which are composed of proliferating initiated cells of large size and deficient in G-6-Pase and bile canalicular ATPase activities. These hypertrophied cells were easily recognized in isolated and cultured cell populations owing to their enzymatic deficiencies. Moreover, cell subpopulations enriched in transformed hepatocytes were obtained by elutriation or counterflow centrifugation [38, 39]. This new methodology based on cell separation according to size and ploidy [23] appears very promising to define biochemical properties of liver parenchymal cells at different stages of neoplasia.

REFERENCES

1. Berry MN, Friend DS (1969) High-yield preparation of isolated rat liver parenchymal cells. J Cell Biol 43:506–520
2. Seglen PO (1973) Preparation of rat liver cells. III. Enzymatic requirements for tissue dispersion. Exp Cell Res 82:391–398
3. Drochmans P, Wanson JC, Mosselmans R (1975) Isolation and subfractionation on ficoll gradients of adult rat hepatocytes. Size, morphology and biochemical characteristics of cell fractions. J Cell Biol 66:1–22
4. Bissell DM, Hammaker LE, Meyer UA (1973) Parenchymal cells from adult rat liver in non-proliferating monolayer culture. I. Functional studies. J Cell Biol 59:722–734
5. Bonney RJ, Becker JE, Walker PR, Potter VR (1974) Primary monolayer cultures of adult rat liver parenchymal cells suitable for study of the regulation of enzyme synthesis. In Vitro 9:399–413
6. Michalopoulos G, Pitot HC (1975) Primary culture of parenchymal liver cells on collagen membranes. Exp Cell Res 94:70–78
7. Jeejeebhoy KN, Phillips MJ (1976) Isolated mammalian hepatocytes in culture. Gastroenterology 71:1086–1096

8. Laishes BA, Williams GM (1976) Conditions affecting primary cell cultures of functional adult rat hepatocytes. I. The effect of insulin. In Vitro 12:521–532
9. Laishes BA, Williams GM (1976) Conditions affecting primary cell cultures of functional adult rat hepatocytes. II. Dexamethasone enhanced longevity and maintenance of morphology. In Vitro 12:821–832
10. Wanson JC, Drochmans P, Mosselmans R, Ronveaux MF (1977) Adult rat hepatocytes in primary monolayer culture. Ultrastructural characteristics of intercellular contacts and cell membrane differentiations. J Cell Biol 74:858–877
11. Bernaert D, Wanson JC, Drochmans P, Popowski A (1977) Effect of insulin on the ultrastructure and the glycogenesis in primary cultures of adult rat hepatocytes. J Cell Biol 74: 878–900
12. Guguen C, Guillouzo A, Boisnard A, Lecam A, Bourel M (1975) Etude ultrastructurale de monocouches d'hépatocytes de rat adulte cultivés en présence d'hémisuccinate d'hydrocortisone. Biol Gastro Enterol 8:223–231
13. Spence JT, Haars L, Edwards A, Bosch A, Pitot HC (1980) Regulation of gene expression in primary cultures of adult rat hepatocytes on collagen gels. In: Williams GM (ed) Conference on differentiation and carcinogenesis in liver cell

cultures. New York: New York Academy of Sciences 349: 99–110

14. Gurr JA, Potter VR (1980) The significance of differences between fresh cell suspensions and fresh or maintained monolayers. In: Williams GM (ed) Conference on differentiation and carcinogenesis in liver cell cultures. New York: New York Academy of Sciences 349:57–66

15. Koch KS, Leffert HL (1980) Growth control of differentiated adult rat hepatocytes in primary culture. In: Williams GM (ed) Conference on differentiation and carcinogenesis in liver cell cultures. New York: New York Academy of Sciences 349:111–127

16. Michalopoulos G, Sattler GL, Pitot HC (1978) Hormonal regulation and the effects of glucose on tyrosine aminotransferase activity in adult rat hepatocytes cultured on floating collagen membranes. Cancer Res 38:1550–1555

17. Wanson JC, Drochmans P, Mosselmans R, Knook DL (1977) Symbiotic culture of adult hepatocytes and sinuslining cells. In: Wisse E, Knook DL (eds) Kupffer cells and other liver sinusoidal cells. Amsterdam: Elsevier, pp 141–150

18. Wanson JC, Mosselmans R, Brouwer A, Knook DL (1979) Interaction of adult rat hepatocytes and sinusoidal cells in co-culture. Biol Cell 36:7–16

19. Wanson JC, Bernaert D, May C (1979) Morphology and functional properties of isolated and cultured hepatocytes. In: Popper H, Schaffner F (eds) Progress in liver diseases, vol 6. New York: Grune and Stratton, pp 1–22

20. Penasse W, Bernaert D, Mosselmans R, Wanson JC, Drochmans P (1979) Scanning electron microscopy of adult rat hepatocytes in situ, after isolation of pure fractions by elutriation and after culture. Biol Cell 34:175–186

21. May C, Bernaert D, Mosselmans R, Popowski A, Penasse W, Wanson JC (1979) Cell aggregates and monolayer cultures of adult rat hepatocytes: models for the study of the ultrastructural behaviour and metabolic functions of parenchymal cells. In: Hommes FA (ed) Models for the study of inborn errors of metabolism. Amsterdam: Elsevier/North-Holland Biomedical, pp 225–238

22. Drochmans P, Wanson JC, May C, Bernaert D (1978) Ultrastructural and metabolic studies of isolated and cultured hepatocytes. In: Whelan J (ed) Hepatotrophic factors. Ciba Foundation Symposium 55. Amsterdam: Elsevier/North-Holland, pp 7–29

23. Bernaert D, Wanson JC, Mosselmans R, De Paermentier F, Drochmans P (1979) Separation of adult rat hepatocytes in distinct subpopulations by centrifugal elutriation. Morphological, morphometrical and biochemical characterization of cell fractions. Biol Cell 34:159–174

24. Wanson JC (1976) Morphological and biochemical characteristics of isolated and cultured hepatocytes. In: Tager JM, Söling HD, Williamson JR (eds) Use of isolated liver cells and kidney tubules in metabolic studies. Amsterdam: North-Holland, pp 185–196

25. Motta PM (1977) The three-dimensional fine structure of the liver as revealed by scanning electron microscopy. Int Rev Cytol 6:347–399

26. Hugon J, Maestracci D, Menard D (1971) Glucose-6-phosphatase activity in the intestinal epithelium of the mouse. J Histochem Cytochem 19:515–525

27. Knook DL, Blansjaar N, Sleyster ECh (1977) Isolation and characterization of Kupffer and endothelial cells from the rat liver. Exp Cell Res 109: 317–329

28. Drochmans P. Sleyster ECh, Penasse W, Wanson JC, Knook DL (1977) Morphology of isolated and cultured sinus-lining cells of rat liver. In: Wisse E, Knook DL (eds) Kupffer cells and other liver sinusoidal cells. Amsterdam: Elsevier, pp 131–139

29. Brouwer A, Wanson JC, Mosselmans R, Knook DL, Drochmans P (1980) Morphology and lysosomal enzymes of primary cultures of rat liver sinusoidal cells. Biol Cell 37: 35–44

30. Wanson JC, Mosselmans R (1980) Coculture of adult rat hepatocytes and sinusoidal cells: a new experimental model for the study of ultrastructural and functional properties of liver cells. Falk Foundation Symposium no. 27: Communications of liver cells. Lancaster: MTP, pp 239–251

31. Mosselmans R, Wanson JC, Brouwer A, Knook DL (1980) Isolation and culture of sinusoidal cells and hepatocytes, extracted from adult and 24 months aged rats. Behaviour of endothelial cells, Kupffer cells and fat-storing cells in single and cocultures. In: Brederoo P, de Priester W (eds) European Congress of Electron Microscopy. Den Haag. Leiden: 7th EUREM Foundation 2:122–123

32. Penasse W, Wanson JC (1980) Cell surface properties of sinusoidal cells and hepatocytes in single and cocultures. In: Brederoo P, de Priester W (eds) European Congress of Electron Microscopy. Den Haag. Leiden: 7th EUREM Foundation 2:36–37

33. Farquhar MG (1978) Recovery of surface membrane in anterior pituitary cells. Variations in traffic detected with anionic and cationic ferritin. J Cell Biol 78:R35–R42

34. Mosselmans R, Wanson JC, Deschuyteneer M (1980) Recycling of plasma membranes in monolayer cultures of adult rat hepatocytes. Second International Congress on Cell Biology (Berlin, 1980). Eur J Cell Biol 22:177

35. Wanson JC, Bernaert D, Lemaire J, Popowski A, Widnell Ch (1980) 5′Nucleotidase activity in isolated and cultured adult rat hepatocytes. Second International Congress on Cell Biology (Berlin, 1980). Eur J Cell Biol 22:267

36. Prieels JP, Deschuyteneer M, May C, Wanson JC (1979) Carbohydrate receptors in primary culture of adult rat hepatocytes. In: Schauer et al (eds) Glycoconjugates. Proceedings Fifth International Symposium Kiel. Stuttgart: G Thieme, pp 502–503

37. Deschuyteneer M, Prieels JP, May C, Perraudin JP, Wanson JC (1980) Presence of galactose and fucose receptors on adult rat hepatocytes in primary monolayer culture. Second International Congress on Cell Biology (Berlin, 1980). Eur J Cell Biol 22:264

38. Wanson JC, Penasse W, Bernaert D, Mosselmans R (1979) Cell surface properties of control and carcinogen-treated hepatocytes, isolated in subpopulations by elutriation. SEM/1979/II, SEM Inc, AMF O'Hare, Il 60666, USA, pp 161–168

39. Wanson JC, Bernaert D, Penasse W, Mosselmans R, Bannasch P (1980) Separation in distinct subpopulations by elutriation of liver cells following exposure of rats to N-nitrosomorpholine. Cancer Res 40:459–471

40. Wanson JC, Bernaert D, May C, Deschuyteneer M, Prieels JP (1980) Isolation and culture of adult rat hepatocytes and preoplastic nodules from diethylnitrosamine treated livers: glucose-6-phosphatase distribution, albumin synthesis and hepatic binding protein activity. In: Williams GM, Borek C (eds) Conference on differentiation and carcinogenesis in liver cell cultures. New York: New York Academy of Sciences 349:413–415

41. Wanson JC, Penasse W, Bernaert D, May C (1980) Ultrastructural properties of adult rat hepatocytes from preneoplastic and neoplastic foci induced in the liver by diethylnitrosamine. SEM/1980 III, SEM Inc, AMF O'Hare, Il 60666, USA, pp 29–35

6. MICROCIRCULATION OF THE LIVER, WITH SPECIAL REFERENCE TO THE PERIBILIARY PORTAL SYSTEM

O. OHTANI, T. MURAKAMI, and A.L. JONES

1. INTRODUCTION

Methods have been developed for making an injection replica for visualization of minute vessels by scanning electron microscopy. These methods have been useful for producing clear three-dimensional images of the vasculature of many organs, including the liver [1–3]. This chapter briefly describes the method and reviews the liver findings in man and in monkey and some other animals [4–6]. Emphasis will be placed on the peribiliary plexus and its connecting vessels. This plexus may have special functional significance in the control of liver microcirculation and bile secretory activity.

2. MATERIALS AND METHODS

The human liver was obtained by necropsy from a Japanese individual who had suffered from chronic renal failure and had been treated with artificial dialysis. Routine H-E stained light microscopy of the tissue demonstrated that the liver had no pathological changes. Monkey (rhesus), rabbit, and rat were killed under anesthesia and portions of their livers were removed. These livers were also found to be normal on light-microscopic examination. In the human liver, catheters were inserted into the hepatic artery and the portal vein. Ringer's solution was perfused through these cannulated vessels to remove as much blood as possible from the liver. Following this procedure, a laboratory-prepared or commercially available low-viscosity methacrylate-resin injection medium (Mercox, Oken-Shoji, Tokyo, Japan) [4, 5] was injected through the cannulated vessels until the hepatic vein was filled with the injected resin. In the animals, the Ringer perfusion and successive resin injection were performed through the thoracic aorta. The resin-injected livers were then placed for several hours in a warm-water bath, corroded overnight in warm 10% NaOH solution, and washed for 8 h or longer in running tap water.

The blood vascular casts thus obtained were frozen in water, cut into appropriate blocks, and air-dried. The dried specimens were mounted on metal specimen stubs, microdissected with sharpened needles and forceps under a binocular stereo-light microscope, coated with a thin layer of gold by evaporation, and observed in a scanning electron microscope with an acceleration voltage of 5 kV. A procedure of dissection followed by scanning electron microscopy was repeated until the most interesting structures were sufficiently exposed.

The resin injection as described produced excellent casts of even the smallest vessels, including the fine capillaries, of the peribiliary plexus, and within the portal canal as well as the hepatic sinusoids. The repeated microdissection and scanning electron microscopy of the vascular casts enabled the detailed analysis of their distributions and connections. The results are described below.

3. GENERAL ASPECTS OF LIVER BLOOD VASCULATURE

Blood enters the liver through the portal vein and hepatic artery and leaves via the hepatic vein. The portal vein runs within the stroma of the portal canal and its terminal branches supply the hepatic sinusoids. The hepatic artery runs with the portal vein in the portal canal, but its terminal branches end not only in the hepatic sinusoids but also in the peribiliary and periportal plexuses. These plexuses drain into the hepatic sinusoids directly or via the

P.M. Motta and L.J.A. DiDio (eds.), Basic and clinical hepatology, pp. 85–96. All rights reserved.
Copyright © 1982 Martinus Nijhoff Publishers, The Hague/Boston/London.

86

portal vein. Therefore, both portal vein and hepatic artery blood flows into the hepatic sinusoids (Table 1 and Fig. 1). Blood in the hepatic sinusoids enters the hepatic vein via the central veins. As an additional blood supply, the liver receives some branches from the subphrenic arteries and veins.

3.1. Portal vein branches and hepatic sinusoids

Terminal branches of the portal vein are classified into the interlobular and periportal venules (Figs. 1–3 and 7). The interlobular venules run into the boundaries of the hepatic lobules, i.e., into the final segments of the portal canal and supply the adjacent two or more lobules. The periportal venules usually run for varying distances in the portal canal along with the distributing veins and only supply the hepatic sinusoids bordering the portal canal. The system of the periportal venules is less developed as the portal canal is traced more proximally toward the liver hilus. Thus, as described by some investigators [19, 20], the hepatic sinusoids around the portal canal are poorly supplied by the portal vein. These sinusoids, however, receive supplementally blood from the periportal and peribiliary plexuses in the portal canal.

The hepatic sinusoids originate at the margin of the lobules in the interlobular and periportal venules. They anastomose freely through the lacunar spaces of the liver plates. The sinusoids radiate toward the central veins. Blood entering the central

Table 1. Abbreviations in Figures 1–9

A:	hepatic artery branch (distributing artery)
B:	bile duct (distributing bile duct)
H:	hepatic vein branch (collecting vein)
P:	portal vein branch (distributing vein)
CV:	central vein
HS:	hepatic sinusoid
PA:	peribiliary afferent arteriole
SV:	sublobular vein
PES:	peribiliary efferent venule (lobular branch)
PEV:	peribiliary efferent venule (prelobular branch)
PbP:	peribiliary plexus
PhP:	perihepatic plexus
PpP:	periportal plexus
ilA:	interlobular arteriole
ppA:	periportal arteriole
ilV:	interlobular venule
ppV:	periportal venule

vein then goes to the sublobular vein, collecting, and finally into the hepatic vein (Figs. 1 and 4).

3.2. Arterial branches

Terminal branches of the hepatic artery are classified into the interlobular, periportal, and peribiliary arterioles (Figs. 1–3 and 5).

The interlobular arterioles run with the interlobular venules into the final segments of the portal canal. They are then divided into fine capillaries at the boundaries of the lobules and merge with the hepatic sinusoids. In man and monkey, some of the interlobular arterioles appear with the interlobular venules on the surface of the liver (Fig. 5). These capsular arterioles are also divided into fine capillaries that flow into the hepatic sinusoids.

The periportal and peribiliary arterioles usually arise in common trunks, and supply the periportal and peribiliary plexuses, respectively.

As confirmed by previous authors [7–13], the interlobular arterioles sometimes give off twigs that continue directly into the accompanying interlobular venules or their parent veins (arterioportal anastomosis) (Figs. 1 and 3). This anastomosis typically occurs in man and rat, but it is not as clear in monkey and rabbit. Some authors described an anastomosis between the branches of hepatic artery and hepatic vein (arteriohepatic anastomosis) [18], and other investigators have reported a so-called intralobular arteriole that penetrates deep into the lobules and joins the hepatic sinusoids near the central veins [14–17]. These arteriohepatic anastomosis and intralobular arterioles have not been demonstrated by our injection replica scanning electron microscope method.

3.3. Periportal and perihepatic plexuses

The portal canal is provided with its own capillary network (periportal plexus), which is characteristically distributed around the branches of the portal vein throughout the portal canal (Figs. 1 and 6).

The periportal plexus is supplied by the periportal arterioles of the hepatic artery, and drained at the periphery of the portal canal into the hepatic sinusoids although it occasionally communicates with the periportal venules and the peribiliary efferent vessels. As in the case of the interlobular

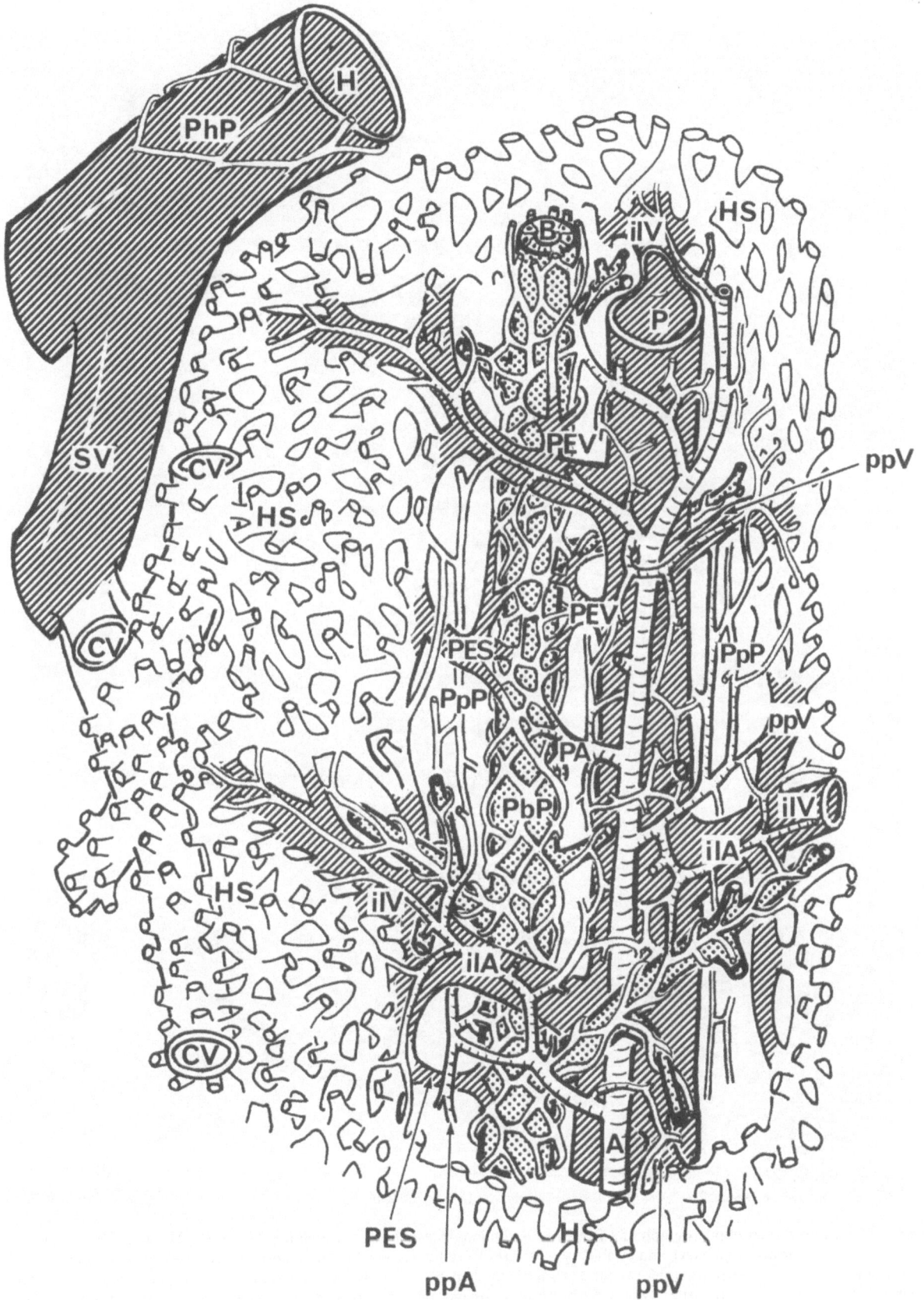

Figure 1. Schematic diagram that shows intrahepatic architectures of blood vessels (see text and Table 1).

88

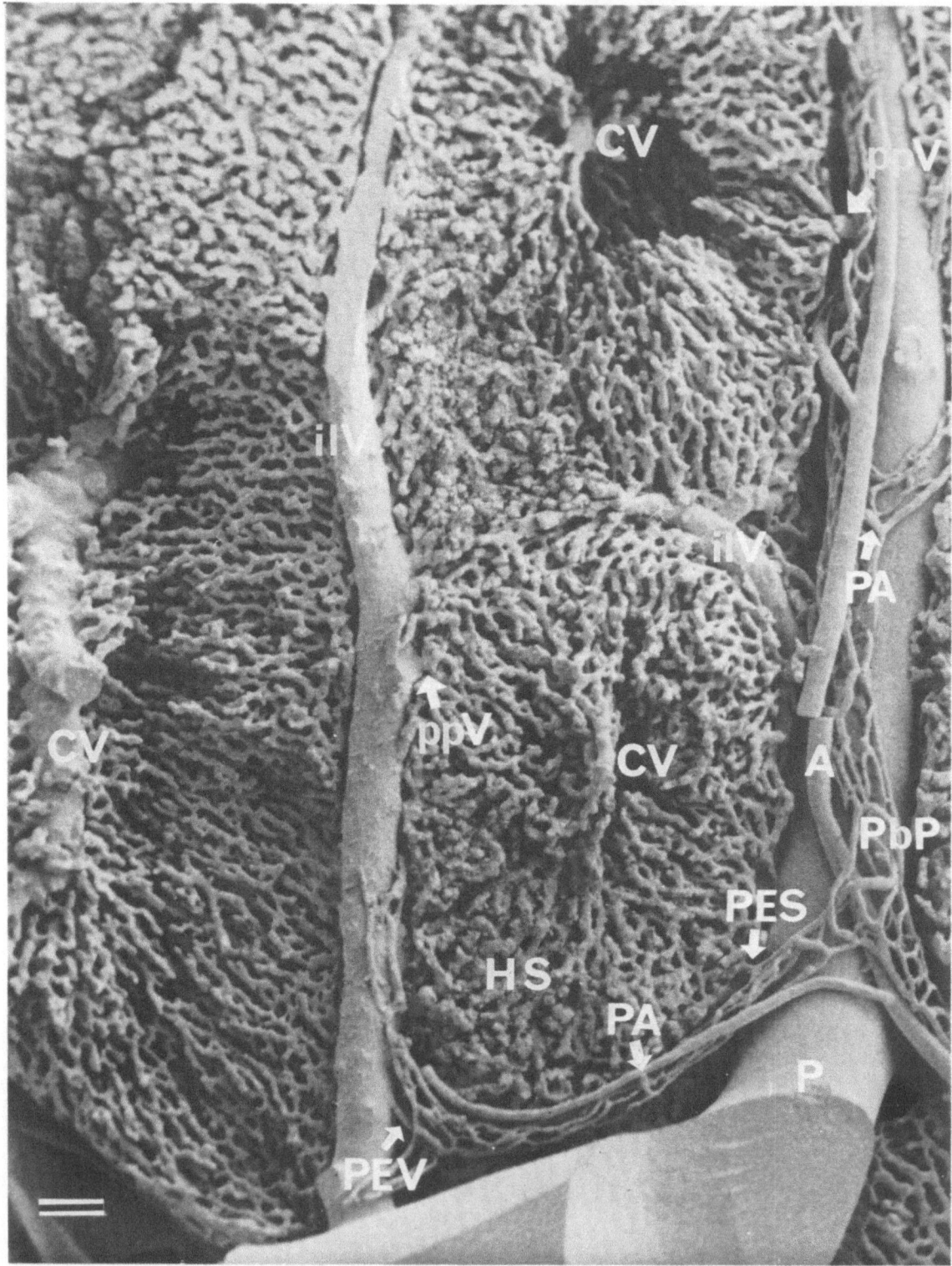

Figure 2. A scanning electron micrograph of a freeze-cut and microdissected blood vascular cast of the rabbit liver. The portal vein branch (P), hepatic artery branch (A), and peribiliary plexus (PbP) run in the portal canal. Note that the portal vein branch gives off the interlobular (ilV) and periportal (ppV) venules to supply the hepatic sinusoids (HS). Note also that the peribiliary plexus (PbP), which is supplied by the hepatic artery twig (PA), has both drainages into the sinusoids (PES) and portal vein branch (PEV). CV, central vein. Bar 100 μm (see Table 1). From O. Ohtani (1979) *Arch. Histol. Jpn.* 42:158 [6].

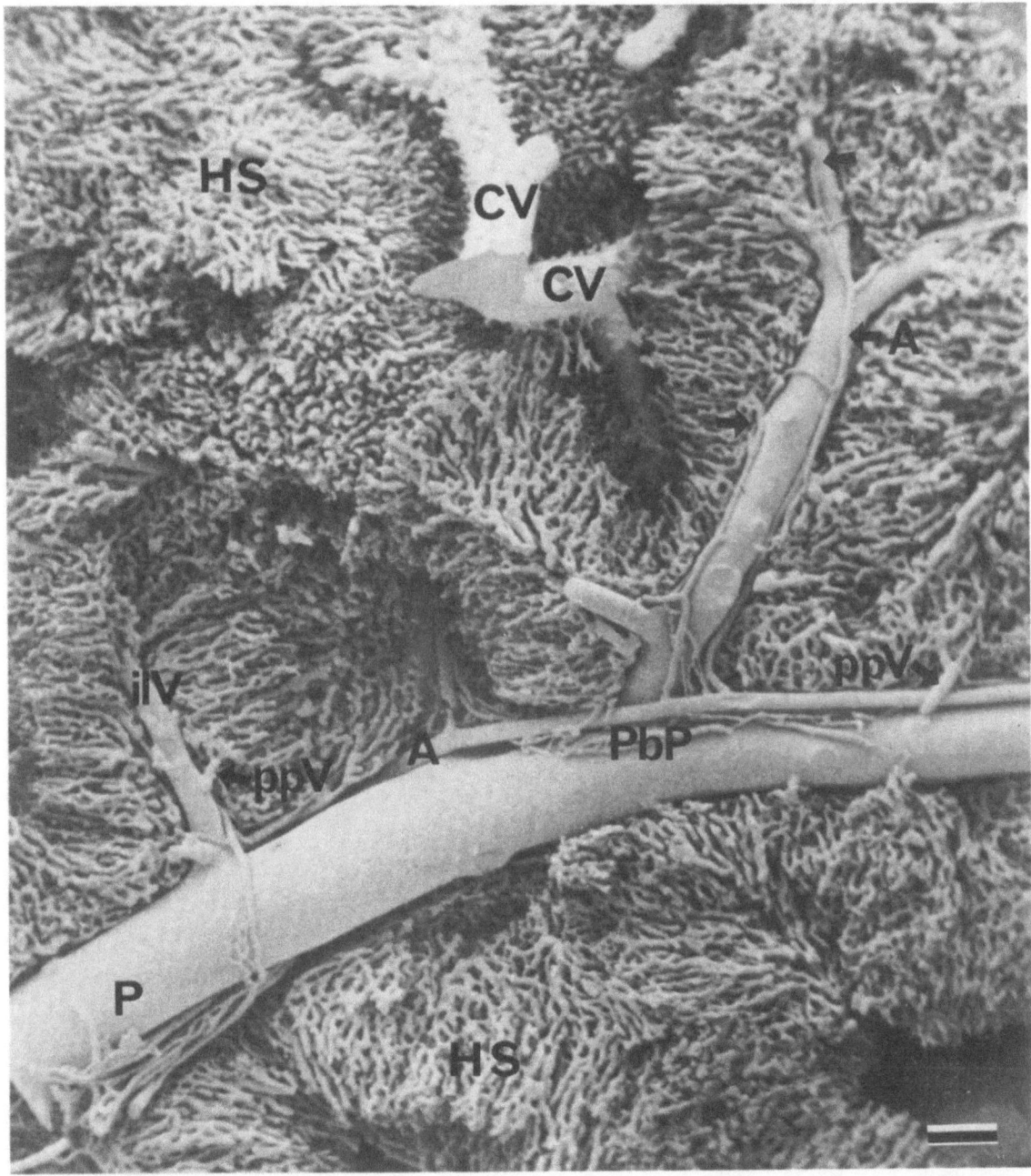

Figure 3. A scanning electron micrograph of a freeze-cut and dissected cast of the rat liver. Arterioportal anastomoses are seen (arrows). A, P, CV, HS, PbP, ppV (see Table 1). Bar 100 μm.

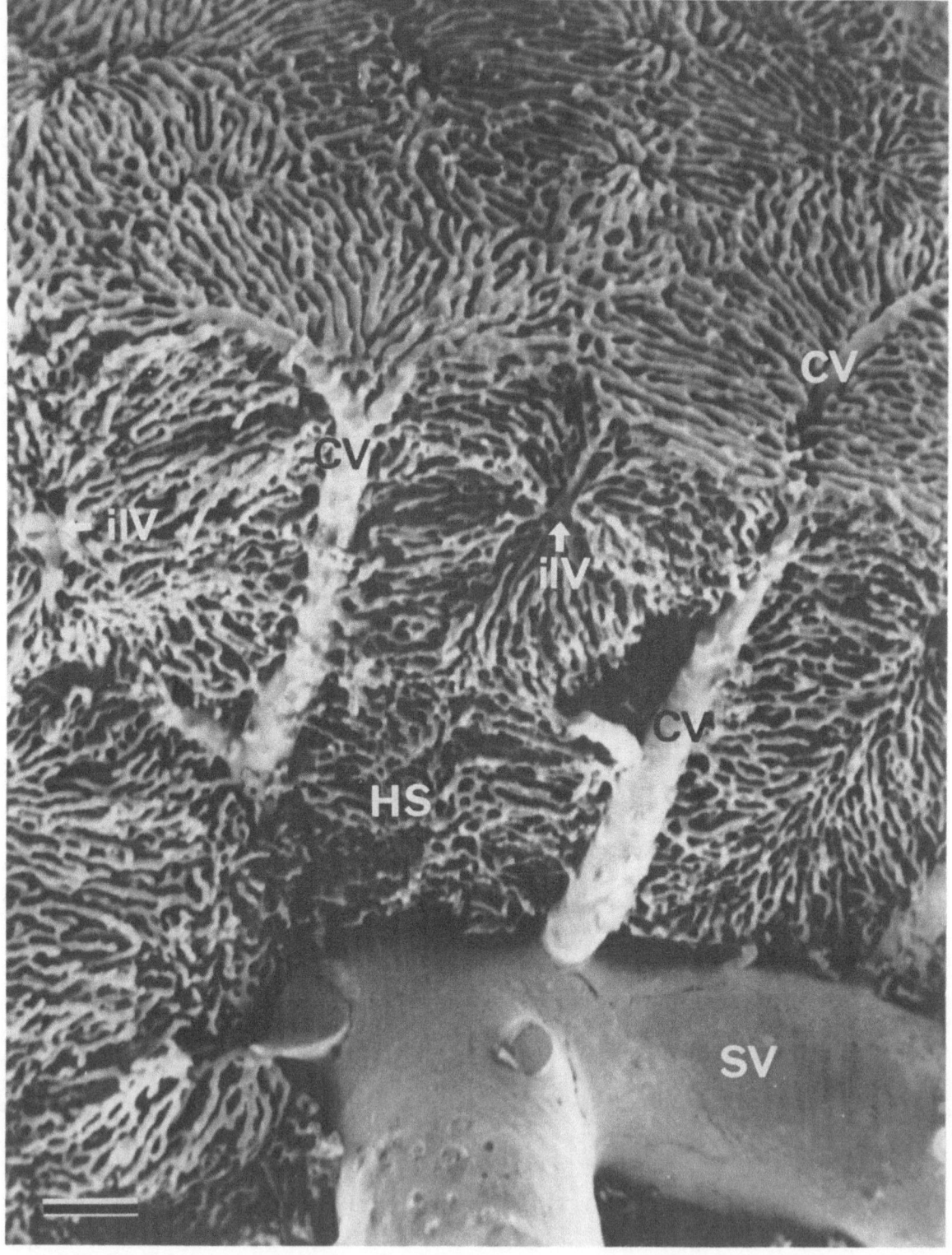

Figure 4. A dissected cast of the rat liver, showing the hepatic venous tree. Hepatic sinusoids (HS) converge into the central veins (CV), which are collected into the sublobular veins (SV). Note that no vascular network is observed in the hepatic canal (see text). ilV, interlobular vein. Bar 100 μm.

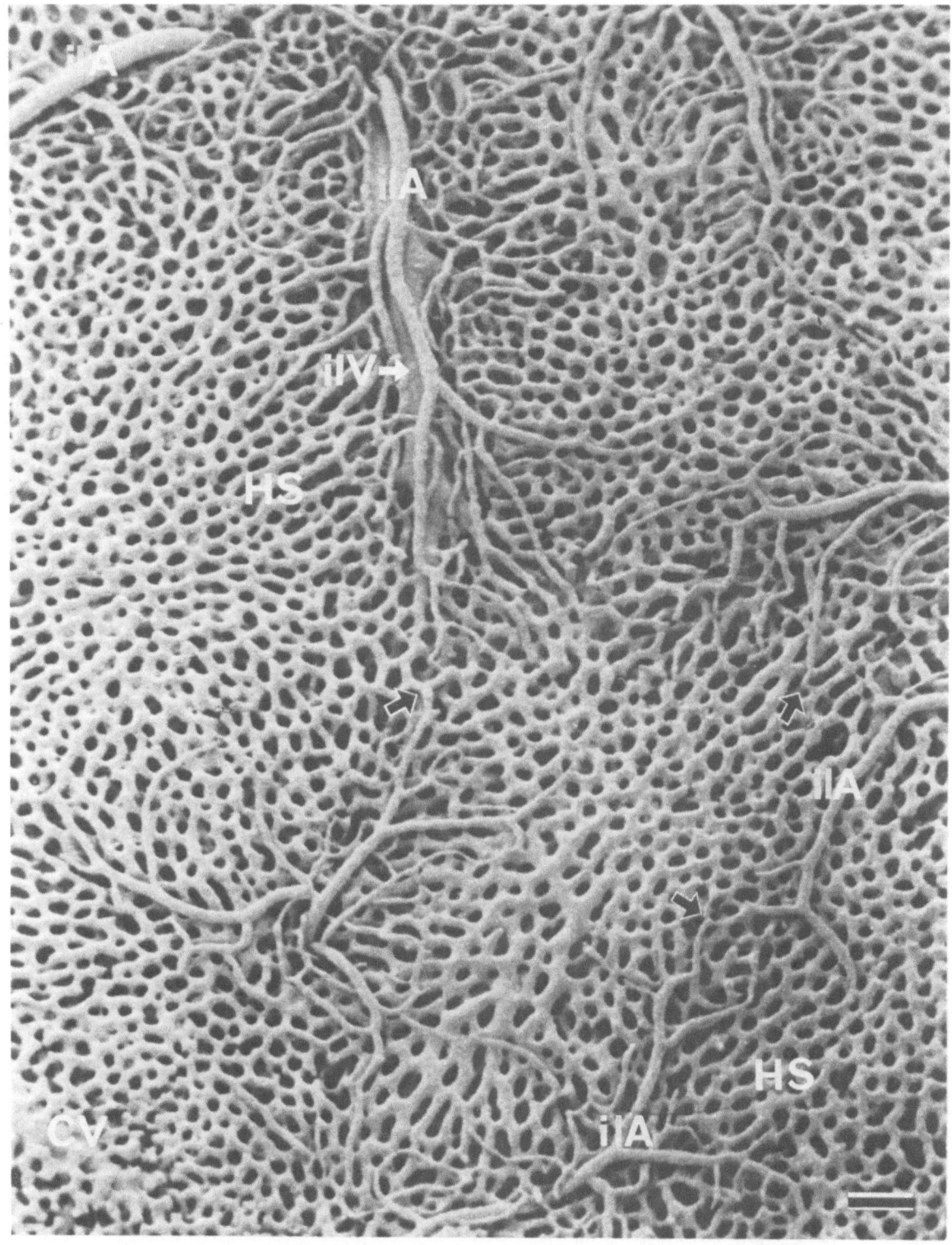

Figure 5. A rhesus monkey liver cast viewed from the surface. Note that the interlobular arterioles (ilA) and venules (ilV) emerge on the surface of the liver. Note also that the terminals of the interlobular arterioles are connected into the liver sinusoids (HS) (arrow). Bar 100 μm. From T. Murakami et al. (1974) *Arch. Histol. Jpn.* 37:426 [4].

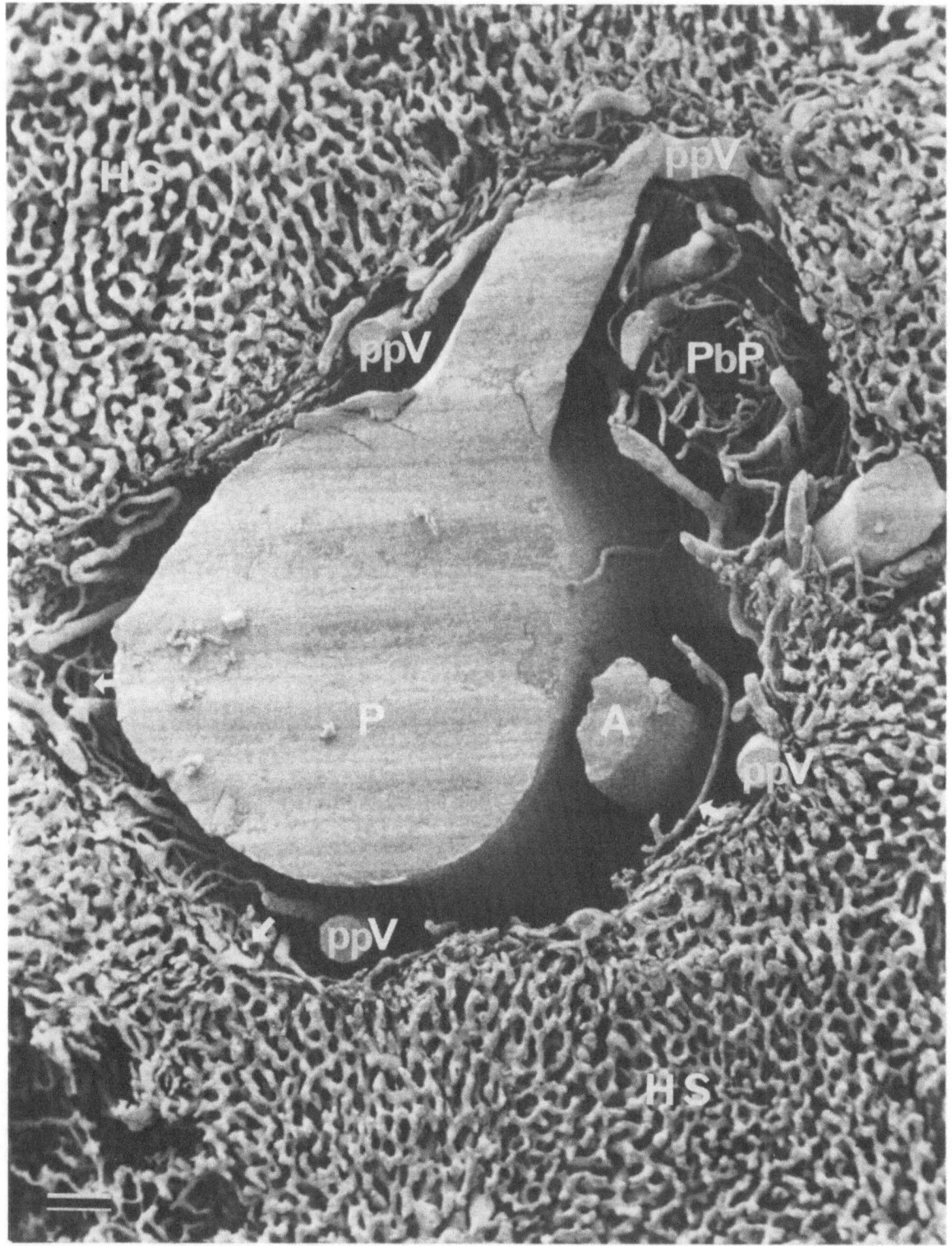

Figure 6. A freeze-cut cast of the human liver. Hepatic artery branch (A), portal vein branch (P), and peribiliary plexus (PbP) are surrounded by coarse capillary networks, which form the so-called which 'periportal plexus' (arrows). Note the direct connections of this plexus with the hepatic sinusoids (HS) (lower-left arrow). Note also that the peribiliary plexus is surrounded by the relatively thick capillaries (outer venous network) (see text). ppV (see Table 1). Bar 100 μm.

arterioles, the periportal arterioles sometimes give off the anastomosing twigs to the neighboring periportal venules of the portal vein. This arterio-portal anastomosis within the portal canal can also be readily observed in man and rat livers.

Some small branches of the subphrenic arteries enter into the hepatic canal, and form very coarse capillary networks that surround the hepatic vein branches (perihepatic plexus). This perihepatic plexus is distributed only in the large hepatic canal, and is drained into the branches of the subphrenic veins.

4. PERIBILIARY PLEXUS OR PERIBILIARY PORTAL SYSTEM

Perhaps the most interesting vascular architecture visualized by using the injection replica scanning electron microscope method is the peribiliary plexus and its connecting vessels (Figs. 1, 2, and 7–9). As discovered by Kiernan (1833) and confirmed by Mall (1906) [21, 22], main branches of the hepatic artery are destined to become peribiliary arterioles to form the peribiliary plexus that supplies the intrahepatic bile ducts.

The large- or medium-sized peribiliary plexus consists of two layers, an inner layer of fine capillaries and an outer layer of venous networks. In this double-layered plexus, the peribiliary afferent arterioles penetrate deep into the plexus to form the inner capillary networks, and the outer venous networks are derived from the inner networks. The small-sized peribiliary plexus consists of a single layer of fine capillaries.

The peribiliary plexus emits fairly independent efferent vessels. In the larger- or medium-sized plexus, the efferent vessels have rather thick calibers that are formed by the confluence of the outer venous networks. In the smaller-sized plexus, the efferent vessels have thin segments that are derived from the fine capillaries. In the most distal segments of the plexus, the peribiliary capillaries become the efferent vessels directly. Regardless of their thickness or position, the peribiliary efferent vessels drain either into the hepatic sinusoids or into the branches of the portal vein branches. We have designated the former drainage into the sinusoids as 'lobular branch,' and the latter ending in the

portal vein branches as the 'prelobular branch' [6].

Occurrence of the lobular and prelobular branches of the peribiliary plexus differs in each animal. In the monkey, the lobular branches occur almost exclusively with few prelobular branches. In the rat, the lobular branches are found with much greater frequency than the prelobular branches. On the other hand, in man and rabbit, the prelobular and lobular branches occur with almost the same frequency.

As described above, the peribiliary efferent vessels are often observed as complicated terminations. At least four differing interpretations of these terminations have been published by the previous authors; (a) The peribiliary plexus has a sole drainage into the portal vein branches [12, 16, 23–26]. (b) The plexus drains into only the hepatic sinusoids [27]. (c) The plexus is provided with both drainages into the sinusoids and portal vein branches [20, 21]. (d) The plexus receives the afferent vessels from the portal vein branches, and emits efferent vessels to the hepatic sinusoids [13, 28]. Our injection replica scanning electron microscope method provides definitive evidence for the third view of Mall [21] and Hase and Brim [20].

Although the details of the blood flow patterns are not completely clear at this time, it is clear that the peribiliary plexus has an exceedingly rich capillary network whose efferent vessels reenter the hepatic sinusoids directly or via the portal vein branches. This route from the peribiliary arterioles to the hepatic sinusoids via the peribiliary plexus is a portal system, and is referred to as the 'peribiliary portal system' [4].

Little is known of the functional significance of the peribiliary portal system. Some studies have confirmed that the so-called basal-granulated cells of the biliary epithelium secrete 'substance P,' which controls the blood flow in the hepatic lobules [29–32]. Other studies have provided evidence that the microvilli of the biliary epithelial cells are rich in ATPase, suggesting reabsorption of bile products through the bile duct [33]. The peribiliary portal system may convey these secreted or absorbed substances to the hepatic sinusoids or cells, to control the microcirculation or bile secretory activity in the liver [4, 5, 34].

94

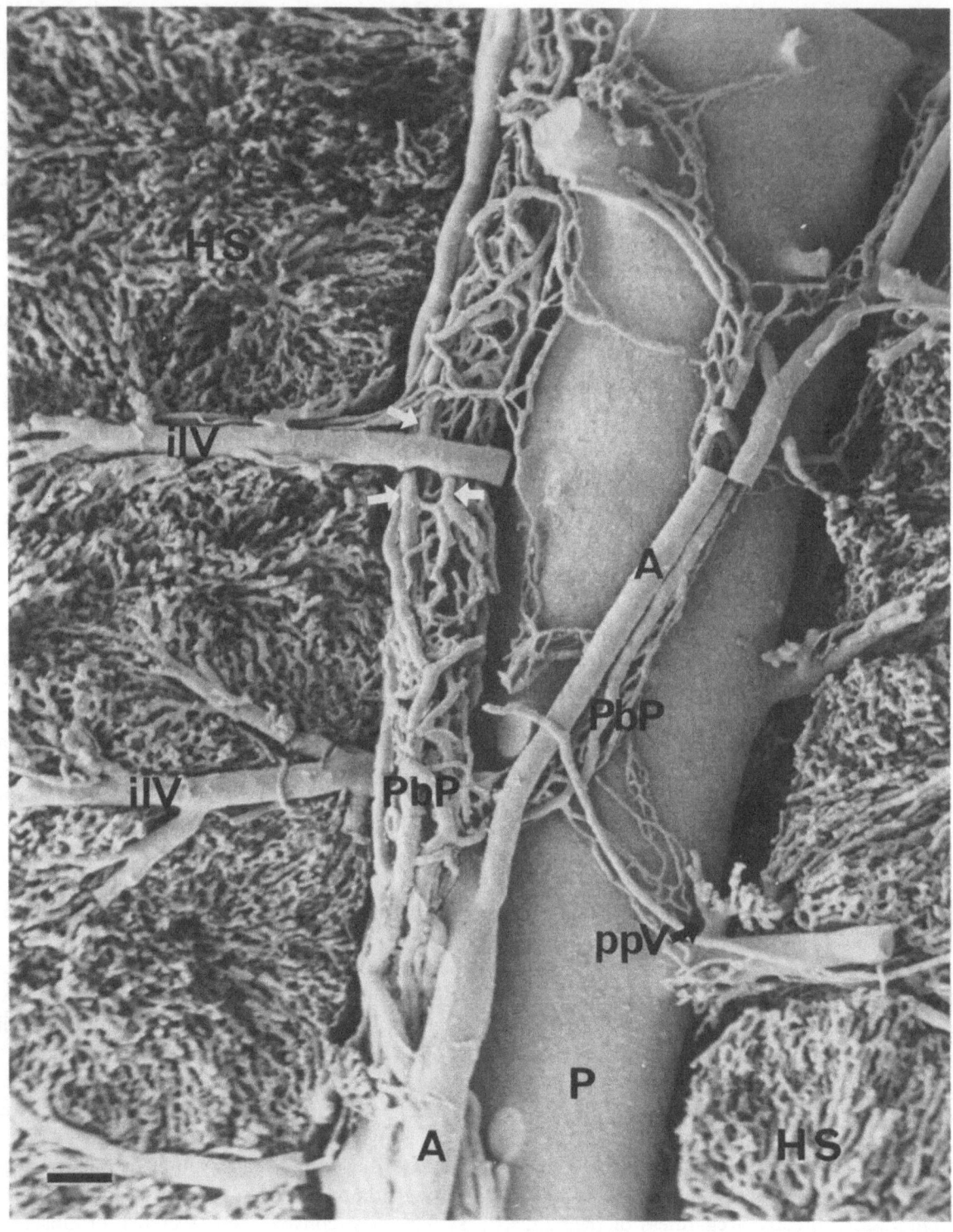

Figure 7. A microdissected cast of the rat liver, showing a peribiliary plexus (PbP) and its connecting vessels. Note that efferent vessels (arrows) join into the portal vein branch (ilV). A, P, ppV, ilV, HS (see Table 1). Bar 100 μm.

95

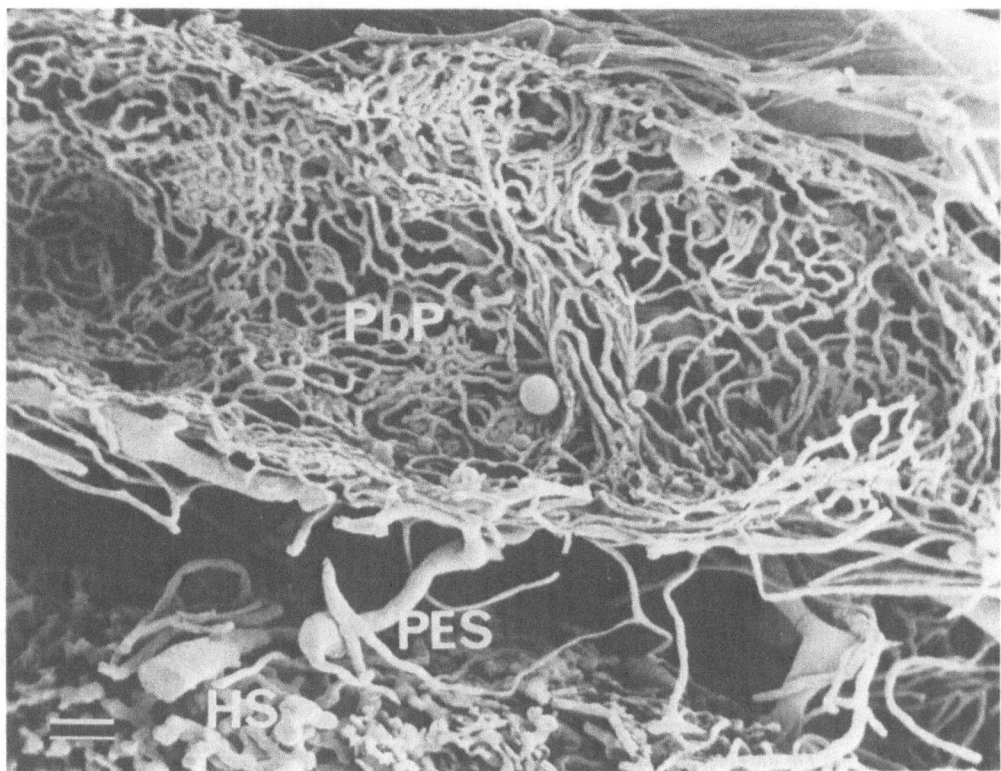

Figure 8. A longitudinally cut peribiliary plexus (PbP) of the human liver, which shows the inner layer of fine capillaries. HS, PES (see Table 1). Bar 100 μm.

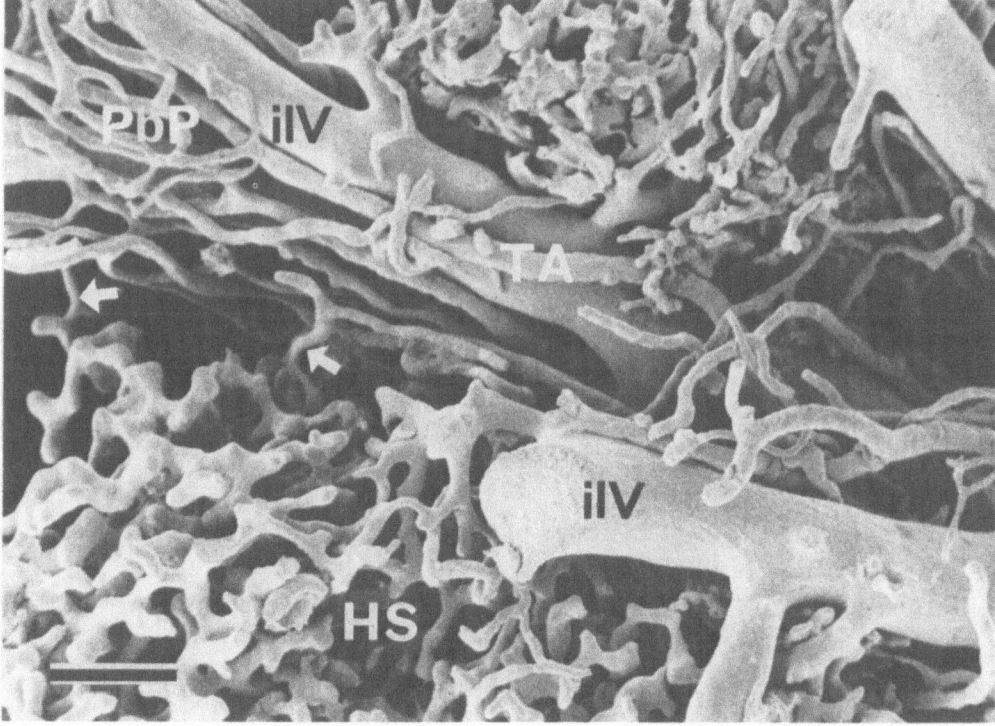

Figure 9. Terminal segment of human peribiliary plexus (PbP). Note the connection of the plexus with the sinusoids (HS) (arrows). TA, arterial twig; ilV (see Table 1). Bar 100 μm.

96

REFERENCES

1. Murakami T (1971) Application of the scanning electron microscope to the study of the fine distribution of the blood vessels. Arch Histol Jpn 32:445–454
2. Murakami T (1972) Vascular arrangement of the rat renal glomerulus. A scanning electron microscope study of corrosion casts. Arch Histol Jpn 34:87–107
3. Fujita T, Murakami T (1973) Microcirculation of monkey pancreas with special reference to the insulo-acinar portal system. A scanning electron microscope study of vascular casts. Arch Histol Jpn 35:255–263
4. Murakami T, Itoshima T, Shimada Y (1974) Peribiliary portal system in the monkey liver as evidenced by the injection replica scanning electron microscope method. Arch Histol Jpn 37:245–260
5. Ohtani O, Murakami T (1978) Peribiliary portal system in the rat liver as studied by the injection replica scanning electron microscope method. In: Becker RP, Johari O (eds) Scanning electron microscopy (1978), vol 2. SEM Inc, AMF O'Hare, IL 60666 USA, pp 241–244
6. Ohtani O (1979) The peribiliary portal system in the rabbit liver. Arch Histol Jpn 42:153–167
7. Bloch EH (1940) Some actions of adrenaline chloride and acetyl-beta-methyl-choline chloride on finer vessels of living frog liver lobules. Anat Rec [Suppl 2] 76:7
8. Wakim KG (1941) The intrahepatic circulation of blood in the intact animal: Preliminary report. Proc Staff Meet Mayo Clin 16:198
9. Wakim KG, Mann FC (1942) The intrahepatic circulation of blood. Anat Rec 82:233–253
10. Knisely MH, Bloch EH, Warner L (1948) Selective phagocytosis. I. Microscopic observations concerning the regulation of the blood flow through the liver and other organs and the mechanism and rate of phagocytic removal of particles from the blood. Biol Str 4:1–93
11. Bloch EH (1955) The in vivo microscopic vascular anatomy and physiology of the liver as demonstrated with the quartz rod method of transillumination. Angiology 6:340–349
12. Mitra SK (1966) The terminal distribution of the hepatic artery with special reference to arterio-portal anastomosis. J Anat 100:651–663
13. Del Rio Lozano I, Andrews WHH (1966) A study by means of vascular casts of small vessels related to the mammalian portal vein. J Anat 100:655–673
14. Chrozonszczewsky N (1866) Zur Anatomie und Physiologie der Leber. Virchows Arch 35:153–165
15. Braus H (1924) Anatomie des Menschen, vol 2. Berlin: Springer
16. Elias H, Petty D (1953) Terminal distribution of the hepatic artery. Anat Rec 116:9–18
17. Tajiri S (1960) The terminal distribution of the hepatic artery. Acta Med Okayama 14:215–226
18. Andrews WHH, Maegraith BG (1953) Anatomical and physiological evidence of anastomosis of the hepatic artery and hepatic vein within the mammalian liver. Nature 171:222–223
19. Elias H, Popper H (1955) Venous distribution in livers. Comparison in man and experimental animals and application to the morphogenesis of cirrhosis. AMA Arch Pathol 59:332–340
20. Hase T, Brim J (1966) Observation on the microcirculatory architecture of the liver. Anat Rec 156:156–174
21. Mall FP (1906) A study of the structural unit of the liver. Am J Anat 5:227–308
22. Kiernan F (1833) The anatomy and physiology of the liver. Phil Trans R Soc Lond [Biol] 123:711–770
23. Cohnheim J, Litten M (1867) Ueber Circulationsstörungen in der Leber. Virchows Arch Pathol Anat 67:153–165
24. Soulie PA (1904) Constitution anatomique et histologique. In: Poirier P, Charpy A (eds) Traite d'Anatomie Humanie, 2nd edn. Paris: Masson, pp 152–203
25. Winternitz MC (1911) The effect of occlusion of the various hepatic vessels upon the liver. Bull Johns Hopkins Hosp 22:396–404
26. Aunap E (1931) Ueber den Verlauf der Arteria hepatica in der Leber. Z Mikrosk Anat Forsch 25:238–251
27. Olds JM, Stafford ES (1930) On the manner of anastomosis of hepatic and portal circulation. Bull Johns Hopkins Hosp 47:176–185
28. Andrews WHH, Maegraith BG, Wenyon CEM (1949) Studies on the liver circulation. II. The micro-anatomy of the hepatic circulation. Ann Trop Med Parasitol 43:229–237
29. Heitz Ph, Polak JM, Kasper M, Timson CM, Pearse AGE (1977) Immunoelectron cytochemical localization of motilin and substance P in rabbit bile duct enterochromaffin (EC) cells. Histochemistry 50:319–325
30. Von Euler US, Gaddum JH (1931) An unidentified depressor substance in certain tissue extracts. J Physiol (Lond) 192:74–87
31. Erspamer V, Melchiorri P (1977) Polypeptides of the amphibian skin active on the gut and their mammalian analoges [Abstr]. In: Speranza V, Basso N, Lezoche E (eds) International Symposium Gastrointestinal Hormones and Pathology of the Digestive System: new trends in pathophysiology, diagnosis and therapy. Rome, pp 14–17
32. Fujita T (1977) Concept of paraneurons. In: Kobayashi S, Chiba T (eds) Paraneurons. New concepts on neuroendocrine relatives. Arch Histol Jpn [Suppl] 40:1–12
33. Gemmels RT, Heath T (1973) Structure and function of the biliary and pancreatic tracts of the sheep. J Anat 115:221–236
34. Motta PM, Muto M, Fujita T, (1978) The liver. An atlas of scanning electron microscopy. Tokyo: Igaku-Shoin

7. LIVER STEREOLOGY

G.C. BUDD

1. INTRODUCTION

Until recently, hepatologists relied on qualitative descriptions of the histology of the liver in almost all studies of liver cytoarchitecture. These studies, while contributing in important ways to our understanding of the relationships between liver structure and function, fail to provide the quantitative data required for statistical correlation of morphological and biochemical observations.

Modern stereological techniques have been developed to provide information about the size and number of cells and intracellular components of the liver. As a result, increasing opportunities for quantitative correlation of morphological observations with physiological and pharmacological data are now available. The application of statistically valid techniques increases the reliability of conclusions concerning structure–function relationships at the cellular and organelle level.

2. STEREOLOGICAL PRINCIPLES AND METHODS

The methods and underlying principles of stereology, or morphometric analysis, in biomedical investigations have been described in a number of publications in the last decade [1–6]. Quantitative information about the three-dimensional structure of an organ such as the liver can be obtained from measurements made on two-dimensional slices cut randomly through the organ. The cross-sectional area of components in a thin slice can be measured to provide data for calculating the volume of the components per unit volume of the organ (volume density). Similarly, the surface area of liver cell membranes per unit volume of liver (surface

density) can be obtained by measuring the profile length of the membranes in a slice of measured area.

The relationship between objects measured in two dimensions and their three-dimensional projections was originally investigated mathematically by the geologist Delesse [7] and investigated further in the studies of Rosiwal [8], Glagoleff [9], and Tomkieff [10].

The application of stereology in biomedicine and in the quantitation of tissue components in microscopic sections has been illustrated in numerous books and reviews [4–6, 11–14].

The fundamental basis for stereology was discovered by Delesse [7] when he showed that the relative area (or areal density) of all the profiles of a component lying in a random section through a rock is equivalent to the relative volume (or volume density) of that component throughout the rock. Using the notation adopted by the International Society for Stereology (Table 1), this relationship can be written:

$$A_A = V_V$$

This relationship has been derived independently on several occasions. A formal presentation will serve to illustrate that measurements made on structures in two dimensions can be extrapolated to provide three-dimensional data.

It is given that a cube of volume V_T has sides of length L such that

$$V_T = L^3 \qquad (7.1)$$

The cube contains a number of irregularly shaped particles (component i) that are randomly distributed within the cube.

Considering a slice through the cube, which has its largest surface parallel to any face of the cube, if the slice is of thickness dx its volume dV_T will be

Table 1. Stereological notation[a]

Definition	Symbol	Alternatives	Dimension
Number of test points	P	—	—
Density of test points on a component (i) in a section (points on (i) per test point)	P_{Pi}	—	—
Number of points in a test grid	P_T	—	—
Length of test line	L	—	cm
Length of line on a component (i) per unit length of test line	L_{Li}	—	—
Total length of test line	L_T	—	cm
Length of test line per unit area	L_A	—	cm/cm^2
Area of profiles on a micrograph or section	A	—	cm^2
Area density of components (i) on a test	A_{Ai}	—	cm^2/cm^2
Area being analyzed (test area)	A_T	—	cm^2
Surface area	S	—	cm^2
Surface density of component (i) per unit volume	S_{Vi}	—	cm^2/cm^3
Volume of component or structure	V	—	cm^3
Volume density of a component (i) per unit volume	V_{Vi}	—	cm^3/cm^3
Volume being analyzed (test volume)	V_T	—	cm^3
Number of particles or features	N	—	—
Numerical density of a component (i) per unit area	N_{Ai}	—	cm^{-2}
Numerical density of (i) per unit volume	N_{Vi}	—	cm^{-3}
Number of intersections of test line with profile boundaries	I	P, N, C	—
Length of profile boundary	B	L	cm
Boundary density of components (i) on a test area	B_{Ai}	—	cm/cm^2
Diameter of a component	D	H	cm
Mean diameter of components (i)	$\bar{D}_i$	$\bar{M}$	cm
Mean volume of a cell	$\bar{v}$	—	cm^3
Section thickness	T	t	cm

[a] Notation based on abbreviations published by Underwood [81] and Weibel [6]. Double symbols (e.g. S$_V$) indicate the measured parameter (e.g., S) referred to a given reference unit (e.g. volume, V) containing the measured parameter.

$$dV_T = L^2 dx \tag{7.2}$$

If $v(x)$ is the fraction of the volume of this slice that contains component i, then the volume dV_i of component i in dV_T at position (x) in the cube will be

$$dV_i = dV_T \cdot v(x) = L^2 dx \cdot v(x) \tag{7.3}$$

If the slice approaches infinite thinness, then

$$L^2 v(x) = A_i(x) \tag{7.4}$$

and

$$dA_i(x) = dx \cdot A_i(x) \tag{7.5}$$

$A_i(x)$, the fraction of the area of the infinitely thin slice that contains component i, will vary with the position (x) of the slice in the cube. The average fractional area $\overline{A}_i(x)$ between one surface of the cube and the opposite surface of the cube separated by a distance L will be

$$\overline{A}_i(x) = \frac{1}{L} \int_0^L dx A_i(x) \tag{7.6}$$

The total volume of component i in the cube (V_i) will be given by

$$V_i = \int_0^L dV_i = L^2 \int_0^L dx \cdot v(x) =$$

$$\int_0^L dx A_i(x) \tag{7.7}$$

From Eqs. 7.6 and 7.7, it follows that

$$V_i = \overline{A}_i(x) \cdot L \tag{7.8}$$

Dividing both sides of Eq. 7.8 by V_T we obtain

$$\frac{V_i}{V_T} = \frac{\overline{A}_i(x) \cdot L}{V_T} = \frac{\overline{A}_i(x)}{A_T} \tag{7.9}$$

The Eqs. 7.1 through 7.9 illustrate that for randomly distributed components in a defined volume, the volume density of i in the test volume $\frac{V_i}{V_T} = V_{Vi}$ is equivalent to the average area density of i on sections through the test volume $\frac{\overline{A}_i(x)}{A_T} = \overline{A}_{Ai}$. The general formula describing this is:

$$V_{Vi} = \overline{A}_{Ai} \qquad (7.10)$$

This demonstration of the Delesse principle for the relationship between area density and volume density can be extrapolated to prove that the surface density of components in a given volume can also be obtained from measurements on sections through the test volume. Further discussion of this and other basic stereological relationships are provided in various publications [1, 4–6, 11].

3. STEREOLOGICAL MEASUREMENTS

The acquisition of stereological data requires careful attention to the sampling procedure for obtaining representative sections of the material to be analyzed. The sections are analyzed by using one or more measuring techniques to obtain estimates of volumetric density, surface density, numerical density, or a combination of these values for the components of interest. The analytical methods will be described in general before discussing the sampling procedures that are appropriate for stereological investigations of the liver.

3.1. Measurement of volumetric density V_{Vi}

The determination of volumetric density requires measurement of the relative area of the components of interest in a section.

It is convenient for some investigations to measure the area of profiles in a section, or a photograph of a section, by tracing around each profile with a planimeter or a cursor on a digitized tablet. The planimeter or digitized tablet is used to obtain the combined area of all the profiles of interest in the section. The combined area of the profiles divided by the area of the section is equal to A_{Ai} and this is equivalent to V_{Vi}. The tracing method is inconvenient if the test area contains a large number of small or irregularly shaped profiles of the component under investigation.

In the intercept method of Rosiwal [8], test lines are superimposed on the section or they may be projected or drawn on a transparent sheet covering the section. The length of the line segments, L_i, included in the profiles of the components, is

measured. The length of this intercept is expressed as a proportion of the total length of the test lines L_T. Rosiwal showed that

$$\frac{L_i}{L_T} = \frac{A_i}{A_T} = A_{Ai} = V_{Vi} \qquad (7.11)$$

The test lines can be placed randomly or in a parallel series on the test area so that this method is useful for automatic instruments using the scanning principle.

A very versatile method of area measurement introduced by Glagoleff [9], originally applied in histological studies by Chalkley [14], uses a regular point lattice superimposed on the section to be analyzed. It can be shown that the ratio of lattice points P_i occurring within the profiles of the component under investigation, compared with the total number of lattice points on the section P_T, is an expression of A_{Ai}

$$\frac{P_i}{P_T} = P_{Pi} = A_{Ai} = V_{Vi} \qquad (7.12)$$

3.2. Determination of surface density S_{Vi}

To the physiologist or biochemist interested in correlating morphology with function, it is often important to measure the surface area of tissue components. For example, the surface area of the plasma membrane or inner mitochondrial membrane may be measured and correlated with the activity of enzymes localized in these membranes.

The surface area of a tissue component, such as a cell or intracellular organelle, is seen in a thin slice as a line tracing the edge of the sectioned profile of the component. The surface area of component S_i contained within a unit volume V_T is defined as the surface density S_{Vi}.

$$S_{Vi} = \frac{S_i}{V_T} \qquad (7.13)$$

On a section through a test volume V_T, the length of profile boundaries per unit area of section is proportional to the surface density S_{Vi}.

Using a single line or a set of test lines with a total length L_T, randomly placed on the section, it can be shown that the number of intersections of the line or lines with the profile boundaries I_i is proportional to both L_T and S_{Vi}. The relationship between I_i and S_{Vi} is given by the formula of Tomkieff [10]:

$$S_{Vi} = 2 \frac{I_i}{L_T} \qquad (7.14)$$

3.3. Surface-to-volume ratio $\frac{S_i}{V_i}$

The surface-to-volume ratio of cells or organelles is often of physiological interest since it is a function of the geometrical shape of the structure and an indicator of the amount of surface area per unit volume available for exchange of water and solutes between the inside and outside of the enclosed structure.

A multipurpose analytical grid introduced for the stereology of electron micrographs consists of a set of short lines of equal length Z, which is superimposed on sections of the structure to be analyzed [12, 15]. The ends of each line are considered as points to determine P_i while simultaneous recording is made of the number of intersections I_i of the test lines with boundary profiles. The surface-to-volume ratio S_i/V_i is obtained by combining the formulae 7.12, 7.13, and 7.14 and substituting

$$L_T = \frac{P_T}{Z} \cdot Z \text{ for } L_T \text{ in formula } 7.14.$$

The absolute volume V_i of component i in the total volume V of the organ is related to the volume density V_{Vi} as follows:

$$V_i = V_{Vi} \cdot V \qquad (7.15)$$

The surface-to-volume ratio is therefore

$$\frac{S_i}{V_i} = \frac{4I_i}{Z \cdot P_i} \qquad (7.16)$$

This formula was derived by Weibel and Knight [15] from an earlier one developed by Chalkley and Cornfield [16].

3.4. Determination of numerical density N_{Vi}

The estimation of the number of particles in a unit volume N_{Vi} from measurements on sections is imprecise because the number of profiles per unit area of a random section N_{Ai} is dependent on the shape and the mean diameter $\overline{D}_i$ of the particle. In addition, if the mean diameter is small, the thickness of the section may influence N_{Ai}.

If the particles are all of the same size and shape, DeHoff and Rhines [11] have shown

$$N_{Vi} = \frac{N_{Ai}}{\overline{D}_i} \qquad (7.17)$$

In practice, $\overline{D}_i$ is not often easily measured due to difficulties in estimating shape, and an alternative method was developed by Weibel and Gomez [18] that requires only an approximate determination of the particle shape. In this formula, N_{Vi} is determined from N_{Ai} and V_{Vi} with the addition of a dimensionless coefficient β that varies with the shape of the particles. This coefficient, which depends on the mean profile area-to-volume ratio of the particles, can be obtained from published graphs [4, 17]

$$N_{Vi} = \frac{K}{\beta} \cdot \frac{N_{Ai}^{3/2}}{V_{Vi}^{1/2}} \qquad (7.18)$$

The factor K is dependent of the size distribution of the particles. It varies from $K = 1$ when all particles are of equal size to 1.37 when the size variation is $\pm 50\%$ of the mean. For most biological particles with a standard deviation of $\pm 25\%$ of the mean or less, the value of K will be between 1.07 and 1.00 and therefore can often be ignored. For the nuclei of normal rat hepatocytes, β has been assumed in published studies to be spherical with a shape coefficient $\beta = 1.38$. The size distribution K was found to have a coefficient of variation of 14% and $K = 1.03$ [18, 19].

3.5. Estimating numerical density and average volume of hepatocytes

The numerical density of hepatocytes is proportional to the hepatocyte volumetric density and inversely proportional to the mean volume of an hepatocyte. It is therefore possible to predict the numerical density if the volumetric density and average hepatocyte volume are given, using the following formula:

$$\frac{V_{Vh} \times 10^{12}}{vh} = N_{VVh} \qquad (7.19)$$

Where V_{Vh} = volume fraction of hepatocytes
vh = mean hepatocyte volume (μm^3)

$N_{V_{Vh}}$ = number of hepatocytes/cm³ liver
10^{12} = one cm³ in μm³

If the volume density and numerical density have been measured, a modification of formula 7.19 can be used to estimate the average hepatocyte volume:

$$\frac{V_{Vh} \times 10^{12}}{N_{V_{Vh}}} = vh \qquad (7.20)$$

A family of curves has been constructed for a range of hepatocyte volumes occupying a range of hypothetical volume fractions (Fig. 1). Using such a family of curves it is possible to predict the concentration of hepatocytes in the liver if the hepatocyte volume fraction and mean cell volume are known. Similar predictions can be made for other types of cells in the liver and for cells in other tissues.

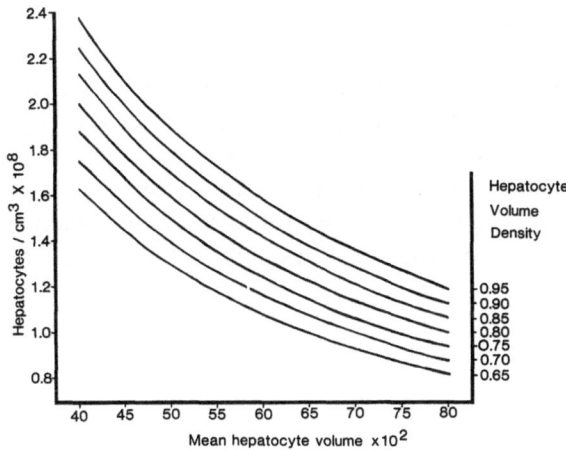

Figure 1. Curves relating hepatocyte volume density to mean cell volume and number of hepatocytes per unit volume in rat liver.

4. STEREOLOGICAL ANALYSIS OF NORMAL LIVER

4.1. Sampling methods

For stereological data to be significant, it is essential that the sampling procedure should be representative of the material under investigation. Careful random-sampling procedures should be adopted including the choice of animal or human subjects, sampling of the tissue, sectioning of the samples, and analysis of the sections. Due to uncertain availability, it is often not possible to obtain ideal samples when human tissues are analyzed. For this reason, careful recording of the sampling procedure is important.

Experimental comparison of various methods indicates that systematic random sampling can result in a smaller standard error than that obtained with simple random sampling [2]. Following the simple random sampling of animals from the population to be analyzed, the systematic random sampling of tissues requires the collection of primary tissue samples at equally spaced sites within the organ. In the sampling of liver tissue, systematic samples may be gathered by first cutting a thin slice of tissue from each lobe of the organ. Each slice can then be placed on plastic sheet enscribed with a square grid of lines. After cutting the slice into equal-sized cubes, a set of equally spaced cubes is removed. Each cube is embedded and one section from each cube is used for stereological analysis. Similar sets of cubes may be removed from each of the other liver lobes. The stereological data obtained from all of the sections can then be pooled to provide representative stereological data for the whole liver. Most published stereological studies of liver tissue have attempted to describe the average composition of liver parenchyma. This is acceptable when the objective is to relate morphological features of the intact liver to structures present in subcellular fractions [20, 21] or when comparisons are to be made between liver samples from animals of differing age, sex, or species [22–27].

Stereological data that represent average information on the liver parenchyma are valuable for comparing control liver with regenerating liver [28] or for describing the morphological effects of specific agents on the liver [29–33].

The stereological analysis of the effects of agents that induce preferential centrilobular or periportal changes are likely to require more extensive sampling procedures of the type employed in other studies [32, 34]. In a comparative study of different zones within hepatic lobules [34], 1-μm-thick sections were used for locating specific sublobular zones of hepatic lobules in the blocks of tissue used for stereological analysis. The position of hepatocytes relative to the portal triad or to the central vein were then tabulated from low-magnification electron micrographs. Finally, electron micrographs at higher magnification were used for stereological quantitation of the general organelle composition of the hepatocytes. The location of each hepatocyte within the lobule was tabulated and the same number of cells was analyzed in each of the peripheral, midzonal, and central zones of the hepatic lobule.

4.2. Stereology of normal rat liver

The liver of the laboratory rat is a convenient source of base-line stereological data for investigations of the mammalian liver. A number of published studies have provided quantitative data on the cellular and organelle composition of the liver in several strains of rat during postnatal development, maturation, and aging [25, 27, 31, 35]. The morphological effects of a number of drugs have also been measured stereologically for correlation with biochemical [30, 36] and histochemical data [37]. In these investigations, the rat liver has been used in the development and testing of stereological methods that may be applied in stereological studies of human liver [38, 39], other species [40], and other organs [41, 42].

A complete quantitative analysis, in which stereological data are related to the whole liver, may be required in comparative studies of animals at different stages of development, or following exposure to drugs, etc. For such analysis, the liver is first weighed or its volume is determined by displacement and then samples of the tissue are analyzed at several resolution levels. After the stereological data have been obtained, the volume, surface, or numerical densities are used together with the liver volume measurement to obtain the total amount of each component in the whole liver.

The relative volumes of lobular and extralobular tissue may be estimated from random sections of liver embedded in paraffin or in large blocks of acrylic or epoxy resin and evaluated at $200 \times$ magnification [19]. The relative volumes of lobular and extralobular tissue obtained in various studies by using a square lattice are shown in Table 2.

The average dimensions of hepatocytes and other cell types and the dimensions and number of nuclei per unit volume of liver tissue have been obtained in a number of investigations by using a square lattice or a linear scanning grid. In these studies, the grid is placed on light micrographs of 1-μm sections of epoxy-embedded tissue or a square lattice graticule is placed in the eyepiece of a light microscope at $1000 \times$ magnification. Data obtained with measurements made at this resolution (approximately 0.1–0.25 μm point-to-point) are presented in Table 3. At the same resolution, the size distri-

Table 2. Volumetric composition of mammalian liver (%)

Component	Species[a]						
	Rats				Dogs		Humans
	(1)	(2)	(3)	(4)	(5)	(6)	(7)
Hepatocytes	83.1	82.6	82.0	87.0	84.0	70.6	77.0
Nucleus	5.0	5.0	8.0	7.0	5.1	—	4.5
Cytoplasm	77.1	—	74.0	80.0	79.0	—	72.5
Intralobular space	16.9	17.2	18.0	13.0	—	—	23.0
Sinusoids	—	—	—	—	15.0	22.3	—
Bile canaliculi	—	—	—	—	0.6	—	—
Extralobular tissue	4.0	—	—	—	—	7.1	—
Portal triads	—	—	—	—	—	4.3	—
Portal veins	—	—	—	—	—	1.8	—
Hepatic arteries	—	—	—	—	—	0.2	—
Bile ducts	—	—	—	—	—	0.3	—
Lymph vessels	—	—	—	—	—	0.1	—
Connective tissue in portal traids	—	—	—	—	—	2.0	—
Central and hepatic veins	—	—	—	—	—	1.4	—
Connective tissue around central and hepatic veins	—	—	—	—	—	1.3	—

[a] References: (1) Weibel et al. [19]; (2) Reith [63]; (3) Schmucker et al. [26], young adults; (4) Schmucker et al. [26], retired breeders; (5) Hess et al. [40], biopsies of liver parenchyma; (6) Hess et al. [40]; (7) Oudea et al. [64], composition of parenchyma.

Table 3. Dimensions of hepatocytes

Species	Diameter (μm)	Volume	References
Rat	—	5100–20,100	Iype et al. [65]
	—	5100	Wiener et al. [29]
	—	5400	Loud [34]
	—	4940	Weibel et al. [19]
	—	6772–8282	Moses et al. [66]
	—	4750	Rohr et al. [67]
	—	4791	Riede et al. [68]
	19	—	Wessel et al. [69]
	—	11,800	Reith [63]
	—	5107	Riede et al. [70]
	—	5511	Riede et al. [71]
	—	4207	Sturgess et al. [72]
	—	4547 (dispersed cells)	Wanson et al. [73]
	—	6027–6536	Jones and Schmucker [74]
	—	4787–8784	Schmucker et al. [35]
Cow	—	4768	Reith [63]
Human	—	4982	De La Iglesia et al. [54]
	—	6341	Calc. from Roessner et al. [38]

bution of nuclear profile diameters may be measured and plotted graphically for comparison with the expected distribution for spherical structures [34]. It has generally been assumed that hepatocyte nuclei are spherical with a shape coefficient = 1.38 [19].

The volumetric and surface density composition of cytoplasmic components can be measured most accurately in electron micrographs with at least two magnifications. Low-magnification electron micrographs (1500–3000× negative magnification) have been analyzed with a square grid [34] or combination point grid and line lattice [19] to obtain both volumetric and surface density data on the same micrograph [43]. Low-magnification electron micrographs are suitable for measuring the volumes of intercellular space, nucleus, and cytoplasm as well as the surface area of the plasma membrane and nuclear envelope.

Higher magnification (7000–10,000× negative magnification) is required for measuring most of the intracellular components. The volumes of smooth and rough endoplasmic reticulum, mitochondria, peroxisomes, lysosomes, lipid droplets, and cytoplasmic ground substance, etc., can be determined within this magnification range and referred to a unit volume of cytoplasm. The surface densities of smooth and rough endoplasmic reticulum, inner and outer mitochondrial mem-

branes, etc., can also be measured at this magnification. The third type of measurement includes the determination of the numerical density of organelles per unit volume of cytoplasm or per unit surface area of membrane, e.g., the number of ribosomes attached per unit area of rough endoplasmic reticulum.

Care must be taken to ensure that all tissue for stereological analysis is fixed, dehydrated, infiltrated, and sectioned under similar, controlled conditions and that all microscopic and photographic enlargement is calibrated with respect to magnification factor. In earlier stereological analyses of intact rat liver by using both light microscopy and electron microscopy, the authors concentrated on collecting data from the hepatocytes, which are the major cell type in the liver parenchyma [19, 34]. The parenchyma has been investigated more extensively with the analysis of the composition of nonhepatocytes and extracellular compartments in addition to the hepatocytes [21]. In this study, the livers of five male Sprague-Dawley rats were fixed by intraportal infusion of phosphate-buffered 1.5% glutaraldehyde. After osmication, dehydration, and infiltration with epoxy resin by standard procedures, a single section from each of 12 random tissue blocks from each liver was used to obtain micrographs for stereological analysis, using a square double-lattice test system. In all, 2520 electron micrographs from the five livers were obtained for analysis. Volumetric and surface densities were estimated from the points and lines intersecting the tissue components, utilizing formulae discussed earlier in this chapter. The hepatocytes were found to occupy 78% of the volume of parenchymal tissue. The nonhepatocytes occupied 6% and the extracellular spaces 16% of the parenchymal volume. Endothelial cells represented 44%, Kupffer cells 34%, and fat-storing cells (lipocytes) 23% of the volume due to nonhepatocyte cells. The extracellular spaces included the sinusoids, 10.6%, and Disse space, 4.9%, of parenchymal volume. The bile canaliculi represented only 0.4% of the parenchymal volume. These data are compared with other published data in Table 4.

Published data for adult rat hepatocytes, presented in Table 5, show both consistent and inconsistent values when results from different laboratories are compared. The data reflect differences in

Table 4. Volumetric composition of rat liver (%)

Component	Volumetric composition[a]						Mean
	(1)	(2)	(3)	(4)	(5)	(6)	
Hepatocytes	77.8	82.6	83.1	82.0	82.2	87.0	82.5
Endothelial cells	2.8	—	—	—	—	—	
Kupffer cells	2.1	—	—	—	—	2.0	
Lipocytes	1.4	—	—	—	—	—	
Disse space	4.9	—	—	—	—		
Sinusoids	10.6	—	—	—	—	11	
Bile canaliculi	0.4	—	—	—	—		
Extrahepatocytic space	22.2	17.2	16.9	18.0	17.7	13.0	

[a] References: (1) Blouin et al. [21]; (2) Reith [63]; (3) Weibel et al. [19]; (4) Schmucker et al. [26]; (5) Oudea et al. [64]; (6) Greengard et al. [75].

fixation procedure, reference volumes, microscopic procedures and resolution of the analyzed images. The volumetric densities of mitochondria, lysosomes, and peroxisomes seem to vary only slightly between different investigations. This may be related to the relative ease with which these structures can be resolved in electron micrographs over a wide magnification range. The rough and smooth endoplasmic reticulum are resolved more easily at moderate or high magnification than at low magnification. In addition, the distinction between what is included or excluded in the endoplasmic reticulum compartments could be interpreted differently in different laboratories. In some instances, the intracisternal space may be included, in others it may be excluded from these two compartments. Differences in the volume of the intracisternal spaces of the rough and smooth endoplasmic reticulum may occur due to diurnal variations or due to the osmotic effects of different fixative or buffer solutions to which the cells are exposed [44].

While it is important and relatively easy to obtain volumetric estimates for liver cells, intercellular spaces, and subcellular components, the measurement of surface density is of equal or greater value for linking histological and cytological features with biochemical data and physiological activity. Recent estimates of surface density for liver membranes take into account the effects of section thickness and compression during sectioning and the effects of electron microscopic magnification on the resolution of the membranes [20, 21, 45]. Over 92% of the surface area of membranes in liver parenchyma was found to be contributed by the hepatocytes. This included the inner and outer mitochondrial membranes (44%), and rough and smooth endoplasmic reticulum (40%), as well as the plasma membrane (6.2%) and the surface area of other membrane-bound organelles (2.8%) [21]. This study reveals that a large part of the total mitochondrial and endoplasmic reticulum membranes in the liver is contained within the hepatocyte. On the other hand, nonhepatocytes contribute significant amounts of other membranes. The endothelial and Kupffer cells contained 19.5% of the plasma membranes, 13.9% of the Golgi membranes, 31.6% of the lysosomal membranes, and 51.9% of the pinocytotic membranes. It is apparent that if the proportions of each membrane type are retained in liver homogenates, then the activity of an enzyme marker attached to one type of membrane (e.g., mitochondrial inner membrane) may reflect the activity in intact hepatocytes, while the activity of an enzyme marker on another component (e.g., lysosomal membranes) may reflect significant activity in nonhepatocytes as well as hepatocytes.

Prior to the studies by Keller [45], published estimates of the surface density of liver membranes rarely included corrections for the effects of section thickness, compression, and resolution. Some authors relate membrane surface area to a unit volume of cell, liver parenchyma, or whole liver, while others present the data as estimates of mean surface area of the measured membrane component per hepatocyte. Many estimates are presented as the combined surface area of both sides of the membrane. It is important to realize this when comparisons of cell surface area to cell volume are made

Table 5. Volumetric densities of adult rat liver organelles (cm³/cm³ × 100)[a]

Ref[c]	Nucleus H	E	K	L	Cytoplasm H	E	K	L	RER H	E	K	L	SER H	E	K	L	Golgi H	E	K	L	Mitochondria H	E	K	L
(1)	9.8	16.4	19.2	20.8	—	—	—	—	—	—	—	—	—	—	—	—	—	—	—	—	28.3	4.26	4.52	4.36
(2)	5.0	—	—	—	—	—	—	—	—	—	—	—	—	—	—	—	—	—	—	—	19.1	—	—	—
(3)	5.0	—	—	—	77.1	—	—	—	7.9	—	—	—	4.9	—	—	—	1.3	—	—	—	18.1	—	—	—
(4)	—	—	—	—	—	—	—	—	6.3	—	—	—	4.4	—	—	—	0.4	—	—	—	21.0	—	—	—
(5)	8.0	—	—	—	—	—	—	—	—	—	—	—	—	—	—	—	—	—	—	—	20.0	—	—	—
(6)	—	—	—	—	74.0	—	—	—	—	—	—	—	—	—	—	—	—	—	—	—	23.0	—	—	—
(7)	8.0 / 7.0	—	—	—	78.0 / 78.0	—	—	—	4.3 / 4.1	—	—	—	6.3 / 6.9	—	—	—	0.2 / 0.1	—	—	—	16.0 / 15.0	—	—	—
(8)	—	—	—	—	—	—	—	—	13.5	—	—	—	20.9	—	—	—	—	—	—	—	18.5	—	—	—
(9)	4.3	—	—	—	—	—	—	—	13.1	—	—	—	20.8	—	—	—	0.4	—	—	—	24.0	—	—	—
(10)	2.5	—	—	—	—	—	—	—	31.8	—	—	—	7.4	—	—	—	0.4	—	—	—	16.5	—	—	—
(11)	—	—	—	—	—	—	—	—	20.1	—	—	—	14.0	—	—	—	—	—	—	—	—	—	—	—
(12)	5.7	—	—	—	—	—	—	—	36.6	—	—	—	14.1	—	—	—	—	—	—	—	23.7	—	—	—
(13)	—	—	—	—	—	—	—	—	4.4	—	—	—	5.5	—	—	—	—	—	—	—	21.3	—	—	—

Ref[c]	Lysosomes H	E	K	L	Peroxisomes H	E	K	L	Granules[b] H	E	K	L	Lipid H	E	K	L	Pinocytotic vesicles H	E	K	L	Cytoplasmic matrix H	E	K	L
(1)	0.82	6.86	13.6	0.23	2.4	—	—	—	0.23	—	—	—	0.37	—	—	25.3	0.18	5.5	1.8	0.16	57.9	66.9	60.9	48.4
(2)	0.3	—	—	—	1.4	—	—	—	—	—	—	—	0.2	—	—	—	—	—	—	—	—	—	—	—
(3)	—	—	—	—	1.2	—	—	—	0.7	—	—	—	—	—	—	—	—	—	—	—	44.4	—	—	—
(4)	0.3	—	—	—	1.1	—	—	—	0.1	—	—	—	1.0	—	—	—	—	—	—	—	—	—	—	—
(5)	0.2	—	—	—	1.2	—	—	—	—	—	—	—	—	—	—	—	—	—	—	—	—	—	—	—
(6)	0.4	—	—	—	1.4	—	—	—	—	—	—	—	—	—	—	—	—	—	—	—	—	—	—	—
(7)	—	—	—	—	1.3 / 1.2	—	—	—	0.1 / 0.1	—	—	—	1.0 / 0.5	—	—	—	—	—	—	—	60.0 / 62.0	—	—	—
(8)	—	—	—	—	—	—	—	—	—	—	—	—	—	—	—	—	—	—	—	—	—	—	—	—
(9)	—	—	—	—	—	—	—	—	—	—	—	—	—	—	—	—	—	—	—	—	—	—	—	—
(10)	0.9	—	—	—	1.0	—	—	—	—	—	—	—	—	—	—	—	—	—	—	—	—	—	—	—
(11)	—	—	—	—	1.3	—	—	—	—	—	—	—	—	—	—	—	—	—	—	—	—	—	—	—
(12)	0.6	—	—	—	1.0	—	—	—	—	—	—	—	—	—	—	—	—	—	—	—	—	—	—	—
(13)	—	—	—	—	1.2	—	—	—	0.2	—	—	—	0.3	—	—	—	—	—	—	—	—	—	—	—

[a] Key: H, hepatocytes; E, endothelial cells; K, Kupffer cells; L, lipocytes.

[b] Granules include: autophagic granules, multivesicular bodies, dense bodies.

[c] References: (1) Blouin et al. [21]; (2) Loud [34]; (3) Weibel et al. [19]; (4) Pfeiffer et al. [76]; (5) Reith [63]; (6) Schmucker et al. [26]; (7) Schmucker et al. [35]; (8) Miller et al. [77]; (9) Miller et al. [77]; (10) Riede et al. [70]; (11) Riede et al. [36]; (12) Christov et al. [78]; (13) Oudea et al. [64].

Table 6. Surface densities of adult rat liver organelles (m²/cm³)[a]

Plasma membrane					RER					SER					Mitochondria outer membrane					Mitochondria inner membrane					Ref[c]
H	E	K	L	Total	H	E	K	L	Total	H	E	K	L	Total	H	E	K	L	Total	H	E	K	L	Total	
0.56	0.12	0.03	0.05	0.77	2.41	0.08	0.06	0.04	2.59	1.39	0.05	0.02	0.01	1.47	1.30	0.02	0.01	0.01	1.34	2.53	0.03	0.02	0.01	2.59	(1)
0.28	—	—	—	—	6.25	(37,900)[b]	—	—	—	4.65	(25,100)[b]	—	—	—	1.46	—	—	—	—	5.88	—	—	—	—	(2)
—	—	—	—	—	25,400[b]	—	—	—	—	16,900[b]	—	—	—	—	8720[b]	—	—	—	—	35,500[b]	—	—	—	—	(3)
—	—	—	—	—	29,200[b]	—	—	—	—	10,600[b]	—	—	—	—	7790[b]	—	—	—	—	32,800[b]	—	—	—	—	(4)
—	—	—	—	—	—	—	—	—	—	—	—	—	—	—	21,300[b]	—	—	—	—	47,000[b]	—	—	—	—	(5)
—	—	—	—	—	2.24	—	—	—	—	4.09	—	—	—	—	—	—	—	—	—	—	—	—	—	—	(6)
—	—	—	—	—	2.14	—	—	—	—	2.42	—	—	—	—	—	—	—	—	—	—	—	—	—	—	(7)
0.50	—	—	—	—	2.86	—	—	—	—	2.00	—	—	—	—	1.07	—	—	—	—	3.04	—	—	—	—	(8)
—	—	—	—	—	4.11	(20,478)[b]	—	—	—	6.87	(34,230)[b]	—	—	—	—	—	—	—	—	—	—	—	—	—	(9)

Golgi					Lysosomes					Pinocytotic vesicles					Total membranes					Ref[c]
H	E	K	L	Total	H	E	K	L	Total	H	E	K	L	Total	H	E	K	L	Total	
0.08	0.02	0.02	0.001	0.12	0.07	0.01	0.02	0.001	0.10	0.01	0.01	0.003	0.0001	0.02	8.44	0.34	0.17	0.12	9.1	(1)
0.17	—	—	—	—	—	—	—	—	—	—	—	—	—	—	—	—	—	—	9.3	(8)
0.38	(1893)[b]	—	—	—	—	—	—	—	—	—	—	—	—	—	—	—	—	—	—	(9)

[a] Key: H, hepatocytes; E, endothelial cells; K, Kuppfer cells; L, lipocytes.

[b] Surface area (μm²) per cell (mononucleate hepatocyte).

[c] References: (1) Blouin et al. [21]; (2) Weibel et al. [19]; (3) Loud [34]; (4) Wiener et al. [29]; (5) Reith [63]; (6) Miller et al. [77]; (7) Oudea et al. [80]; (8) Bolender et al. [20]; (9) Schmucker et al. [35].

and when stereological data are being compared with biochemical or other functional data. Current available estimates of surface density are presented in Table 6.

4.3. Comparisons of published stereological data on adult rat liver

Published estimates of the volume density of hepatocytes in adult rat liver are presented in Table 4. There is good agreement between authors working with different strains of laboratory rat. The mean volume density is about 0.83.

Estimates of the mean hepatocyte volume (Fig. 2) are variable due, in part, to differences between hepatocytes with a centrilobular, intermediate, or peripheral location within the liver lobule. There may also be variability in hepatocyte volume due to factors that include strain, sex, age, and diet. The mean volume of an adult rat hepatocyte according

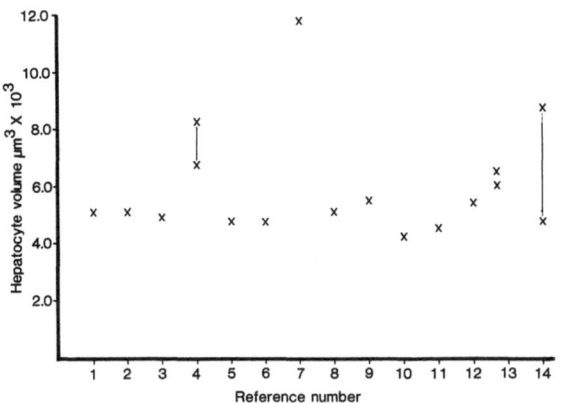

Figure 2. Published estimates of the volume of an adult rat (mononuclear) hepatocyte. References: (1) Iype et al. [65]; (2) Wiener et al. [29]; (3) Weibel et al. [19]; (4) Moses et al. [66]; (5) Rohr et al. [67]; (6) Riede et al. [36]; (7) Reith [63]; (8) Riede et al. [70]; (9) Riede et al. [71]; (10) Sturgess et al. [72]; (11) Wanson et al. [73]; (12) Loud [34]; (13) Jones and Schmucker [74]; (14) Schmucker et al. [35].

to most authors is about 4,900 μm^3. Some estimates diverge considerably from this value.

A survey of the published estimates for the surface density of various hepatocyte membranes (Table 6) leads to the following general conclusions about rat liver cell membranes. The surface density of rough-surfaced endoplasmic reticulum exceeds the smooth-surfaced endoplasmic reticulum. The combined surface density of rough- and smooth-surfaced endoplasmic reticulum is similar to the combined surface densities of inner and outer mitochondrial membranes. Together, the endoplasmic reticulum and mitochondrial membranes represent most of the hepatocyte membranes. The plasma membrane and remaining internal membranes (Golgi complex, peroxisomes, etc.) constitute less than 10% of the total surface area of hepatocyte membranes.

Only a few estimates of plasma membrane surface density have been published in studies that also include estimates of the volumetric density of the same hepatocytes. Because surface density estimates include both surfaces of a membrane, to calculate the surface-to-volume ratio it is necessary to divide the surface density measurement by 2 before calculating the surface area of the average hepatocyte according to the following formula:

$$\frac{\frac{S_{Vh}}{2} \cdot 12^{12}}{N_{Vh}} = Sh \qquad (7.21)$$

Where $S_{Vh}/2$ = one-half the surface density of plasma membrane

N_{Vh} = numerical density of hepatocytes/cm³ liver

10^{12} = one cm³ in μm^3

S_h = surface area of the average hepatocyte (μm^2)

The surface-to-volume ratios obtained from published estimates of the surface area and volume of hepatocytes may be compared with predicted ratios for various geometrical structures. When such comparisons are made (Table 7), it is apparent that hepatocytes in sections of liver parenchyma closely resemble cuboidal or polygonal structures while isolated hepatocytes resemble spheres. This conclusion is in agreement with SEM observations of liver tissue in which polygonal hepatocytes are clearly seen [46, 47].

The numerical density, or number of hepatocytes per unit volume, of parenchymal tissue in the adult rat liver has been estimated by some authors (Table 8). The numerical density of hepatocytes can also be predicted from the volume density of hepatocytes and the mean hepatocyte volume by using the formula 7.19 and compared with the published estimates.

Table 7. Calculated surface-to-volume ratios for rat hepatocytes

	Surface area (μm^2)	Volume (μm^3)	Surface volume	References[a]
Sectioned liver parenchyma	1680	4940	0.34	(1)
Isolated hepatocytes	1296	4547	0.29	(2)
Calculated sphere	1403	4940	0.28	(1)
Calculated sphere	1327	4547	0.29	(2)
Calculated cube	1740	4940	0.35	(1)
Calculated cube	1647	4547	0.36	(2)

[a] References: (1) Weibel et al. [19]; (2) Wanson et al. [73].

Table 8. Numerical density of hepatocytes in rat liver

Numerical density (number/cm^3)	Volume density	Hepatocyte volume (μm^3)	Calculated[a] numerical density (number/cm^3)	References[b]
1.69×10^8	0.83	4940	1.68×10^8	(1)
0.07×10^8	0.83	11,800	0.70×10^8	(2)
1.66×10^8 (30 month portal hepatocytes)	0.85	4787	1.78×10^8	(3)
1.33×10^8 (6 month portal hepatocytes)	0.88	6532	1.35×10^8	(3)
2.76×10^8 (8 days)	0.87	3183	2.73×10^8	(4)
1.85×10^8	—	5608	—	(5)
1.68×10^8	0.79	4926	1.60×10^8	(6)
—	0.86	4791	1.80×10^8	(7)
—	0.83	4860	1.71×10^8	(8)

[a] Numerical density was calculated by using the formula:

$$N_{VVh} = \frac{V_{Vh} \times 10^{12}}{vh}$$

[b] References: (1) Weibel et al. [19]; (2) Reith [63]; (3) Schmucker et al. [35]; (4) Rohr et al. [24]; (5) De la Iglesia et al. [54]; (6) Budd et al. [43]; (7) Riede et al. [36]; (8) Jones and Schmucker [74].

4.4. *Liver stereology in developing and aging rats*

Stereological studies of the liver of normal rats at various stages of pre- and postnatal development, or during aging, help to further define our quantitative knowledge of the normal liver (Table 9).

In studies of stereological parameters from three days before birth to eight days postnatally [24, 25], it was observed that for a day or two following birth, the rate of increase in liver weight is reduced in many species, including the rat. The liver volume ratio gradually changes from about 10 cc/100 g body weight at three days before birth in the rat, to

the same as the adult liver volume ratio (3.4 cc/100 g) by the 8th postnatal day. This is associated with quantitative cellular changes including a reduction in intrahepatic hemopoietic cells so that the volume density of hepatocytes per unit volume of liver is increased from about 0.5 to 0.8 during this perinatal period. The studies agree that an increase in the volume of an average hepatocyte is observed during the few days before birth, followed by a reduction during the 2–3 days after birth.

A marked increase in the volumetric density of rough endoplasmic reticulum and decrease in the volume density of cytoplasmic area containing free

Table 9. Composition of pre- and postnatal rat liver (per ml tissue and per cm^3 cytoplasm)

Age (days)	Prenatal				Postnatal							Ref.[a]
	15–18	18–19	20	21–22	1	2	3	118	13	28	100	
Hepatocytes												
Volume density	—	0.5	—	0.76	0.88	—	0.81	0.87	—	—		(1)
Mean volume (μm^3)	—	1392	—	5161	3612	—	2713	3183	—	—	—	
Number (per ml × 10^8)	—	3.62	—	1.44	2.26	—	2.99	2.75	—	—	—	
Mitochondria												
Volume (per ml)	—	0.05	—	0.10	0.21	—	0.22	0.21	—	—	—	
Number (per ml × 10^9)	—	76.18	—	42.83	61.47	—	124	132	—	—	—	
Rough E.R.												
Volume (per ml)	—	0.14	—	0.20	0.21	—	0.20	0.19	—	—	—	
Smooth E.R.												
Volume (per ml)	—	—	—	0.02	0.03	—	0.11	0.13	—	—	—	
Mitochondria												(2)
Volume (per cm^3)	0.135	0.143	0.134	0.132	—	0.230	—	—	0.190	0.214	0.200	
Number (per cm^3 × 10^9)	96.4	94.4	70.0	90.5	—	221	—	—	180	258	199	
Mean volume	1.40	1.50	1.90	1.46	—	0.96	—	—	1.06	0.83	1.00	
Rough E.R.												
Surface (m^2/cm^3)	4.04	4.15	4.33	5.05	—	4.70	—	—	4.43	3.31	3.44	
Smooth E.R.												
Surface (m^2/cm^3)	0.59	0.51	0.77	0.74	—	0.59	—	—	2.42	3.83	2.29	

[a] References: (1) Rohr et al. [24]; (2) Herzfeld et al. [25]

ribosomes occurs in late fetal life. Most of the volumetric density of rough endoplasmic reticulum represents dilatation of the cisternae, which is prominent at about the time of birth [24]. The volume density of rough endoplasmic reticulum does not change during the eight days following birth, but the smooth endoplasmic reticulum volume density increases significantly during this time [24, 25] due to increased metabolic activity at the time of birth. Other evidence of increased hepatic metabolism includes an increase in the volume density of autophagic vacuoles, microbodies, and Golgi elements within 24 h postnatally [24]. Within this period, a marked mitotic activity in the hepatocyte population results in a reduction in the mean hepatocyte volume from that found at birth. Associated with this is an increase in the volume of individual mitochondria and a transient decrease in the number of mitochondria per cell. It has been proposed [24] that when hepatocytes divide during the 24 h after birth, the daughter cells each receive half the mitochondria from the parent cell. These mitochondria then double in volume and divide shortly thereafter to restore the number of mitochondria per cell that existed prior to birth. Eventually the adult number of mitochondria per cell is achieved by growth and division of some or all of the total population.

The subcellular compartments mature at different rates (Table 9). Rough endoplasmic reticulum surface density approaches the adult level during fetal life. Mitochondrial volume density approaches the adult level during the first week of postnatal life, but smooth endoplasmic reticulum surface density requires an additional week before it resembles the adult quantity [25].

Stereological analysis of the liver of rats during maturation and aging indicates that the volume density of hepatocytes does not change much during 30 months [35]. However, individual hepatocytes increase in volume during the first 12–16 months and then decline until, at 30 months, the average hepatocyte volume resembles that in the one-month-old group [35]. In contrast, Pieri [27, 48] observed a continued increase in hepatocyte volume throughout 27 months.

The surface density of rough endoplasmic reticulum either does not change through the lifespan [35] or it steadily declines between one and 27 months [27, 48]. On the other hand, the surface area of the smooth endoplasmic reticulum was observed to increase up to 16 months of age [35]. During senescence, a significant loss of smooth endoplasmic reticulum may occur. In another study, the amount of smooth endoplasmic reticulum declines significantly during the first 12 months of life, but then increases so that 27-month-old rats contain significantly greater amounts than young rats [27, 48].

A decrease in the number of mitochondria in the liver of aged animals has been observed in a number of studies [35, 49, 50]. In rat liver analyzed stereologically from one to 30 months after birth, the mitochondrial volume density increased in portal hepatocytes by 23% between six and ten months, but declined by 30 months to less than the volume density in one-month-old animals [35]. In centrilobular hepatocytes, the mitochondrial volume density also increased during maturation but declined by 30 months. The volume density of microbodies (peroxisomes) was reduced in senescent animals over 20–25 months old, but the specific volume and volume density of dense bodies (secondary lysosomes) increased between one and 30 months [35]. This age-dependent increase is in agreement with other studies showing an accumulation of lysosomes with age [51].

4.5. Comparisons between species

Stereological data from the liver of mammals other than the rat is relatively sparse, but nevertheless valuable for assessing quantitative similarities and differences between species. Data accumulated from published and previously unpublished sources are included in Table 10.

4.6. Human liver

Stereological analysis of human liver has been the subject of relatively few investigations. Some of the observed variations may be due to age-related changes in fine structure or to genetic differences. Other factors that could produce quantitative variations include diet, hormonal balance, and previous drug exposure. In a study of 14 needle liver

Table 10. Composition of the liver of various species[a]

Species		Dog (1)	Dog (2)	Cow (3)	Human (4)	Human (5)
Extrahepatic space	V_{Vex}	0.15	0.16	—	0.22	0.19
Hepatocytes						
Volume	V_{Vh}	0.85	0.84	—	0.78	0.81
Surface	S_{Vh}	0.29	0.30	—	—	—
Nuclei volume	V_{Vn}	0.051	0.047	—	0.056	0.06
Number	$N_{Vn}(\times 10^8)$	—	—	—	1.23	—
Cytoplasm	V_{Vcyt}	0.80	0.79	—	0.73	—
Mitochondria	V_{Vm}	0.21	0.22	0.23	0.14	0.15
Outer membrane	S_{Vmo}	1.08	1.09	—	1.16	—
Inner membrane and cristae	S_{Vmc}	—	—	—	2.17	—
Endoplasmic reticulum						
Rough ER	V_{Vrer}	0.063	0.063	0.093	—	0.12
	S_{Vrer}	2.51	2.57	—	1.71	—
Smooth ER	V_{Vser}	0.077	0.090	0.210	—	0.43
	S_{Vser}	3.31	3.94	—	1.98	—
Peroxisomes	V_{Vmb}	0.040	0.036	0.032	0.01	—
	$N_{Vmb}(\times 10^9)$	295	281	—	55.5	—
Lysosomes	V_{Vlys}	0.0076	0.0069	0.016	0.0056	0.02
	$N_{Vlys}(\times 10^9)$	18	14	—	—	—
Lipid droplets	V_{Vlip}	0.0018	0.0042	0.0018	0.0045	0.008

[a] References: (1) Hess et al. [40], blocks of liver tissue; (2) Hess et al. [40], needle biopsies; (3) Reid [79]; (4) Roessner et al. [38]; (5) Budd (unpublished).

biopsies, obtained from normal volunteers of different ages, before breakfast, it was shown that the surface density of the smooth endoplasmic reticulum was significantly greater than that for the rough endoplasmic reticulum [38]. This observation is in agreement with other reports [39, 52–54]. In other respects, the human liver data resemble the data from rat liver and the liver of other species. The volume density of hepatocytes per milliliter of liver tissue is 0.78–0.81 in human liver compared with 0.78–0.87 in rat liver, and 0.85 in dog liver (Table 10). The number of hepatocyte nuclei per milliliter of liver tissue is 1.23×10^8 in human liver [38] and 1.69×10^8 in rat liver [19]. Using formula 7.20 (described previously), the calculated volume for an average human hepatocyte is about 6000 μm^3. The stereological data for organelles in human hepatocytes is compared with the data for various animals in Table 10.

4.7. Stereology and histochemistry

In an effort to correlate cellular morphology with functional activity, as reflected in an enzyme histochemical reaction, Böcking and Riede [37] quantified the distribution of reaction products formed from two substrates for liver esterases in fructose-fed and control mice. The percent surface area of smooth and rough endoplasmic reticulum membranes on which enzyme reaction product occurred in hepatocytes decreased after fructose loading. At the same time the amount of esterase-positive surface on cytoplasmic lipid droplets increased. With o-acetyl hydroxyquinoline as substrate, the surface density of SER that stains for esterase is 53% of the control surface density after fructose loading. However, because the surface density of the total SER is reduced to 54% of the control value, the fraction of SER membrane that is esterase positive is not changed when the total SER is reduced in surface density. In the same cells, the surface density of fat droplets increases 7.7. times after fructose treatment and the esterase-positive surface of the fat increases 7.6 times. Like the SER, the fraction of fat-droplet surface that is esterase positive with o-acetyl hydroxyquinoline is unchanged after fructose loading. On the other hand, using S-acetyl mercaptoquinoline as substrate, the fraction of fat surface area that is esterase positive

increases more than ten times from 0.02 in control animals to 0.24 in fructose-loaded animals. It was concluded that the combined histochemical and quantitative stereological results demonstrate the presence of two (or more) esterases at the surface of fat droplets in hepatocytes that behave differently in response to fructose loading [37].

4.8. Stereology and autoradiography

It is not generally feasible to measure the amount of histochemical reaction product to obtain an absolute measure of enzyme activity in intracellular organelles. This is due in part to variations in the availability of substrate to the enzyme, resulting from permeability differences between subcellular compartments. In addition, a buildup of reaction product increasingly interferes with substrate availability.

These difficulties in measuring the quantity of enzyme can be overcome with the use of readily diffusible agents that attach irreversibly to specific enzyme-active centers at their locations within the tissue. Using an irreversible enzyme inhibitor labeled with a radioactive marker, it is feasible to combine quantitative autoradiography with stereology to measure the absolute concentration of enzyme-active centers in defined compartments within the liver (Fig. 4) and other tissues [43, 55].

Using ^{3}H-diisopropyl fluorophosphate (^{3}H-DFP), an irreversible inhibitor of certain esterases and proteases, it can be shown by combined light- and electron-microscopic autoradiography and stereology that in the adult rat liver, fluorophosphate-reactive esterase molecules are located in rough and smooth endoplasmic reticulum and in cytoplasmic granules [43]. The concentrations of fluorophosphate-reactive esterase-active centers (FPR sites) were found to be $24.9 \times 10^5/\mu m^3$ in the cytoplasmic granules, $6.7 \times 10^5/\mu m^3$ in the smooth endoplasmic reticulum and $4.9 \times 10^5/\mu m^3$ in the rough endoplasmic reticulum. Although the concentration was highest in the granules, most of the FPR sites ($\sim 2 \times 10^9$ per cell) were present in the smooth and rough endoplasmic reticulum that together represented 58% of the volume of the hepatocytes. The granules only occupied 3% of the hepatocyte volume ($\sim 0.4 \times 10^9$ FPR sites per cell). The concentrations of FPR sites per unit volume of labeled

112

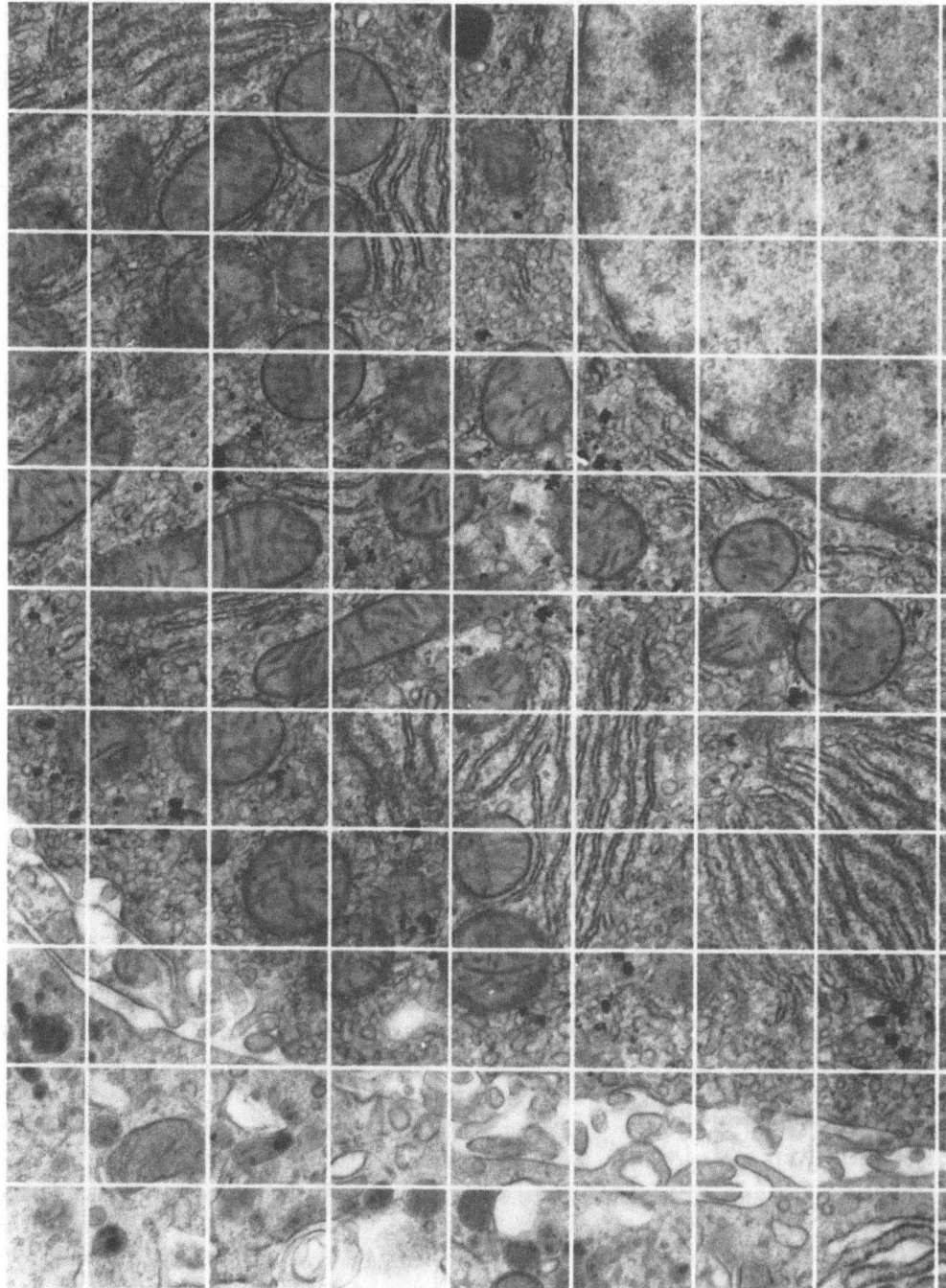

Figure 3. Electron micrograph of rat liver with superimposed square lattice for stereological analysis. Intersections of the lattice are used as grid points and the lines connecting grid points are used to measure intersections with organelle boundaries; × 16,500.

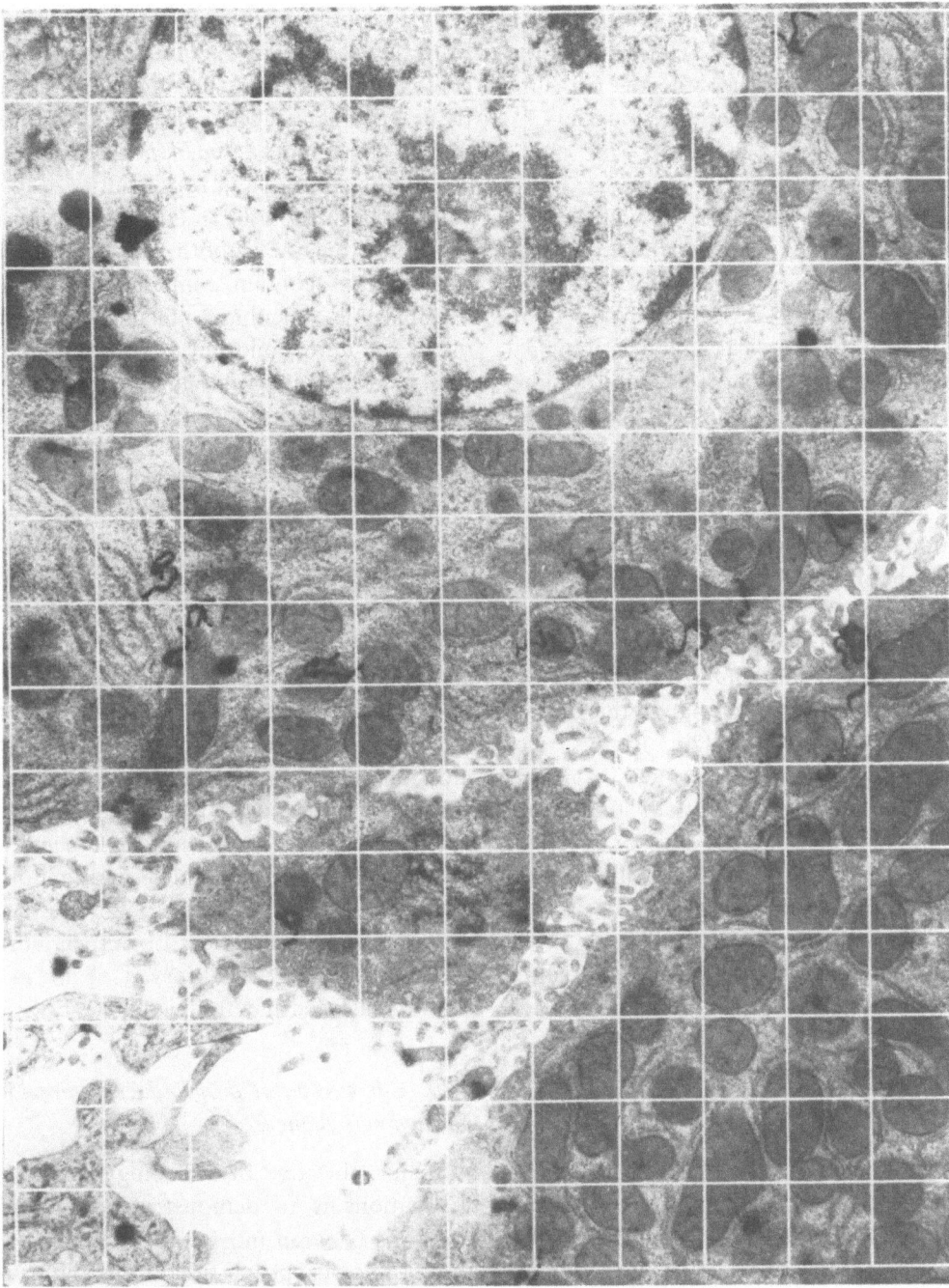

Figure 4. Electron-microscopic autoradiograph of rat liver. The superimposed square lattice is used for obtaining volumetric and surface density data. In addition, the density of developed autoradiographic grains is obtained by dividing the number of grains over each compartment by the number of grid points over the same compartment; ×13,000.

organelle can be combined with stereological data on the same liver sections, to obtain estimates of the number of FPR sites per hepatocyte, per unit volume (cm^3) of liver and in the whole liver [43].

4.9. Stereology of subcellular fractions

The stereological analysis of hepatocyte membranes and other cellular components need not be limited to the analysis of intact tissue sections. Wibo et al. [56] applied both biochemical and stereological methods in the analysis of microsomal fractions from homogenized liver. This is a more direct correlative approach than those studies in which stereological analyses are performed on intact tissue while biochemical analyses are made on microsomal fractions that represent only a part of the homogenate obtained from a region of liver adjacent to the region used for stereology [30].

The recoveries of tissue components have recently been assessed in subcellular fractions by the use of stereological methods to analyze the surface area of recovered membranes [20]. Because stereological analysis can be performed on intact tissue, whole homogenates, and individual fractions, it is possible to calculate recoveries of all three preparations and estimate how well the membranes found in intact liver are recovered in both the homogenate and the fractions.

According to the method of Bolender [20], after homogenizing the liver, known amounts of each fraction obtained by differential centrifugation are collected as pellicles on filters, fixed, dehydrated, and embedded in epoxy resin. The diameter of each pellicle is measured and thin sections are cut perpendicular to the surface of the pellicle. The volume of each pellicle is determined from its diameter and its thickness measured in electron micrographs. After measuring the surface area of each type of membrane per unit volume of pellicle, using stereological methods, these surface areas are related to 1g liver. The surface densities of each class of membrane in sections of intact liver tissue are also converted to membrane area per 1 g liver. After correcting for section thickness and compression, and accounting for the contribution of nonhepatocyte membranes to the total membrane area [21], the membrane areas per gram of whole tissue, homogenate, and each fraction are calculated.

Of the 9.3 m^2 of membrane surface area per 1 g liver, the recovery in fractions compared with tissue (F/T) averaged 80.5%, homogenate compared with tissue (H/T) averaged 84.3%, and fractions compared with homogenate (F/H) averaged 95.5% [20]. The mitochondrial and rough-surfaced membranes can be identified in the fractions and in corresponding tissue, but the smooth-surfaced membranes in the fractions contain contributions from smooth endoplasmic reticulum, plasma membrane, fragments of mitochondria, and Golgi components. The recovery of rough and smooth membranes together in the homogenate (H/T) and fractions (F/T) is about 100%, but there is a loss of mitochondrial membranes of over 40% in both compartments. The recoveries of membranes were compared by Bolender [20] with the recoveries of marker enzymes including cytochrome oxidase ($F/H = 83\%$), glucose-6-phosphatase 5'-nucleotidase, monoamine oxidase, and protein (F/H for all about 95%). Significant amounts of marker enzymes are present in fractions other than the fraction with the most activity, including 14% of monoamine oxidase activity and 3% of the cytochrome oxidase activity in the microsomal fraction. Fragmentation of mitochondrial membranes followed by their formation into small smooth vesicles could explain, in part, this shift in the enzyme activities and also the loss of mitochondrial membrane area and the observed slight increase in smooth-surfaced membranes [20].

4.10. Correlation of drug-induced stereological and biochemical changes

A major objective of stereology in biological investigations is to demonstrate quantitative relationships between morphological and biochemical or physiological properties of cells and tissues. Such correlations have been obtained in studies involving the effects of phenobarbital on the liver [30, 57].

Phenobarbital, together with a number of other compounds, characteristically induces an increase in the activity of microsomal enzymes including NADPH-cytochrome C reductase and cytochrome P-450 [58]. In addition, phenobarbital causes an increase in liver weight and a marked proliferation of the smooth-surfaced endoplasmic reticulum membranes [59, 60].

In a stereological study of the liver in phenobarbital-fed rats, Staubli et al. [30] showed that there is a significant increase in the relative liver weight at two and five days after oral administration of 100 mg phenobarbital per kg body weight per day. This increase reflects a proportionate increase in the volume of hepatocyte cytoplasm. The major contributor to the volume increase is the hepatocyte endoplasmic reticulum. The volume and surface densities of both the rough-surfaced and smooth-surfaced endoplasmic reticulum increase in response to the phenobarbital treatment. The most pronounced change occurs in the surface area of the smooth-surfaced endoplasmic reticulum during the first 16 h of treatment (58% increase), but the surface area of the rough-surfaced endoplasmic reticulum also increases significantly (23%) during this time. Later, the surface area of the SER continues to increase to 130% above the control level on the fifth day of treatment, while after two days, the surface area of the RER returns to the control level. In the same animals, the activity of the microsomal enzymes NADPH-cytochrome C reductase, N-demethylase, and cytochrome P-450 increases approximately linearly with the time of phenobarbital treatment. The increments in surface density of the endoplasmic reticulum membranes, with respect to controls, increase colinearly with increases in enzyme activity. The volume density of mitochondria does not change during the treatment but the dense bodies (lysosomes) increase significantly on the fifth day of treatment when compared with controls. Although the mitochondrial volume density does not change, the number of mitochondria per hepatocyte increases significantly. The mean mitochondrial volume decreases between two and five days. The number of microbodies doubles and the mean volume of a microbody is significantly reduced without any change in the volume density during the first two days of treatment and remains at this level.

One to three days after the end of phenobarbital treatment (100 mg/kg/day for five consecutive days), the liver increases in volume but returns to the control volume in five to seven days. During this time the activities of microsomal enzymes also return to normal in correlation with changes in membranes during the recovery period [57, 61]. No changes occur during recovery in the volume densities of mitochondria, peroxisomes, or dense bodies, but a significant increase in the volume density of autophagic vacuoles is observable at two and five days after the end of phenobarbital treatment. The increase in autophagic activity may be associated with the removal of cytoplasmic membranes. The presence of ER membranes enclosed in autophagic vacuoles suggests that such vacuoles are formed nonrandomly for the removal of excess ER membranes [57].

The effects of numerous other agents on the smooth- and rough-surfaced endoplasmic reticulum have been investigated stereologically. Proliferation of endoplasmic reticulum and microsomal enzyme induction is a frequent adaptive response of liver parenchymal cells to such agents. In stereological analyses of the effects of ethanol, it has been observed that a single dose (6 k/kg body weight intragastrically) in rats results in a marked increase in the volume and surface area of SER per hepatocyte within 12 h [62]. The RER volume and surface densities do not change during the same time period.

Acknowledgments. The author acknowledges the assistance of Sharon (Mattimoe) Fitzgerald, Judy Perry, and Mary Jo Swartzberg in the preparation of this manuscript. This work was supported by NIH grant AM-21380.

REFERENCES

1. Underwood EE (1970) Quantitative stereology, Reading MA: Addison-Wesley
2. Elias H, Hennig A, Schwartz DE (1971) Stereology: applications to biomedical research. Physiol Rev 51:158–200
3. Mayhew TM (1972) A comparison of several methods for stereological determination of the numbers of organelles per unit volume of cytoplasm. J Microsc 96:37–44
4. Weibel ER, Bolender RP (1973) Stereological techniques for electron microscopic morphometry. In: Hayat MA (ed) Principles and techniques of electron microscopy, vol 3. New York: Van Nostrand Reinhold, pp 237–296
5. James NT (1977) Stereology. In: Meek GA, Elder HY (eds) Analytical and quantitative methods in microscopy. Cambridge: Society for Experimental Biology Seminar Series, Cambridge University
6. Weibel ER (1979) Stereological methods: vol 1. Practical methods for biological morphometry. New York: Academic Press
7. Delesse A (1847) Procede mechanique pour determiner la composition des roches. CR Acad Sci [D] (Paris) 25:544
8. Rosiwal A (1898) Uber geometrische Geskeins analysen Verhandel. Geol Reichsaustalt Wien 143

9. Glagoleff AA (1933) On the geometrical methods of quantitative mineralogic analysis of rocks. Trans Inst Econ Miner (USSR) 59:1–18

10. Tomkeieff SI (1945) Linear intercepts, areas and volumes. Nature 155:24–26

11. DeHoff RT, Rhines FN (1961) Determination of the number of particles per unit volume from measurements made on random plane sections: the general cylinder and ellipsoid. Trans Am Inst Miner Met Eng 221:975

12. Weibel ER, Kistler GS, Scherle WF (1966) Practical stereological methods for morphometric cytology. J Cell Biol 30:23–38

13. Weibel ER, Elias H (1976) Quantitative methods in morphology. Berlin: Springer

14. Chalkley HW (1943) Method for the quantitative morphologic analysis of tissue. J Natl Cancer Inst 4:47–53

15. Weibel ER, Knight BW (1964) A morphometric study on the thickness of the pulmonary air-blood barrier. J Cell Biol 21:367–384

16. Chalkley HW, Cornfield J, Park H (1949) A method for estimating volume-surface ratios. Science 110:295–297

17. Weibel ER, Gomez DM (1962) A principle for counting tissue structures on random sections. J Appl Physiol 17: 343–348

18. Knight BW, Weibel ER, Gomez DM (1963) Effect of size distribution on a principle of counting on sections, structures contained in a volume. In: Haug H (ed) Proc 1st Int Congr Stereol Wien, pp 18–24

19. Weibel ER, Stäubli W, Gnägi HR, Hess FA (1969) Correlated morphometric and biochemical studies of the liver cell. I. Morphometric model, stereological methods and normal morphometric data for rat liver. J Cell Biol 42:68–91

20. Bolender RP, Paumgartner D, Losa G, Muellener D, Weibel ER (1978) Integrated stereological and biochemical studies on hepatocytic membranes. I. Membrane recoveries in subcellular fractions. J Cell Biol 77:565–583

21. Blouin A, Bolender RP, Weibel ER (1977) Distribution of organelles and membranes between hepatocytes and non-hepatocytes in the rat liver parenchyma. J Cell Biol 72:441–455

22. Schmucker DL, Mooney JS, Jones AL (1977) Age-related changes in the hepatic endoplasmic reticulum: a quantitative analysis. Science 197:1005–1007

23. Lang CA, Herbener GH (1972) Quantitative comparison of the mitochondrial populations in the livers of newborn and weanling rats. Dev Biol 29:176–182

24. Rohr HP, Wirz A, Henning LC, Riede UN, Bianchi L (1971) Morphometric analysis of the rat liver cell in the perinatal period. Lab Invest 24:128–139

25. Herzfeld A, Federman M, Greengard O (1973) Subcellular morphometric and biochemical analyses of developing rat hepatocytes. J Cell Biol 57:475–483

26. Schmucker DL, Jones AL, Mills ES (1974) Morphometric analysis of the ultrastructural changes in the liver of aging rats. J Gerontol 29:506–513

27. Pieri C, Nagy IZ, Mazzufferi G, Giuli C (1975) The aging of rat liver as revealed by electron microscopic morphometry. I. Basic parameters. Exp Gerontol 10:291–304

28. Pfeiffer U (1979) Inhibited autophagic degredation of cytoplasm during compensatory growth of liver cells after partial hepatectomy. Virchows Arch [Cell Pathol] 30:313–333

29. Wiener J, Loud AV, Kimberg DV, Spiro D (1968) A quantitative description of cortisone-induced alterations in the ultrastructure of rat liver parenchymal cells. J Cell Biol 37:47–61

30. Stäubli W, Hess R, Weibel ER (1969) Correlated morphometric and biochemical studies on the liver cell. II. Effects of phenobarbital on rat hepatocytes. J Cell Biol 42:92–112

31. Rohr HP, Michel HJ, Bianchi L (1971) Ultrastrukturell-morphometrische Untersuchungen an der Rattenleberparenchymzelle nach akuter Alkoholintoxikation. Pathol Eur 6:322–341

32. Jones AL, Schmucker DL, Mooney JS, Adler RD, Ockner RK (1976) Morphometric analysis of rat hepatocytes after total biliary obstruction. Gastroenterology 71:1050–1060

33. Moody DE, Reddy JK (1976) Morphometric analysis of ultrastructural changes in rat liver induced by peroxisome proliferator SAH 42:348. J Cell Biol 71:768–780

34. Loud AV (1968) A quantitative stereological description of the ultrastructure of normal rat liver parenchymal cells. J Cell Biol 37:27–46

35. Schmucker DL, Mooney JS, Jones AL (1978) Stereological analysis of hepatic fine structure in the Fischer 344 rat. J Cell Biol 78:319–337

36. Riede UN, Strässle H, Bianchi L, Rohr H (1971) Ultrastructural-morphometric analysis of rat liver after orotic acid administration. Exp Mol Pathol 15:271–280

37. Böcking A, Riede UN (1979) Morphometric analysis of an ultrahistochemical demonstration of nonspecific esterases in hepatocytes of mice after fructose overload. J Histochem Cytochem 27:967–974

38. Roessner A, Kolde G, Stahl K, Blanke G, Van Husen N, Themann H (1978) Ultrastructural morphometric investigations on normal human liver biopsies. Acta Hepatogastroenterol Belg 25:119–123

39. Jézéquel AM, Koch M, Orlandi F (1974) A morphometric study of the endoplasmic reticulum in human hepatocytes: correlation between morphological and biochemical data in subjects under treatment with certain drugs. Gut 15:737–747

40. Hess FA, Gnägi HR, Weibel ER, Preisig R (1973) Morphometry of dog liver: a comparison of wedge and needle biopsies. Eur J Clin Invest 3:451–458

41. Loud AV, Anversa P, Giacomelli F, Wiener J (1978) Absolute morphometric study of myocardial hypertrophy in experimental hypertension. I. Determination of myocyte size. Lab Invest 38:586–596

42. Mori H, Christensen AK (1980) Morphometric analysis of Leydig cells in the normal rat testis. J Cell Biol 84:340–354

43. Budd GC, Barnard EA, Porter C, Mattimoe S (1980) Fluorophosphate-sensitive esterases in mammalian liver: the radioactive localization and measurement of fluorophosphate-reactive sites in adult rat liver. J Histochem Cytochem 28:533–542

44. Chedid A, Nair V (1972) Diurnal rhythm in endoplasmic reticulum of rat liver: electron microscopic study. Science 175:176–180

45. Keller HJ, Friedli HP, Gehr P, Bachofen M, Weibel ER (1975) The effects of optical resolution on the estimation of stereological parameters. Proc 4th Int Cong Stereol, Washington DC: US Natl Bureau Standards, pp 409–410

46. Motta P, Porter KR (1974) Structure of rat liver sinusoids and associated spaces as revealed by scanning electron microscopy. Cell Tissue Res 148:111–125

47. Motta P, Muto M, Fujita T (1978) The liver: an atlas of scanning electron microscopy. Tokyo: Igaku-Shoin

48. Pieri C, Nagy IZ, Giuli C, Mazzufferi G (1975) The aging of rat liver as revealed by electron microscopic morphometry. II. Parameters of regenerated old liver. Exp Gerontol 10:341–349

49. Herbener GH (1976) A morphometric study of age-de-

pendent changes in mitochondrial populations in mouse liver and heart. J Gerontol 31:8–12

50. Tate EL, Herbener GH (1976) A morphometric study of the density of mitochondrial cristae in heart and liver of aging mice. J Gerontol 31:129–134

51. Knook DL, Bezooijen CE van (1975) Age-related phenomena in liver cells isolated from young and old rats: Respiratory capacity and lysosomal activities. Scand J Clin Lab Invest [Suppl] 43:30–31

52. Budd GC (1974) Quantitative aspects of hepatocyte fine structure in human liver compared with rat liver. 32nd Annu Proc Electron Microsc Soc Am 204–205

53. Rohr HP, Lüthy J, Gudat F, Oberholzer M, Glysin C, Bianchi L (1976) Stereology of liver biopsies from healthy volunteers. Virchows Arch [Pathol Anat] 371:251–263

54. De la Iglesia FA, Sturgess JM, McGuire EJ, Feuer G (1976) Quantitative microscopic evaluation of the endoplasmic reticulum in developing human liver. Am J Pathol 82:61

55. Jacob J, Budd GC (1975) Application of electron microscope autoradiography to the localization of enzymatic activity. In: Hayat MA (ed) Electron microscopy of enzymes: principles and methods, vol 4. New York: Van Nostrand Reinhold, pp 217–266

56. Wibo M, Amar-Costesec A, Berthet J, Beaufay H (1971) Electron microscope examination of subcellular fractions. III. Quantitative analysis of microsomal fractions isolated from rat liver. J Cell Biol 51:52–71

57. Bolender RP, Weibel ER (1973) A morphometric study of the removal of phenobarbital-induced membranes from hepatocytes after cessation of treatment. J Cell Biol 56:746–761

58. Remmer H (1970) The role of the liver in drug metabolism. Am J Med 49:617–629

59. Remmer H, Merker HJ (1963) Enzyminduktion und Vermeturung von endoplasmatischen Retikulum in der Leberzell wahrend der Behandlung mit Phenobarbital. Klin Wochenschr 41:276–282

60. Jones AL, Fawcett DW (1966) Hypertrophy of the agranular endoplasmic reticulum in hamster liver induced by phenobarbital (with a review of the function of this organelle in the liver). J Histochem Cytochem 14:215–232

61. Orrenius S, Ericsson JLE (1966) Enzyme-membrane relationship in phenobarbital induction of synthesis of drug-metabolizing enzyme system and proliferation of endoplasmic membranes. J Cell Biol 28:181–198

62. Rohr JP, Michel HJ, Bianchi L (1971) Ultrastrukturell-morphometrische Untersuchungen an der Rattenleber-parenchymzelle nach akuter Alkoholintoxikation. Pathol Eur 6:322–341

63. Reith A (1975) The influence of triiodothyronine and riboflavin deficiency on the rat liver with special reference to mitochondria. A morphologic, morphometric and cytochemical study by electron microscopy. Lab Invest 29:216–228

64. Oudea MC, Dedien P, Oudea P (1973) Morphometric study of the ultrastructure of human alcoholic fatty liver. Biomedicine 19:455–459

65. Iype PT, Bhargava PM, Tasker AD (1965) Some aspects of the chemical and cellular composition of adult rat liver. Exp Cell Res 40:233–251

66. Moses HL, Stein JA, Tschudy DP (1970) Hepatocellular changes associated with allylisopropyl acetamide-induced hepatic porphyria in rats. Lab Invest 22:432–442

67. Rohr HP, Strebel J, Bianchi L (1970) Ultrastrukturell-morphometrische Untersuchungen an der Rattenleberparenchymzelle in der Frühphase der Regeneration nach partieller Hepatektomie. Beitr Pathol Anat 141:52–74

68. Riede UN, Roth M, Molnar JJ, Bianchi L, Rohr HP (1971) Penicillamine induced changes in growing rats. II. Liver parenchymal cells. Experientia 27:794–797

69. Wessel W, Cerny J, Segschneider I, Paquet KJ (1972) Elektronenmikroskopische, morphometrische und histologische Untersuchungen an Rattenlebern nach Unterbindung eines Astes der Vena portae. Beitr Pathol 145:119–148

70. Riede UN, Hodel J, Matt CV, Rasser Y, Rohr HP (1973) Einfluss des Hungers auf die quantitative Cytoarchitektur der Rattenleberzelle. II. Chronischer partieller Hunger. Beitr Pathol 150:246–260

71. Riede UN, Kreutzer W, Robansch T, Kiefer G, Sandritter W (1974) Einfluss der partiellen Exsiccose auf die quantitative Cytoarchitektur der Rattenleberzelle. (Eine cytophotometrische und morphometrische Studie.) Beitr Pathol 153:379–394

72. Sturgess JM, Minaker E, Mitranic M, Moscarello MA (1974) The Golgi complex. II. The effects of aminonucleoside on ultrastructure and glycoprotein biosynthesis. Lab Invest 31:6–14

73. Wanson JC, May G, Penasse W, Popowski A (1975) Isolation of centrolobular and perilobular hepatocytes after phenobarbital treatment. J Cell Biol 66:23–41

74. Jones AL, Schmucker DL (1977) Current concepts of liver structure as related to function. Gastroenterology 73:833–851

75. Greengard O, Federman M, Knox WE (1972) Cytomorphometry of developing rat liver and its application to enzymic differentiation. J Cell Biol 52:261–272

76. Pfeiffer U (1973) Cellular autophagy and cell atrophy in the rat liver during long term starvation. A quantitative morphological study with regard to diurnal variation. Virchows Arch [B] 12:195–211

77. Miller ML, Murphy L, Basom CR, Petering HG (1974) Alterations in hepatocytes after manipulation of the diet: copper, zinc and cadmium interactions. Am J Anat 141:23–40

78. Christov K, Riede UN, Helin H, Rohr HP (1974) Ultrastructural morphometric studies on the effect of irradiation on hepatic parenchymal cells in rats. Pathol Eur 9:11–15

79. Reid IM (1973) An ultrastructural and morphometric study of the liver of the lactating cow in starvation ketosis. Exp Mol Pathol 18:316–330

80. Oudea MC, Colette M, Oudea P (1973) Morphometric study of ultrastructural changes induced in rat liver by chronic alcohol intake. Digest Dis 18:398–402

81. Underwood EE (1975) Basic stereology. In: Underwood EE, de Wit R, Moore GA (eds) Proc 4th Int Congr Stereol, p 509

8. LIVER PHYSIOLOGY AND BIOCHEMISTRY

G.C. BUDD

1. INTRODUCTION

Because the major functions of the liver are essential components in the homeostatic machinery of the organism, the liver is essential for the maintenance of life in man and other vertebrates. The liver functions as a digestive gland by synthesizing bile salts from cholesterol and transporting these substances as conjugates with amino acids into the bile. After bile has been secreted into the small intestine, the bile salts assist in the digestion and absorption of fat for use as an energy source and for incorporation into cell membranes. Newly formed bile also carries with it bilirubin and other substances removed from plasma by the hepatic cells. Biliburin is excreted into the bile after conjugation with glucuronate in the liver cells.

The liver has a very important role in metabolizing the absorbed products of digestion and regulating the systemic dispersal of monosaccharides, fatty acids, and amino acids. In addition, the liver stores minerals and vitamins and produces considerable amounts of heat from metabolism. Much of our present knowledge concerning oxidative metabolism, glycogenesis, gluconeogenesis, lipogenesis, and other biochemical pathways demonstrates that the liver has a major role in storing and releasing metabolic energy for utilization in the activities of the whole organism.

The liver has an additional vital role in protecting the organism from endogenous and exogenous toxic substances. Hormones, neurotransmitters, and foreign substances, including microorganisms, endotoxins, ammonia, and drugs are generally inactivated by reticuloendothelial (Kupffer) cells or detoxified by the hepatocytes. This activity is essential for protecting the organism and its sensitive tissues from the products of its own metabolism

and also from harmful factors incorporated from the environment.

The liver is uniquely suited to carry out its secretory, excretory, metabolic, and protective functions due to its strategic location between the gastrointestinal tract and the heart. Two-thirds of the blood supply to the liver is *via* the portal vein which drains the intestines and spleen and carries most of the absorbed products of digestion directly to the liver. The remaining blood reaches the liver from the heart via the abdominal aorta and hepatic artery. As blood flows through the liver to the hepatic vein and heart, albumin and most of the other plasma proteins, including coagulation factors, which are produced exclusively by the liver, are added to the plasma and the products of digestion are removed. The liver performs other important circulatory and hematologic functions including erythropoiesis in the fetus and neonate and the formation of large quantities of lymph.

Each of the functional properties of the liver has been subjected to close investigation in recent years. In part this is due to the development of new methods, but continued investigation is also stimulated by the increasing importance of an understanding of how the liver functions after exposure to drugs and environmental pollutants. The purpose of this chapter is to review the physiological and biochemical properties of developing and mature liver with emphasis on recent contributions to knowledge.

2. HEPATIC CIRCULATION AND THE FORMATION OF LYMPH

Approximately 1.5 liters of blood per minute flow into the sinusoids of the average human liver from the portal vein and hepatic artery. Most of this blood enters from the portal vein (two-thirds to four-fifths of the total flow) at a pressure of 5–13 mmHg. The remaining blood is supplied at high pressure (90–100 mmHg) from the hepatic artery. The resistance in the hepatic arterial inflow is 30–40 times that in the portal inflow. The portal blood is well saturated with oxygen ($\sim 78\%$ of fully saturated blood) except during alimentation when the oxygen saturation may be reduced due to increased intestinal oxygen utilization. About 70% of the hepatic oxygen requirement is supplied by portal blood. The remaining oxygen is carried in fully saturated hepatic arterial blood. About 60% of the portal venous blood flow is from the superior mesenteric vein, which drains the small intestine, head of the pancreas, and part of the large intestine. The other 40% of portal blood flows to the liver from the spleen, stomach, body of the pancreas, and large intestine.

The liver in the fetus has a third source of blood supply, the umbilical vein which carries well-oxygenated blood from the placenta at moderately high pressure (~ 25 mmHg at term). The small diameters of the hepatic artery and trunk of the portal vein indicate that they contribute relatively little to the prenatal blood supply to the liver. On the other hand, the left main branch of the portal vein is in direct continuity with the umbilical vein and receives about 50% of the blood flow from the placenta [1].

The relative significance of portal flow and hepatic arterial flow in the postnatal liver has been clarified as a result of studies on the effects of vascular occlusion and diversion of blood flow. The serious vascular congestion in the splanchnic vasculature which follows acute occlusion of the portal vein can be avoided by the production of an Eck's fistula or portacaval shunt, which diverts portal blood so that it bypasses the liver without inducing splanchnic vascular congestion. Following this procedure, liver function is sufficient for life to continue even though there may be a diminished tolerance to a high-protein diet and a tendency for the liver to atrophy and have a reduced capacity for regeneration. A reduction in portal blood flow can result in up to a 100% increase in hepatic arterial blood flow. If the hepatic artery is disrupted or occluded following traumatic abdominal injury while portal flow and oxygenation are maintained,

the liver may recover [2]. In experimental gradual occlusion of the hepatic artery in animals with a diverted portal venous supply, the development of a collateral supply to the liver from the phrenic, intercostal, and adrenal arteries can occur to maintain the minimal blood supply to the liver that is needed for survival [3]. Such observations indicate that 50% or less of normal blood flow and oxygen delivery to the liver is sufficient for maintenance of liver functions.

Lymph provides an alternative route for the transfer of water and solutes from the liver to the blood pool. Lymphatic capillaries in the interlobular connective tissue of the liver drain into lymphatics in the portal tracts. The lymph flows into intrathoracic lymph nodes associated with the inferior vena cava and esophagus and also into abdominal lymph nodes associated with the hilus [4].

Hepatic lymph contains a high concentration of plasma proteins (80%–90% of the plasma concentration), which suggests that relatively unaltered plasma is transferred from the blood into the subendothelial Disse space and then into the lymphatics in the interlobular connective tissue and portal tracts. This concept has received support from scanning and transmission electron-microscopic studies showing the existence of fenestrae in the sinusoidal endothelium in sufficient quantity to permit the bulk flow of plasma through the endothelial wall [5, 6]. A pressure gradient between the already low sinusoidal pressure (3–7 mmHg) and the subendothelial space must exist if outward movement occurs, but this has not been measured. In the dog, ligation of the hepatic artery has relatively little effect on the protein concentration of liver lymph, indicating that hepatic arterial pressure or blood flow contributes little to the formation of lymph. Also in the dog, the ratio of concentration of some plasma proteins in lymph compared with plasma is inversely dependent on their molecular weights [7]. These findings suggest that there is a semipermeable barrier between the blood and lymph which effectively acts as a molecular sieve for the plasma proteins. The interstitial fluid may be considered the source for the fluid present in the lymphatic capillaries and larger vessels, but the contributions to interstitial fluid are by no means certain. One source of interstitial fluid appears to be fluid resulting from a net difference in fluid outflow from the hepatic sinusoids under the influence of hydrostatic pressure and inflow into the sinusoids due to oncotic pressure and tension imposed by the containing capsular wall of the liver. Another factor to be considered is the possibility that water and solutes exchange between the interstitium and bile. Fluid may leak out of the interstitium into bile at the complex junctions between hepatocytes adjacent to the bile canaliculi [8]. Alternatively, there could be a normal low-level movement of bile constituents into the interstitium and from there into both blood and lymph. The observation that plasma proteins occur in human bile supports the concept of a movement of interstitial fluid into bile channels. It has been observed that such a·movement is increased or decreased in parallel with changes in bile salt secretion [9]. On the other hand, retrograde movement of whole bile into the interstitium, blood, and lymph occurs if there is an interference with bile drainage.

3. BILE FORMATION

Bile is an aqueous digestive secretion produced by hepatocytes and released into canaliculi for transfer through the bile ducts to the lumen of the duodenum. The main organic constituents of bile are conjugated bile acids, cholesterol, and phospholipids associated in mixed micelles in an aqueous solution of inorganic cations and anions. The inorganic ions are sodium, potassium, calcium, magnesium, chloride, and bicarbonate in similar concentration to their plasma concentrations. Bile also contains small quantities of albumin and other proteins and serves as an important excretory pathway out of the body for a number of metabolic products and drugs (especially bilirubin and anionic dyes).

Bile is modified in the bile ducts by the addition and reabsorption of water and inorganic ions, but it remains almost isosmotic with plasma. The organic constituents in the micelles contribute little to the osmotic activity of bile.

Most of the bile is secreted into canaliculi in amounts that are dependent on the transport of bile acids into the canaliculi (bile-salt-dependent bile flow). The remaining bile is formed independently

of bile acid secretion, partly in the canaliculi and also in the ducts, where secretin and other hormones can influence bile formation and composition. While chloride concentration in bile is influenced by bile salts [10], the bicarbonate concentration is less affected by salts but depends on hormones. Recently a bicarbonate pump has been implicated in the formation of a large fraction of canalicular bile [11].

An accepted method for estimating bile flow is to measure the clearance of erythritol or mannitol from plasma. In this technique it is assumed that the test solute enters bile by simple diffusion at a rate governed by the rate of bile secretion. It is also inferred that the solute is unable to cross the duct epithelium. In several species, including man, erythritol clearance is strongly correlated with bile acid secretion. Extrapolation of the generally linear plot of erythritol clearance against bile acid excretion rate to zero bile-acid excretion is now accepted as defining the bile-acid-independent component of canalicular bile flow. Within the ductular system, secretin stimulates the addition of HCO_3^- and Cl^- to bile. Similar modifications to bile have been observed with cholecystokinin (CCK), gastrin, and cerulein, which share an identical sequence of the C-terminal amino acids. The ductular system can also reabsorb electrolytes, water, and glucose.

3.1. Bile-salt synthesis and recirculation

The important dependence of physiological bile secretion on the secretion of conjugated bile acids has stimulated research on the biochemistry of these steroid compounds and on the mechanisms of conjugation, secretion, and enterohepatic circulation of primary and secondary bile acids [12].

The major pathway for conversion of cholesterol to the primary 24-carbon atom bile acids, cholic acid, and chenodoeoxycholic acid has been known since 1943 [13] (Fig. 1). The initial reaction is the hydroxylation of cholesterol in the 7-alpha-position by the enzyme 7-alpha-hydroxylase, a microsomal enzyme which requires NADPH, oxygen, and cytochrome P-450 to function. Next, the 3-beta-hydroxy group is oxidized by incompletely characterized microsomal enzymes to a 3-keto group to form 7-alpha-hydroxy-4-cholesten-3-one, a substrate for microsomal 12-alpha-hydroxylase. At this point the

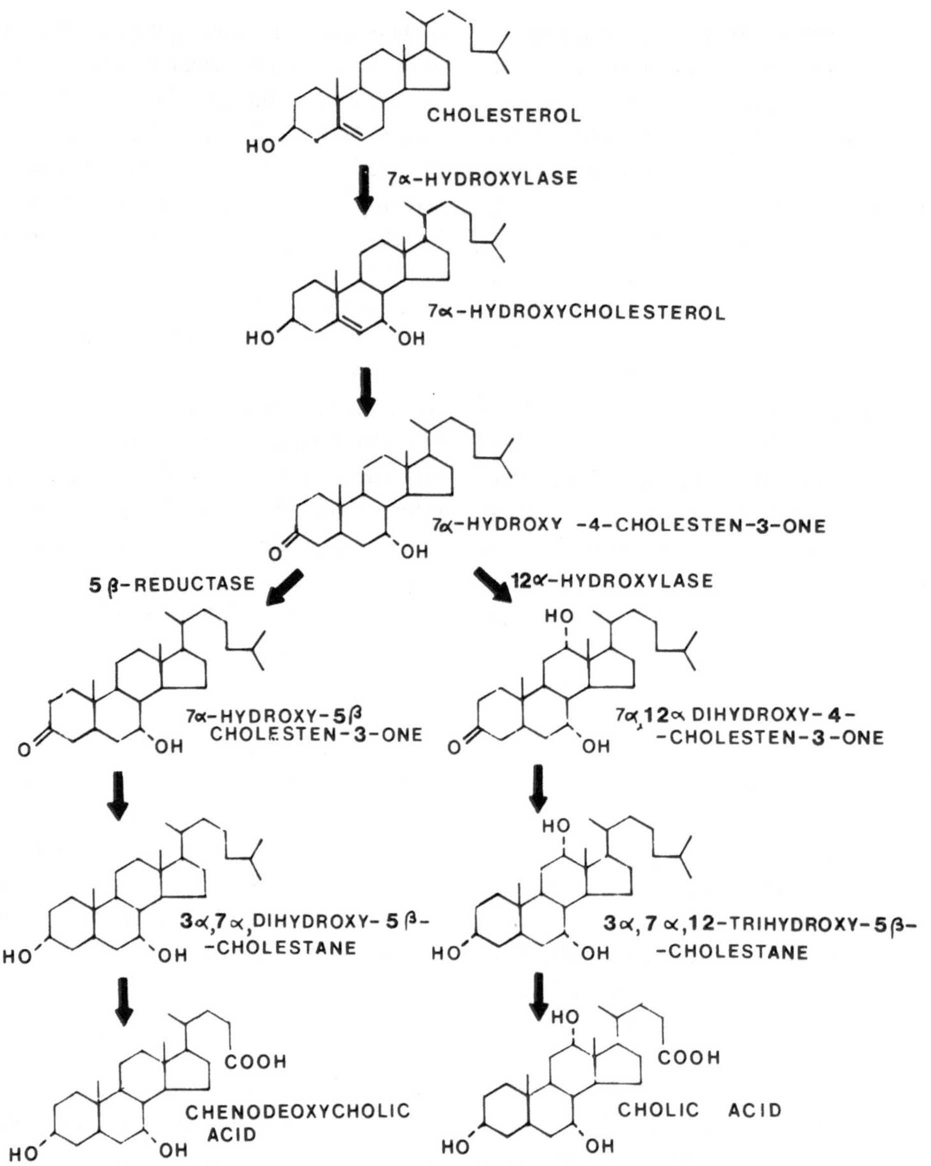

122

Figure 1. The major pathway for the formation of primary bile acids from cholesterol.

pathway splits and the 7-alpha-hydroxy-4-cholesten-3-one is metabolized into both cholic acid and chenodeoxycholic acid. The 3-keto group is reduced by enzymes in the cytosol to a 3-alpha-hydroxy group and the Δ 4-double bond is also reduced. The dihydro- and trihydro-cholestanes produced in these reactions are then hydroxylated in the 26-position and oxidized to corresponding carboxylic acid groups in this position. The 26-alpha-hydroxylation reactions occur predominantly in the hepatocyte mitochondria but may also take place in the endoplasmic reticulum (microsomal fraction). In

the final synthetic step, the dihydro- and trihydrocholestanoic acids are rapidly converted into cholic acid and chenodeoxycholic acid in mitochondria and microsomes.

In addition to this major pathway for synthesis of primary bile acids, there is an alternative pathway contributing significantly to chenodeoxycholate synthesis in human and rat liver mitochondria [14, 15]. A 26-hydroxylase acts on cholesterol to form 26-hydroxycholesterol. This compound is then converted sequentially into 3-beta-hydroxy-5-cholenoic acid and lithocholic acid before being converted to chenodeoxycholic acid (Fig. 2). Both the 3-beta-hydroxy-5-cholenoic acid and lithocholic acid are hepatotoxic and have been shown to contribute to fetal or infant hepatic disease, including some cases of extrahepatic biliary atresia and neonatal hepatitis. It is probable that most lithocholic acid is detoxified in man by excretion following conjugation with sulfate in the liver and kidney. Jenner and Howard [16] have suggested that impairment of hepatic sulfation may allow accumulation of toxic acids and contribute to the etiology of biliary atresia and neonatal hepatitis.

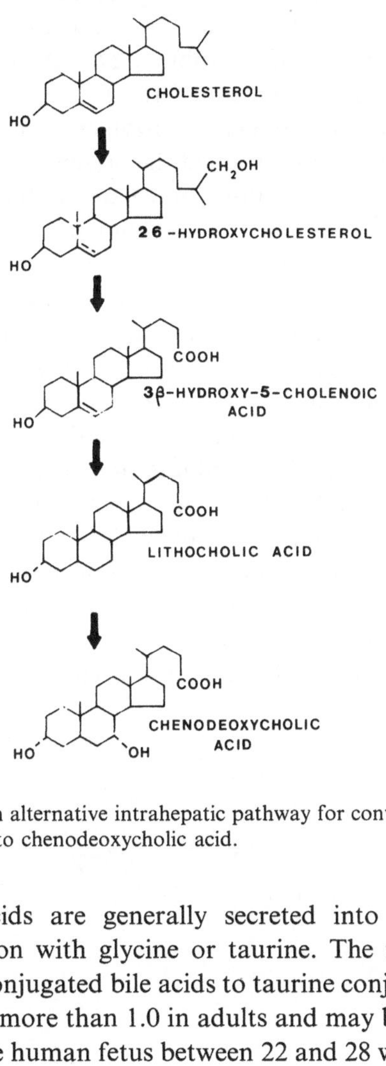

Figure 2. An alternative intrahepatic pathway for conversion of cholesterol to chenodeoxycholic acid.

Bile acids are generally secreted into bile in conjugation with glycine or taurine. The ratio of glycine-conjugated bile acids to taurine conjugate is normally more than 1.0 in adults and may be up to 6.0. In the human fetus between 22 and 28 weeks of gestation, the glycine–taurine ratio of gallbladder bile is less than 0.10. Even at term, taurine conjugation predominates, but by ten days of postnatal age, glycine conjugation approaches the adult ratio. The reason for the change in glycine–taurine ratio

in development is not clear, but it may reflect changes in diet or a relative immaturity of taurine-catabolizing activity in the fetus and neonate [17].

The secretion of newly synthesized bile acid (or bile salts, as they are called when conjugated with glycine or taurine) probably involves active transport across the canalicular membrane. Conjugated bile salts are secreted more efficiently than unconjugated bile acids. Following its secretion in bile, up to one-fifth of the glycocholate pool in adults is deconjugated by intestinal bacteria with the release of glycine, which is absorbed and metabolized, and cholic acid, which is absorbed and returned to the liver to be reconjugated. Several bacterial species remove the 7-alpha-hydroxyl group from cholic acid and chenodeoxycholic acid to produce the secondary bile acids, deoxycholic acid, and lithocholic acid, respectively. Other bacterial changes in bile acids lead to many other secondary bile acids which occur in the feces.

The conjugated bile acids are actively reabsorbed in the ileum, probably in a sodium-coupled transport process. In addition, some glycine-conjugated bile acids are passively absorbed in the proximal small intestine. After absorption into the portal blood, the bile acids, at a concentration 40–100 times higher than in the systemic circulation, are carried to the liver where an efficient sodium-dependent transport mechanism for their uptake into hepatocytes resides. Bile-acid uptake from plasma into liver is more rapid than the rate of secretion into bile, showing that the hepatic uptake system is probably not rate limiting in the entero-hepatic circulation of bile acids [18]. In adults, the bile salts recycle through the intestine two or more times during digestion of a meal and are contained in a total bile salt pool of 2–4 g. Daily losses of 15%–20% of the pool have been estimated.

Bile-salt secretion is associated with the appearance of cholesterol and lecithin in bile. The mechanism of cholesterol and phospholipid transfer to bile is not understood. Based on studies with colchicine in rats, the microtubular and vesicular route for secretion is not involved [19], but a more recent study indicated that microtubules are involved in the transport of lipids into the bile [20]. Cholesterol and phospholipids synthesized in the microsomal membranes move rapidly to the canalicular membranes of hepatocytes [21] prior to their transfer to

124

bile under the influence of bile salts. It has been proposed that the detergent action of bile salts causes the secretion of phospholipids into bile [22], but such a proposal cannot account for the differing phospholipid composition [23] and higher specific activity of phospholipids [21] in bile relative to the canalicular membrane. Cholesterol and lecithin are aggregated together with other phospholipids in mixed micelles in bile. The composition of micelles is critical for stabilizing lecithin and cholesterol at concentrations much higher than their maximum solubility in water. Deviation from the ideal micellar composition may be a major factor in the formation of cholesterol gallstones [24]. The lowest concentration of bile salts at which stable micelles are formed (the critical micellar concentration) in human bile is about 1.45 mmol/l, but this concentration may depend on the phospholipid content of the bile [25].

3.2. Bilirubin

Bilirubin is the major excretory component of bile. It is a product of heme metabolism in the hepatic and extrahepatic reticuloendothelial cells engaged in the destruction of erythrocytes. The uptake, metabolism, and excretion of bilirubin by hepatycotes involves specific carriers and enzymes which are subject to alteration by congenital or induced pathological and therapeutic influences. Jaundice may result from the interruption of any of these steps.

Bilirubin bound to plasma albumin is delivered to the liver in the portal and hepatic arterial circulations. After passing through the fenestrated sinusoidal endothelium into Disse space, most of the bilirubin is detached from the albumin to enter the hepatocytes. Bilirubin uptake involves a carrier-mediated transport system in the hepatocyte plasma membrane. Bilirubin within the hepatocytes is passively dispersed among various subcellular compartments containing binding sites. Within the cytosol, two heat-labile anion-binding proteins, Y and Z proteins, bind bilirubin. Y protein, also called ligandin, is identical with glutathione S-transferase B [26, 27]. This enzyme, which represents up to 5% of the protein in hepatic cytosol, catalyzes the conjugation of the dye, bromosulfothalein (BSP), with glutathione, but also binds

albumin, indocyanine green, and fatty acids, none of which are conjugated with glutathione. The binding of ligandin with bilirubin may help to increase the intracellular concentration of bilirubin above that which would be present in solution or it may facilitate the presentation of bilirubin to its conjugating enzyme. In addition, ligandin protects mitochondrial respiration from the depressant effects of bilirubin [28]. Z protein appears to be more important in fatty-acid transport.

Bilirubin is rapidly conjugated via the carboxyethyl side chains to uridine diphosphoglucuronic acid (UDPGA) and UDP-sugars, including UDP-glucose and UDP-xylose (Fig. 3). The major conjugating enzyme is bilirubin UDPGA transferase (bilirubin glucuronyl transferase). The existence of other bilirubin-conjugating enzymes in the liver and other tissues is uncertain at the present time. Under physiological conditions, most of the bilirubin in the body is eliminated by excretion into bile following hepatic conjugation. In mice, guinea pigs, rabbits, sheep, pigs, calves, and chickens the mono-conjugated bilirubin predominates in bile, but in man, rats, dogs , and cats diconjugated bilirubin is the main product in bile [29, 30]. An alternative mechanism which is relatively inefficient has been observed in newborn infants and in infants with Crigler-Najjar syndrome in which there is a congenital deficiency in bilirubin glucuronyl transferase. Under these conditions, bilirubin is degraded to more hydrophilic derivatives which are excreted in bile and urine. The Gunn rat, which in the homozygous condition lacks bilirubin glucuronyl trans-

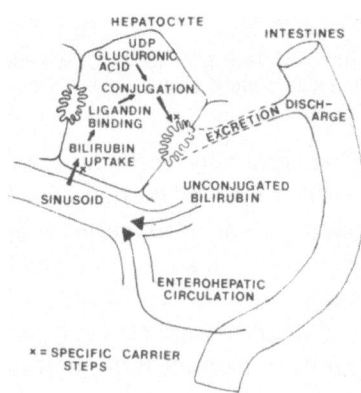

Figure 3. Diagrammatic summary of the steps in the hepatocytic uptake, conjugation, excretion, and recirculation of bilirubin.

ferase, is an animal model for the Crigler-Najjar syndrome.

The transfer of conjugated bilirubin into bile involves a carrier-mediated transport process at the canalicular membrane. Bilirubin is concentrated in bile to over 100 times the plasma concentration, almost all of it being conjugated with glucuronide. Unconjugated bilirubin is poorly excreted into bile. The rate of bilirubin transport into bile is increased by bile salts except at very high rates of bilirubin infusion when the transport maximum (T_m) for bilirubin is decreased, possibly due to cytotoxic effects. It remains uncertain whether there is one discrete system for canalicular transport of conjugated bile acids into bile and another system or systems for the transport of bilirubin and other anions into bile [31]. It is possible that the active transport of bile acids into the bile canaliculus is related in a cotransport process to the transport of anions into bile.

Conjugated bilirubin is carried in the bile through the intralobular and interlobular bile ducts to the extrahepatic ducts and the gallbladder. Bile is generally stored in the gallbladder between meals, where it undergoes concentration of the organic constituents as electrolytes and water are reabsorbed. Cholecystokinin released during food intake causes gallbladder contraction and relaxation of the sphincter of Oddi. There is a resultant forceful ejection of gallbladder bile into the duodenal lumen.

Within the intestine, the conjugated bilirubin is partially deconjugated by the action of bacterial, hepatic, and intestinal mucosa β-glucuronidase. About half of the bilurubin is converted into a group of chromogens, or urobilinogens, by the intestinal flora. Some of these compounds (about 20%) are reabsorbed passively together with unconjugated bilirubin into the portal blood and later are reexcreted into bile. Approximately 2%–5% of the recirculating urobilinogens are filtered by the kidneys to be excreted in the urine every 24 h.

Bilirubin is efficiently removed from the fetus by transplacental transfer of the unconjugated pigment into the maternal circulation. Conjugated bilirubin is not generally transferred back to the fetus even if it rises to high levels in the maternal circulation. At birth there is a moderate accumulation of unconjugated bilirubin in the plasma of the newborn to a concentration of 6–7 mg/dl; a phenomenon that is commonly called 'physiologic' or 'developmental' jaundice. A number of processes have been considered as contributory factors to developmental jaundice. The shorter life-span of fetal erythrocytes, less efficient erythropoiesis, and greater total hemoglobin mass in the late fetus all contribute to an increased bilirubin production rate in the neonate relative to the adult. Immature and low-birth-weight infants often have a relative hypoalbuminemia which would lead to a low proportion of albumin-bound bilirubin in relation to free bilirubin in the circulation. A moderate to severe acidosis is common in association with respiratory distress in the newborn. This can cause dissociation of bilirubin from plasma albumin below pH 7.0. Organic anionic drugs, including antibiotics and salicylates, may displace bilirubin from albumin-binding sites and contribute to an increased unbound bilirubin fraction [32]. These factors combined with the immaturity of the bilirubin-UDPGA glucuronyl transferase and low intrahepatocytic ligandin in the newborn appear to cause physiologic or developmental jaundice. Additional contributory factors may include inhibitory steroid hormones in maternal milk, and immaturity of the bilirubin uptake, intracellular binding and excretion mechanisms in the neonatal liver.

4. SINUSOIDAL CELL FUNCTIONS

Estimates of the cellular composition of mammalian liver indicate that sinusoidal cells comprise numerically about 33% of the population of cells in the liver and about 6.3% of the volumetric composition of the liver [33, 34]. For comparison, the hepatocytes represent about 60% of the number of cells in the liver and 78% of the liver volume [33, 34].

The sinusoidal cell population is composed of two distinct subpopulations, the endothelial cells and Kupffer cells. The endothelial cells are thin squamous cells with a nucleus which causes a localized bulging of the cell into the sinusoidal lumen. The cytoplasm contains a small quantity of granular endoplasmic reticulum and a large number of small pinocytotic vesicles. The most notable feature, distinguishing these endothelial cells from most others in the body, is the existence of large holes and multiple fenestrations which permit the ready passage of plasma solutes and proteins between the sinusoidal and Disse spaces. The main distinguishing functional characteristic of the Kupffer cell is its phagocytic activity. Volumetrically and numerically, Kupffer cells constitute about 2% of the liver [33, 34]. It has been estimated that these cells comprise 80%–90% of the functional mass of the reticuloendothelial system in the body [35].

Scanning electron microscopy has confirmed and extended earlier observations with transmission electron microscopy in demonstrating the stellate morphology of Kupffer cells [5, 36, 37]. These cells are usually found attached to the lumenal surface of the sinusoidal endothelium, or they may be embedded in the endothelial lining with long microvilli projecting into the sinusoid lumen. The cell surface of Kupffer cells bears F_c and C_3 receptors and opsonins belonging to the alpha-2-macroglobulin group. These receptors are involved in attachment and uptake of antigenic material into the cytoplasm, where a varied population of lysosomal particles is found. Erythrocytes and partially digested fragments of erythrocytes are present in many Kupffer cells.

The Kupffer cells appear to monitor the intravascular contents of the sinusoids and guard the hepatocytes and the rest of the body from toxic agents entering the liver in portal blood. Their location near the fenestrations in the sinusoidal endothelial wall may permit the Kupffer cells to ameliorate the activity of toxic substances on the other side of the endothelial boundary.

Kupffer cells can synthesize urea and bind insulin at rates comparable to the hepatocytes. In some species (e.g., the rat and mouse) the nuclear envelope and endoplasmic reticulum of Kupffer cells contain peroxidase activity which may have a detoxifying function [38], and it has been suggested that this enzyme could be used as a marker for the identification of mononuclear phagocytes (Kupffer cells) in rat liver [39]. It has been shown, however, that in the mouse, weak to moderate peroxidase activity also occurs in the sinusoidal endothelial cell endoplasmic reticulum, making this enzyme unsuitable as a specific Kupffer cell marker in this species [40].

The phagocytic role of Kupffer cells in various liver diseases and experimental conditions has been studied. The number and size of Kupffer cells and their complement of cytoplasmic projections are increased in acute viral hepatitis. In time-sequence studies of Kupffer cell activity after injection of colloidal carbon or murine hepatitis virus, a rapid phagocytosis was revealed. No immediate Kupffer cell changes occurred after virus administration, but after 24–72 h, virus particles were found in necrotic hepatocytes and in Kupffer cells. Cellular debris resulting from hepatocyte destruction was also seen in Kupffer cells following murine hepatitis virus administration.

Kupffer cells are hypertrophic and markedly increased in number in reticuloendotheliosis. Following the administration of Thorotrast, a radioactive radiocontrast agent which was widely used in the 1940s and 1950s, this material accumulates in the reticuloendothelium and has been implicated in the induction of reticuloendotheliosis. The presence of radioactive Thorotrast deposits in Kupffer cells has been detected in autoradiographs of human liver sections obtained about 30 years after administration of Thorotrast [41].

The possible role of Kupffer cells in modulating the spread of metastatic tumor cells to the liver is under active investigation. Recently, Roos and Dingemans [42] introduced several types of tumor cells into perfused liver in vitro or in vivo. They observed that some tumor cell lines were actively phagocytized by Kupffer cells, including an adenocarcinoma subline which also produced few metastatic lesions. By contrast, another adenocarcinoma subline which was not so actively removed by the phagocytic activity of Kupffer cells was observed to produce profound metastatic lesions in the liver. These observations, suggesting that phagocytic activity may influence liver metastasis, need to be followed with additional studies to establish whether Kupffer cells possess tumor cell cytotoxicity comparable to other phagocytic cells.

The importance of Kupffer cells in removing endotoxins in the human liver has been demonstrated recently. With the Limulus lysate gelation test, it has been shown that systemic endotoxemia, which is uncommon in the absence of liver disease, was present in 50% of a group of patients with cirrhosis [43]. In another study of 259 patients, all of those with hepatic failure or chronic alcoholic hepatitis had a positive result in the Limulus test for endotoxin. About half the population with chronic active hepatitis were endotoxin positive [44]. Individuals with portacaval collateral circulation had a high frequency of endotoxemia compared with those without collateral development. Liehr and Grun [44] suggested that Kupffer cell removal of endotoxins is depressed in liver disease and that this permits the development of endotoxemia. Recognized sequelae include intravascular coagulation and renal failure.

Recent evidence suggests that the Kupffer cells are involved in the response to hemorrhagic shock. Initial effects included stickiness of lymphocytes and leucocytes and their attachment to endothelial and Kupffer cells. The resulting retention of leucocytes by the liver resulted in a significant systemic leucopenia. Not only did leucocytes adhere to Kupffer cells, but they were also ingested into Kupffer cell cytoplasmic particles. In later stages, degeneration and loss of Kupffer cells was observed. It was suggested that the irreversible stage of shock may result from degeneration and loss of Kupffer cells prior to alterations in endothelial cells and centrolobular necrosis of the hepatic lobules [45].

Two mechanisms for the renewal of Kupffer cells have been demonstrated in rodents. Transplantation studies have suggested that they are derived from bone marrow precursor cells while other studies have demonstrated a local proliferation of Kupffer cells within the liver. Recently, two male patients were studied after receiving bone marrow transplants after high-dose chemotherapy and whole body irradiation. In both cases, Kupffer cells were shown to be present in the liver with characteristics specific to the donor cells [46].

Investigations of the origin of Kupffer cells in mice have confirmed that these cells are derived mainly from bone marrow cells [47]. At any given time, only about 1% of the Kupffer cells divide in the liver. Most Kupffer cells are derived from monocytes migrating from the sites of production in the bone marrow. In mice, the total population of Kupffer cells is replaced in about 21 days.

5. HOMEOSTATIC AND METABOLIC FUNCTIONS

The liver occupies a strategic position in the metabolism of all the major constituents of food and serves a vital role in regulating the availability of energy sources and metabolic precursors required throughout the body.

5.1. Carbohydrate metabolism

The liver is an important supplier of glucose to the cells that depend on it for metabolism, particularly the cells in the central nervous system. This glucose results from the glycogenolysis of glycogen which is deposited in the hepatocytes following the absorption of glucose from the intestines when carbohydrates are digested. The glucose concentration in blood plasma is subject to regulation by hormones and the availability of substrates. During fasting, the glucose supply may be augmented by gluconeogenesis within the hepatocytes. Absorbed glucose is transported from portal blood in the hepatic sinusoids and Disse space into hepatocytes by a specific membrane transport system. The intracellular glucose concentration in liver cells is about 128 mg/100 ml intracellular water compared with 90 ml/100 ml plasma [48]. The intracellular glucose is phosphorylated to glucose-6-phosphate (G6P) by at least four hexokinase enzymes with high affinity for glucose. At physiological glucose concentrations, the hexokinases are saturated and this is the rate-limiting step in glycogen synthesis. Between 25% and 100% of administered glucose is retained by the liver. The amount retained is dependent on the dose administered, route of administration (oral administration or intravascular infusion), insulin response, and species of mammal. Infusion of ^{14}C-labeled glucose into dogs, followed by measurement of ^{14}C-uptake into hepatic glycogen, results in about 50% of the glucose taken up by the liver appearing in glycogen. This represents 26%–34% of the uptake in all of the tissues [48]. In rats, liver glycogen formed after oral administration of ^{14}C-glucose may account for 27% of the absorbed glucose [49].

Liver G6P is utilized for glycogen synthesis or it is oxidized directly or through the Embden-Meyerhof pathway. The current concept of the steps in

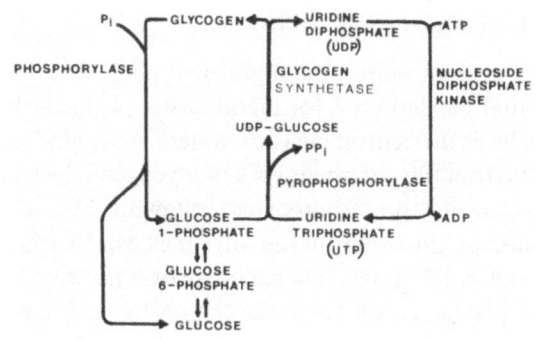

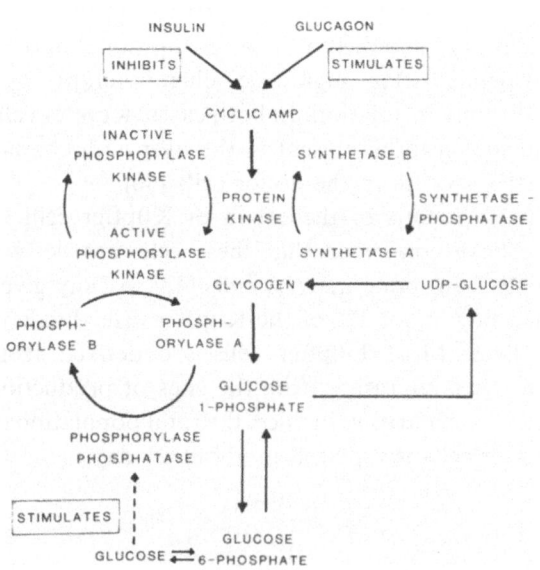

of phosphorylase phosphatase may result from exposure of liver cells to glucocorticoids. The phosphorylase phosphatase tends to decrease phosphorylase *a* and diminish its inhibitory effect on synthetase phosphatase.

The glycogenolysis and hepatic glucose output induced by hypoglycemia is assumed to be due to the direct effects of epinephrine and glucagon on hepatocytes. These hormones stimulate adenylcyclase, which increases the synthesis of cyclic AMP. Protein kinase stimulation by cyclic AMP causes an increase in the activation of phosphorylase kinase and a subsequent increase in the phosphorylase *a* concentration and glycogenolysis. At the same time, synthetase is inactivated by protein kinase and glycogen synthesis is relatively inhibited.

The utilization of glucose by the tissues and the hepatic output of glucose is 150–180 mg/kg/h in the basal conditon in man and in the dog. The regulation of glucose output by glucagon and epinephrine requires a significant hypoglycemia, and it is likely that an intrinsic hepatic mechanism is involved in regulating small changes in glucose output. A direct relationship between hepatic glycogen levels and glucose output has been demonstrated in dogs [48]. Insulin decreases (or prevents an increase) in the output of glucose while deficiency of insulin, as in acute exclusion of the pancreas from the circulation, results in an increase in hepatic output of glucose.

Glucose is also used as an energy source for the metabolic activity of the liver cells. In addition, it is required as a reducing agent and in the synthesis of polysaccharides and plasma lipids. Glucose is also required in the formation of bile salts and serum proteins. Glucuronic acid formed from glucose is important for conjugating steroids and other substances prior to excretion in bile. Glucose catabolism in the liver occurs mainly in the Embden-Meyerhof glucolytic pathway to produce pyruvate and lactate as end products.

5.2. Pyruvate oxidation and the TCA cycle

Pyruvate is oxidized in liver mitochondria to form acetyl coenzyme A, which is the donor of acetyl groups to the tricarboxylic acid (TCA) cycle. Two molecules of CO_2 are formed and four molecules of NAD are reduced to $NADH_2$ with the oxidation of

each acetyl group. The $NADH_2$ conserves energy by entering the electron transport chain. Each $NADH_2$ molecule contributes to the formation of three ATP molecules during oxidative phosphorylation. The metabolism of a glucose molecule generates 38 molecules of ATP.

5.3. Phosphogluconate pathway

Up to 50% of the glucose used by the liver involves the degradation of G6P to fructose-6-phosphate and glyceraldehyde-3-phosphate. In the process, NADP is reduced to $NADPH_2$, which is essential for fatty-acid synthesis, bile-salt production, and steroid metabolism. In addition, glutathione oxidation utilizes $NADPH_2$. Pentose phosphate, an additional product of this pathway, is used in RNA synthesis.

5.4. Glucuronic acid production

The formation of glucuronic acid from glucose is important in the liver for utilization in conjugation reactions and in mucopolysaccharide synthesis.

5.5. Fructose and galactose metabolism

Fructose enters the glycolytic pathway after absorption from the intestine, where it occurs as an equal constituent with glucose in the dietary sugar sucrose. The liver contains a fructokinase for phosphorylating fructose to fructose-1-phosphate (F1P). Unlike muscle, there are no liver enzymes for converting F1P into fructose 1,6-diphosphate for direct entry into the glycolytic pathway. For fructose to enter the glycolytic pathway, it must first be cleaved by aldolase to dihydroxyacetone phosphate, which is an intermediate in the glycolytic pathway, and glyceraldehyde, which can be phosphorylated to glyceraldehyde 1-3-phosphate, another intermediate in glycolysis. Hereditary fructose intolerance is a condition in which aldolase activity is impaired. The resultant fructosemia and accumulation of F1P may inhibit glycogenolysis and gluconeogenesis. Fructose can also be converted by sorbitol dehydrogenase to sorbitol, which is then converted to G6P. Galactose is formed from lactose, especially in infants. The galactose is then phosphorylated by galactokinase to galactose-1-

phosphate (Gal.1P). Gal.1P reacts with uridine diphosphoglucose (UDP-glucose) in the presence of Gal.1P uridyl transferase to form UDP-galactose and G1P. The UDP-galactose is then converted to UDP-glucose by the enzyme UDP-galactose-4-epimerase (Fig. 7).

In classic galactosemia, the uridyl transferase enzyme is deficient and Gal.1P accumulates. Some of the Gal.1P is converted to galactitol (an alcohol), which is probably sufficiently toxic to account for the cataracts observed in galactosemic patients.

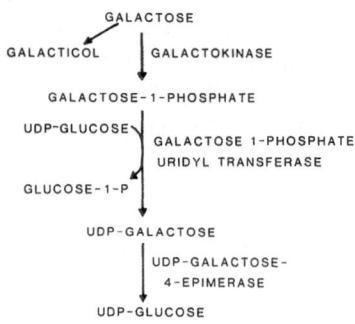

Figure 7. Pathway for the conversion of galactose to glucose in the liver.

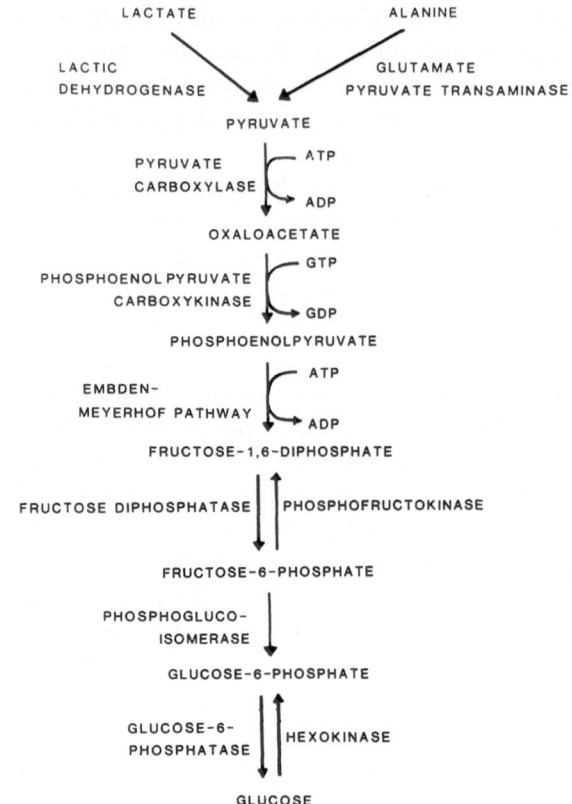

Figure 8. The stepwise pathway for conversion of lactate, pyruvate, and alanine to glucose in the liver.

5.6. Gluconeogenesis

Glucose may be formed from nonglucose sources in a series of gluconeogenic reactions. Gluconeogenic sources include lactate, pyruvate, oxaloacetate by the enzyme pyruvate carboxylase. The oxaloacetate is then converted reversibly to phosphoenolpyruvate by the enzyme phosphoenolpyruvate carboxykinase (PEPCK) in the presence of guanosine triphosphate (GTP) (Fig. 8). Pyruvate conversion to phosphoenolpyruvate is in delicate balance with the alternative reaction which converts pyruvate to acetylcoenzyme A, which is utilized in the TCA cycle. During starvation, diabetes, or glucocorticoid treatment, the synthesis of PEPCK is increased and acetylcoenzyme A tends to accumulate. This results in a preferential conversion of pyruvate to phosphoenolpyruvate and glucose. In other reactions analogous to the Cori cycle, alanine and glutamine are transported to the liver from muscle and other tissues. Within the liver they are deaminated. Alanine is thereby converted to pyruvate, which is utilized for glucose synthesis. Within the

liver, the amino groups are converted into urea, which cannot be produced in other tissues. The amino acid cycles are completed when glucose is converted into these amino acids in muscle [50].

5.7. Lipid metabolism

The major energy source for metabolism in liver cells is derived from fatty acids. These fatty acids are present in the blood as free fatty acids and are synthesized in the hepatocytes from carbohydrates and amino acids. The supply of free fatty acids in the circulation is normally high. Some is derived from the digestion of dietary fat and the rest comes from the mobilization of stored lipid in adipose tissue.

Fatty acids are oxidized within hepatic mitochondria by ß-oxidation to yield acetyl-CoA. Two ATP molecules are utilized in the oxidation of each molecule of stearic acid to acetyl-CoA, but 40 molecules of ATP and nine molecules of acetyl-CoA are produced. The acetyl-CoA is available for oxidation in the tricarboxylic acid (TCA) cycle to yield 12 additional ATP molecules for each acetyl-CoA unit that is oxidized. Thus, the complete oxidation of one stearic acid molecule can yield up to 146 ATP molecules.

Within the liver, the ß-oxidation reactions yield acetyl-CoA and sufficient ATP for most of the energy needs of this organ, especially when supplemented by ATP produced during carbohydrate metabolism and oxidation of some of the acetyl-CoA. Most of the acetyl-CoA is condensed to form acetylacetate instead of being oxidized within the liver. This acetylacetate is then partially converted to ß-hydroxybutyrate and acetone. The acetylacetate and ß-hydroxybutyrate are liberated into the blood as ketone bodies to be transported to muscle and other tissues where they can be used as energy sources.

Only a fraction of the fatty acid molecules entering the liver cells are oxidized to supply energy for other metabolic activities in the liver. Most of the fatty acid molecules are esterified with a-glycerophosphate to form triglycerides. The triglycerides are then combined with phospholipids, cholesterol, cholesterol esters, and protein in the endoplasmic reticulum and Golgi complex of the hepatocytes to produce complex lipoproteins. The lipoproteins are released into blood, where further modifications to their structure occur. Plasma lipoproteins are considered to be composed of cell membrane lipoproteins derived from intracellular membranes sequestered in secretory granules by the Golgi complex [51, 52]. The lipoproteins appear to be released at the cell surface as the secretory granules fuse with the plasma membrane. Within the blood, several lipoprotein fractions, differing in density from the very low (VLDL) to the high-density lipoproteins (HDL), are found. The major component, VLDL, releases fatty acids under the influence of lipoprotein lipase, for local utilization in adipose tissue and other sites.

Most, or all, of the fatty acids synthesized from nonlipid dietary sources are formed in the liver and in adipose tissue. The synthesis of fatty acids is dependent on carbohydrate intake in the diet and is favored by increased tissue utilization of glucose and a reduction in circulating free fatty acids. A high-carbohydrate diet results in increased glucose uptake into hepatocytes under the stimulating in-fluence of insulin. Increased production of a-glycerophosphate occurs and this is utilized in the esterification of fatty acids to form triglycerides.

Liver lipid metabolism is very sensitive to toxins including ethanol, ethionine, and orotic acid, which have been investigated in detail. Ethionine interferes with the synthesis of apoprotein B, an essential component of VLDL. This results in accumulation of fat droplets in the hepatocyte cytoplasm. The rate of accumulation of fat droplets influenced by the plasma free fatty acid concentration which in turn may be dependent on the rate of lipolysis in adipose tissue. Ethionine induction of fatty liver can be reduced or prevented by adenine which lowers the plasma free fatty acid concentration [53] and reduces the rate of triglyceride uptake and accumulation within hepatocytes.

In cholestasis, an abnormal lipoprotein designated 'lipoprotein X' may appear in plasma [54]. Probably this lipoprotein is formed from a precursor which is normally secreted into bile. In cholestasis, this material spills over into the plasma where it becomes attached to albumin as lipoprotein. The appearance of this lipoprotein in plasma can help in the differentiation of biliary atresia from neonatal hepatitis [55].

5.8. Protein synthesis and secretion

The liver plays a strategic role in regulating amino acid available to the rest of the body and in the utilization of absorbed amino acids from the digestive tract. In a study of dogs, 57% of amino acid nitrogen absorbed after a large protein meal was converted to urea in the liver, 15% was retained as liver protein and 6% was used in the synthesis of plasma proteins in the hepatocytes. Those protein were then secreted. Only 23% entered the circulation as free amino acids to be utilized by other tissues [56].

The protein synthetic capacity of the liver is impressive. All of the plasma proteins except most of the immunoglublulins are synthesized in the liver. In man, hepatic protein synthesis has been studied with labeled amino acids. In addition, uptake studies have utilized nonmetabolized amino acids including alpha-amino isobutyric acid. The general process involves transcription of specific RNA species by nuclear DNA; release of three types of RNA into the cytoplasm; messenger RNA which provides the code for the specific protein to be synthesized; ribosomal RNA which reads the messenger RNA: and transfer RNA species which transfer activated amino acids to the growing peptide chain. Ribosomes containing ribosomal RNA are connected in a chain on a single messenger RNA molecule to form polysomes. Some polysomes are attached to endoplasmic reticulum membranes, while others are free in the cytoplasm. Secretory proteins, including albumin, appear to be synthesized by the attached polysomes. Intracellular proteins, e.g., ferritin, are synthesized by free polysomes.

The major protein synthesized in the liver is albumin, which is released into the serum. At any time, about 30% of hepatocytes appear to be synthesizing albumin. In an adult man, the average production of albumin is 100–200 mg/kg/day. The circulating half-life is about 18–20 days. The normal serum albumin concentration is 3.5–5.0 g/100 ml. Hyperalbuminemia is only seen clinically in acute dehydration or occasionally in heroin or methadone addicts. Reduced albumin synthesis may occur in cirrhosis, although not always. Factors influencing albumin synthesis include: (a) nutritional uptake of amino acids, (b) plasma oncotic pressure, (c) circulating hormone levels, and (d) general homeostatic state.

Nutrition is the most important regulator of albumin synthesis. Dietary insufficiency of essential amino acids results in impaired protein synthesis. The balance of individual amino acids as well as the total availability of amino acids are important. Because tryptophan is the least abundant amino acid in the intracellular liver pool of amino acids, rats fed a tryptophan-deficient diet show a more pronounced depression of ^{14}C-leucine incorporation into peptides in the liver than they do with diets deficient in other essential amino acids.

The serum albumin level is depressed in malnutrition and albumin synthesis falls to 50–100 mg/kg/day. This depression in albumin synthesis in response to reduced amino acid intake occurs despite the recycling of amino acids during protein catabolism in the body.

The metabolism of dietary protein is not significantly altered in patients with stable cirrhosis, indicating that absorption, digestion, and utiliza-

tion of protein remains adequate [57]. Cirrhotic patients maintained on a low-protein diet (2 g) for 8–10 days can conserve nitrogen normally, but a high-protein diet (120 g/day) for the same time period can result in an unusually high retention of nitrogen and low urea synthesis. Although average total body nitrogen is often within normal limits, the distribution between the liver and other organs may be altered, suggesting that regeneration and healing processes in the liver may cause nitrogen to be removed from other tissues. This could explain the muscle wasting often associated with cirrhosis.

In kwashiorkor, where there is severe protein deprivation and moderate calorie insufficiency, fatty liver associated with edema and ascites is consistently observed. The fatty change in the liver is associated with low plasma cholesterol, triglyceride, and phospholipid concentrations and increased free fatty acid levels. The hypothesis that there is a reduced synthesis of the apoproteins for very low density lipoproteins (VLDL) and impaired release of triglycerides in kwashiorkor has been proposed to account for the observed intrahepatic accumulation of lipids. Experimental studies with primates lends support for this concept]58].

An imbalance in the relative abundance of aromatic amino acids (phenylalanine, tyrosine, and tryptophane) and methionine compared with the branched chain amino acids (leucine, isoleucine, and valine) has been observed in a variety of liver disorders. The aromatic amino acids and methionine are catabolized mainly in the liver while the branched chain amino acids are catabolized predominantly in muscle and other tissues. In patients with fulminant hepatitis and those with cirrhosis and hepatic encephalopathy, the plasma levels of aromatic amino acids are elevated, but the branched chain amino acids are normal or decreased in plasma concentration. By influencing the entry of phenylalanine and tryptophan into the central nervous system, it has been suggested that these severe liver disorders indirectly lead to increased neural synthesis of serotonin and decreased catecholamine formation]59]. A depression of neural function produced in this way could conceivably be corrected by appropriate amino acid infusion to reduce the tendency toward the development of hepatic coma.

It would be helpful to be able to assess the general status of protein metabolism in the liver with appropriate markers. Recent tests include the ratio of plasma alpha-amino butyric acid to leucine (A:L) and the measurement of maximal rate of urea synthesis (MRUS). The A:L ratio is affected by a number of factors including dietary protein intake, the presence of hepatocellular disease, and chronic alcohol consumption [60]. The MRUS is reduced early in the development of cirrhosis before the development of hyperammonemia and it may predict the level of tolerance for dietary protein in cirrhotics. Measurement of MRUS may be helpful in evaluating the risk of encephalopathy [61].

After infection or inflammation, the plasma levels of a number of alpha-globulins are raised. These include haptoglobulin, ceruloplasmin, and alpha$_1$-acid glycoprotein. The liver is the only known site for the synthesis of these 'acute-phase' proteins. Other proteins produced predominantly in the liver include transferrin, high-density and low-density lipoproteins, fibrinogen, and pro-thrombin. The Kupffer cells in mammalian liver are known to synthesize complement components C_2, C_3 and C_4. Other components may also be formed in the liver.

At least nine inhibitors of proteolytic enzymes are found in normal human plasma. They are essential for normal control of enzymatic processes and are synthesized, apparently exclusively, in the liver. The plasma levels of these proteins are elevated or unchanged in almost all patients with liver disease unless hepatocellular destruction is almost complete. Exceptions include a reduction in anti-thrombin levels in most adult cirrhotic patients, probably due to utilization in response to thrombin activation. Alpha$_1$-antitrypsin deficiency can occur due to an inherited deficiency [62].

Alpha$_1$-antitrypsin represents 80%–90% of the trypsin inhibitory capacity of serum. This protein is the predominant alpha-1-globulin band in serum electrophoretograms stained with routine protein stains. At least 18 genetic variants of alpha-1-antitrypsin have been recognized electrophoretically at pH 4.95. The most common phenotype, protease inhibitor PiMM, occurs in over 92% of American caucasians and blacks. A decreased plasma antitrypsin level is found with four Pi alleles, and at least one, the PiZ protein, may be reduced in the circulation due to decreased release from hepatocytes. Because the synthesis of PiZ alpha-1-anti-trypsin is not decreased relative to PiM, there is a pronounced intrahepatic accumulation of this protein.

Genetic deficiency of alpha-1-antitrypsin has been associated with childhood cirrhosis and also with chronic obstructive pulmonary disease. In both conditions the PiZ protein has been demonstrated in serum. Between 10% and 20% of children with PiZZ alpha-1-antitrypsin develop liver disease in childhood. Most of these children develop so-called neonatal giant-cell hepatitis and cholestasis during the first two months of life. Some of these children develop severe liver failure and die before six years of age. Many, however, recover, but develop cirrhosis after a latent period of weeks to years. Chronic obstructive pulmonary disease associated with PiZZ alpha-1-antitrypsin is seen in 25%–30% patients with early onset emphysema. Usually no pulmonary changes are seen in most individuals with PiZZ alpha-1-antitrypsin until after puberty, and children with liver disease and alpha-1-antitrypsin deficiency do not usually develop obvious pulmonary changes. Although some reports of simultaneous hepatic and pulmonary disease in adults with alpha-1-antitrypsin deficiency have appeared, there is no evidence that a patient with hepatic disease associated with PiZZ protein will necessarily develop pulmonary disease or vice versa.

Although accumulation of PiZZ protein inside hepatocytes has been demonstrated with electron microscopy and immunocytochemistry, it seems unlikely that this is the major cause of the hepatocellular disease because similar accumulations occur in PiZZ patients without evidence of hepatic pathological changes. Normally alpha-1-antitrypsin is distributed randomly among the hepatocytes, but in individuals with the PiZ gene, most of the protease inhibitor is in the periportal cells. The pathogenesis of the hepatic disease remains obscure.

5.9. Metabolism of hormones and drugs

The liver is a major site for the degradation of hormones, especially steroids, and many drugs. It was pointed out by Williams [63] that enzymatic reactions catalyze the metabolic transformation of drugs in two general phases. The first phase, which is characterized by oxidation, reduction, or hydrolytic reactions, may modify a drug by converting one functional group into another, or by adding polar groups to nonpolar compounds. The second phase includes reactions that conjugate the drug or its first-phase product with glucuronate, sulfate, or amino acids. Acylation and methylation may also occur as a phase-two reaction.

The oxidative metabolism of drugs is catalyzed by oxygen and NADPH-requiring enzymes (mixed-function oxidases) in the hepatocyte endoplasmic reticulum. The drug combines with a carbon-monoxide-sensitive hemoprotein 'cytochrome P-450' in its oxidized form. The complex is then reduced by NADPH-cytochrome-C-reductase. The reduced complex then reacts with oxygen and an electron from NADPH of NADH to form an unstable complex which breaks down to form oxidized cytochrome P-450 and oxidized drug.

Alcohols appear to be oxidized in the liver in at least three processes [64, 65]. The main pathway for ethyl alcohol oxidation utilizes alcohol dehydrogenase which is generally located in the portal areas of the hepatic lobules and requires NAD^+ as a hydrogen acceptor. The alcohol is converted to an aldehyde by the NAD^+ enzyme complex.

Ethyl alcohol may also be oxidized to acetaldehyde by catalase in liver peroxisomes. This pathway is not the main oxidation route for ethyl alcohol but it may be the main one for methanol. The catalase reaction requires a source of H_2O_2 to oxidize ethanol. This can be provided in peroxisomes by various oxidases including xanthine oxidase [65]:

$$\text{hypoxanthine} \xrightarrow[\text{H}_2\text{O} + \text{O}_2]{\text{xanthine oxidase}} \text{uric acid} + \text{H}_2\text{O}_2$$
$$\text{(xanthine)}$$

$$H_2O_2 + CH_3CH_2OH \xrightarrow{\text{catalase}} 2H_2O + CH_3CHO$$

The importance of ethanol metabolism by catalase in man has not been established. It may be minor under normal circumstances but could be significant after prolonged ethanol ingestion.

The third mechanism for oxidizing alcohols in the liver has been the subject of considerable research in the last decade, following its postulation in the 1960s. This mechanism implies that there is a microsomal ethanol-oxidizing system (MEOS) analogous or identical to the NADPH-requiring microsomal drug-metabolizing system. While the evidence for the operation of a MEOS is persuasive, its quantitative significance is uncertain. According to Lieber and DeCarli [66], about 25% of ingested ethanol can be metabolized by this system normally, but the role of the MEOS may be much greater after prolonged ethanol consumption.

Enzymes catalyzing the hydrolysis of amides and esters are present in mammalian, including human, liver. They are localized in the endoplasmic reticulum of hepatocytes. Included in this group are the so-called nonspecific esterases with varying substrate specificity to aliphatic and aromatic esters. The number of such enzyme species is unknown, but studies with a variety of substrates and inhibitors have demonstrated broad categories and number of enzyme species within each category.

Phase-two reactions involve the conjugation of the polar groups of a drug or drug metabolites with glucuronate, sulfate from the foreign compound or from an energy-rich phosphate source. Microsomal glucuronyl transferases in hepatocytes conjugate UDPGA to phenols, alcohols, carboxylic acids, and many other substances in a reaction resembling the conjugation of UDPGA with bilirubin. A number of sulfuryl transferases also conjugate phenols, alcohols, and aromatic amines with 3'-phosphoadenosine-5'-phosphosulfate (which itself is formed from ATP and sulfate). In addition, different enzymes catalyze the conjugation of glutathione with epoxides, halides, hydroxylamines, and other compounds. Methylation reactions are catalyzed by a number of enzymes utilizing S-adenosylmethionine, formed from ATP and methionine as substrate. With such an array of transferases in the endoplasmic reticulum and cytosol of hepatocytes, it is not surprising that a foreign compound may be converted by several different enzymes in several reactions to a variety of different metabolic products.

Acknowledgments. The author gratefully acknowledges the expert assistance of Mary Jo Swartzberg and Sharon (Mattimoe) Fitzgerald in the preparation of this manuscript. This work was supported by NIH grant AM-21380.

REFERENCES

1. Walsh SZ, Lind J (1978) In: The fetal circulation and its alteration at birth. In: Stave U (ed) Perinatal physiology. New York: Plenum Medical, pp 129–180
2. Madding GF, Kennedy PA (1971) Trauma to the liver, 2nd edn. Philadelphia: WB Saunders
3. Bengmark S, Rozengren K (1970) Angiographic study of the collateral circulation to the liver after ligation of the hepatic artery in man. Am J Surg 119:620–624
4. Bradley SE (1979) Hepatic lymph formation – basic mechanisms and dysfunctions. In: Davidson CS (ed) Problems in liver disease. New York: Stratton Intercontinental Medical, pp 53–65
5. Motta P, Porter K (1974) Structure of rat liver sinusoids and associated tissue space as revealed by scanning electron microscopy. Cell Tissue Res 148:111–125
6. Wisse E (1970) An electron microscopic study of the fenestrated endothelial lining of rat liver sinusoids. J Ultrastruct Res 31:125–150
7. Dive C, Nadalini RA, Heremans JF (1974) Origin and nature of the proteins of bile. II. A comparative analysis of serum, hepatic lymph and bile proteins in the dog. Eur J Clin Invest 4:241–246
8. Layden TJ, Elias E, Boyer JL (1978) Bile formation in the rat. The role of the paracellular shunt pathway. J Clin Invest 62:1375–1385
9. Bradley SE, Morris TQ, Baker KJ (1974) Characterization of taurocholate-induced proteobilia in the dog. In: Matern S, Hackenschmidt J, Back P, Gerok W (eds) Advances in bile acid research. III. Bile acid meeting. Stuttgart: Schattauer, pp 74–78
10. Barnhart JL, Combes B (1978) Erythritol and manitol clearances with taurocholate and secretin induced choleresis. Am J Physiol 234:E146–E156
11. Hardison WGM, Wood CA (1978) Importance of bicarbonate in bile salt independent fraction of bile flow. Am J Physiol 235:E158–E164
12. Hanson RF, Pries JM (1977) Synthesis and enterohepatic circulation of bile salts. Gastroenterology 73:611–618
13. Bloch K, Berg BN, Rittenberg D (1943) The biological conversion of cholesterol to cholic acid. J Biol Chem 149:511–517
14. Mitropoulus KA (1974) The biosynthesis of bile acids and its control. In: Matern S, Hackenschmidt J, Back P, Gerok K (eds) Advances in bile acid research. III Bile acid meeting. Stuttgart: Schattauer, pp 53–59
15. Anderson KE, Kok E, Javitt NB (1972) Bile acid synthesis in man. Metabolism of 7-alpha hydroxycholesterol-^{14}C and 26-hydroxycholesterol-^{3}H. J Clin Invest 51:112–117
16. Jenner RE, Howard ER (1975) Unsaturated monohydroxy bile acids as a cause of idiopathic obstructive cholangiopathy. Lancet 2:1073–1075
17. Jacobson JG, Smith LH (1968) Biochemistry and physiology of taurine and taurine derivatives. Physiol Rev 48:424–511
18. Reichen J, Paumgartner G (1976) Uptake of bile acids by the perfused rat liver. Am J Physiol 231:734–742
19. Steiner O, Sanger L, Stein Y (1974) Colchicine-induced inhibition of lipoprotein and protein secretion into serum and lack of interference with secretion of biliary phospholipids and cholesterol by rat liver in vivo. J Cell Biol 62:90–103
20. Gregory DH, Vlahcevic ZR, Prugl MF, Swell L (1978) Mechanism of secretion of biliary lipids: role of a microtubular system in hepatocellular transport of biliary lipids in the rat. Gastroenterology 74:93–100
21. Gregory DH, Vlahcevic ZR, Schatzki P, Swell L (1975) Mechanism of secretion of biliary lipids I. Role of bile canalicular and microsomal membranes in the synthesis and transport of biliary lecithin and cholesterol. J Clin Invest 55:105–114
22. Wheeler HO (1972) Secretion of bile acids by the liver and their role in the formation of hepatic bile. Arch Int Med 130:533–541
23. Evans H, Kremmer T, Culvenor JG (1976) Role of membranes in bile formation. Comparison of the composition of bile and a liver bile canalicular plasma membrane subfraction. Biochem J 154:589–595
24. Small DM (1975) The formation and treatment of gallstones. In: Schiff L (ed) Diseases of the liver. Philadelphia: Lippincott, pp 146–162
25. Carey MC, Small DM (1970) The characteristics of mixed micellar solutions with particular reference to bile. Am J Med 49:590–608
26. Habig WH, Papst MJ, Gleischner G, Gatmaitan Z, Arias IM, Jakoby WB (1974) The identity of glutathione S-transferase B with ligandin, a major binding protein of liver. Proc Natl Acad Sci USA 71:3879–3882
27. Wolkoff AW (1980) The glutathione S-transferases: their role in the transport of organic anions from blood to bile. Int Rev Physiol 21:151–169
28. Kamisaka K, Gatmaitan Z, Moore CL, Arias IM (1975) Ligandin reverses bilirubin inhibition of liver mitochondrial respiration in vitro. Pediatr Res 9:903–905
29. Fevery J, Van Dawne B, Michiels R, DeGroote J, Heirwegh KPM (1972) Bilirubin conjugates in bile of man and rat in the normal state and in liver disease. J Clin Invest 51:2482–2492
30. Fevery J, Van de Vijver M, Michiels R, Heirwegh KPM (1977) Comparison in different species of biliary bilirubin IX conjugates with the activities of hepatic and renal bilirubin IX uridine diphosphate glycosyltransferases. Biochem J 164:737–746
31. Forker EL (1977) Mechanisms of hepatic bile formation. Annu Rev Physiol 39:323–347
32. Sisson TRC (1978) Blood volume. In: Stave U (ed) Perinatal physiology. New York: Plenum Medical, pp 181–198
33. Daust R (1958) The cell population of liver tissue and the cytological reference bases. In: Brauer RW (ed) Liver function. Washington DC: Am Inst Biol Sci, pp 3–23
34. Blouin A (1977) Morphometry of liver sinusoidal cells. In: Wisse E, Knook EL (eds) Kupffer cells and other liver sinusoidal cells. Amsterdam: Elsevier/North-Holland, pp 61–71
35. Salky NK, DiLuzio NR, P'Pool DB, Sutherland AJ (1964) Evaluation of reticuloendothelial function in man. JAMA 187:744–748
36. Wisse E (1972) An ultrastructural characterization of the endothelial cell in the rat liver sinusoid under normal and various experimental conditions, as a contribution to the distinction between endothelial Kupffer cells. J Ultrastruct Res 38:528–562
37. Motta P (1977) Kupffer cells as revealed by scanning electron microscopy. In: Wisse E, Knook DL (eds) Kupffer cells and other liver sinusoidal cells. Amsterdam: Elsevier/North-Holland, pp 93–103
38. Fahimi HD (1970) The fine structural localization of endogenous and exogenous peroxidase activity in Kupffer cells of rat liver. J Cell Biol 47:247
39. Widmann JJ (1972) Mononuclear phagocytes (Kupffer cells)

136

and endothelial cells. Identification of two functional cell types in rat liver sinusoids by endogenous peroxidase activity. J Cell Biol 52:159

40. Stohr G, Deimann W, Fahimi HD (1978) Peroxidase-positive endothelial cells in sinusoids of the mouse liver. J Histochem Cytochem 26:409–411

41. Sindelar WF, Costa J, Ketcham AS (1978) Osteosarcoma associated with therotrast administration. Cancer 42:2604–2609

42. Roos E, Dingemans KP (1977) Phagocytosis of tumor cells by Kupffer cells in vivo and in the perfused mouse liver. In: Wisse E, Knook DL (eds) Kupffer cells and other sinusoidal cells. Amsterdam: Elsevier/North-Holland, pp 183–190

43. Prytz H, Holst-Christensen J, Korner B, Liehr H (1976) Portal venous and systemic endotoxemia in patients without liver disease and systemic endotoxemia in patients with cirrhosis. Scand J Gastroenterol 11:857–863

44. Liehr H, Grun M (1977) Clinical aspects of Kupffer cell failure in liver diseases. In: Wisse E, Knook DL (eds) Kupffer cells and other liver sinusoidal cells. Amsterdam: Elsevier/North-Holland, pp 427–436.

45. Kajihara H, Yokoro K, Mochizuki T (1977) Structural changes of sinusoidal cells of the dog liver in hemorrhagic shock. In: Wisse E, Knook DL (eds) Kupffer cells and other liver sinusoidal cells. Amsterdam: Elsevier/North-Holland, pp 201–212

46. Gale RP, Sparkes RS, Golde DW (1978) Bone marrow origin of hepatic macrophages (Kupffer cells) in humans. Science 201:937–938

47. Crofton RW, Diesselhoff-den Dulk MMC, Furth R van (1978) The origin, kinetics, and characteristics of the Kupffer cells in the normal steady state. J Exp Med 148:1–17

48. Altszuler N, Finegold MJ (1974) Glucose metabolism. In: Becker FF (ed) The liver, normal and abnormal functions. Part A. New York: Marcel Dekker, pp 463–529

49. Jeffcoate SL, Moody AJ (1969) The role of the liver in the disposal of orally administered ^{14}C-glucose in the normal rat. Diabetologia 5:293–299

50. Ruderman NB (1975) Muscle aminoacid metabolism and gluconeogenesis. Annu Rev Med 26:245–258

51. Eisenberg s, Levy RI (1975) Lipoprotein metabolism. Adv Lipid Res 13:1–89

52. Villa-Trevino S, Shull KH, Farber E (1963) The role of adenosine triphosphate deficiency in ethionine-induced inhibition of protein synthesis. J Biol Chem 238:1757–1763

53. Glaser G, Mager J (1972) Biochemical studies on the mechanism of action in liver poisons: II. Induction of fatty livers. Biochem Biophys Acta 261:500–507

54. Seidel D, Alaupovic P, Furman RH (1969) A lipoprotein characterising obstructive jaundice. I. Method for quantitative separation and identification of lipoproteins in jaundiced subjects. J Clin Invest 48:1211–1223

55. Poley JR, Magnani HN (1976) Cholestatic jaundice in infancy. Diagnosis, differential diagnosis and treatment. Aust Paediatr J 12:134–153

56. Elwyn DH, Parikh HC, Shoemaker WC (1968) Aminoacid movements between gut, liver and periphery in unanesthetized dogs. Am J Physiol 215:1260–1275

57. Chopra S, Schimmel EM (1979) The precarious balance – protein metabolism in liver disease. In: Davidson CS (ed) Problems in liver diseases. New York: Stratton Intercontinental, pp 64–79

58. Kumar V, Deo MG, Ramalingaswamy V (1972) Mechanism of fatty liver in protein deficiency. Gastroenterology 62:445–451

59. Freund H, Yoshimura N, Fischer JE (1979) Chronic hepatic encephalopathy. Long-term therapy with a branched-chain amino-acid-enriched elemental diet. JAMA 242:347–349

60. Shaw S, Lieber CS (1978) Plasma aminoacid abnormalities in the alcoholic. Gastroenterology 74:667–682

61. Rudman D, DiFulco TJ, Galambos JT (1973) Maximal rates of excretion and synthesis of urea in normal and cirrhotic subjects. J Clin Invest 52:2241–2249

62. Johnson M (1974) Antiproteases and the liver. In: Becker FF (ed) The liver; normal and abnormal functions. Part A. New York: Marcel Dekker, pp 103–128

63. Williams RT (1959) Detoxification mechanisms, 2nd edn. New York: John Wiley and Sons

64. Comporti M (1978) Ethanol-induced liver injury. In: Slater TF (ed) Biochemical mechanisms of liver injury. New York: Academic, pp 469–516

65. Khanna JM, Israel Y (1980) Ethanol metabolism. Int Rev Physiol 21:275–315

66. Lieber CS, DeCarli LM (1972) The role of hepatic microsomal ethanol oxidizing system (MEOS) for ethanol metabolism in vivo. J Pharmacol Exp Ther 181:279–288

9. ELECTRON MICROSCOPY IN HUMAN LIVER PATHOLOGY

R. Laschi and C.A. Busachi

1. INTRODUCTION

The liver was the first human organ to be studied by electron microscopy owing to the fact that it is easy to obtain bioptic samples. The liver cell immediately represented an admirable model of complex macromolecular organization in which structure could be identified with function. A great deal of data and information emerged from this, followed by critical comment and reexamination, given the overlap of different aspecific factors and the difficulty in defining a description of the 'normal liver' within precise limits (due to technical problems, functional and topographical modifications, and not wholly valid deductions between the liver of experimental animals and the human liver).

However, the contribution of electron microscopy has enabled a thorough study of the many pathogenetic mechanisms in liver diseases. In different situations this contribution has led to a better understanding of earlier data supplied by light microscopy and in some, albeit limited, cases it has proved a valid diagnostic tool [1].

2. CHOLESTASIS

The electron microscope enables a state of cholestasis to be identified even in the absence of manifest signs of jaundice. In fact, characteristic subcellular features can be detected at an early stage, corresponding to changes in the bile secretion apparatus.

The morphological patterns detectable during both intra- and extrahepatic cholestasis can be divided into essential and secondary [2, 3]. The essential ones involve the bile secretion apparatus and consist of:

– Dilatation of the canalicular lumen in varying degrees depending on the canaliculus, and along the course of the canaliculus itself (Fig. 1).

– Reduction in the number of microvilli in the biliary canaliculus to the point of disappearance. The residual microvilli appear irregular in various ways (stumpy, shortened, etc.) and sometimes resemble edematous microvillar blebs which may obstruct the actual canaliculus (Fig. 2).

– Increase in the winding course of the canaliculus, often combined with focal dilatations in the form of pockets, invaginations, and diverticula (canalicular diverticulosis). This combination of images of tortuosity and diverticulosis is called canalicular varicosis.

– Partial or total canalicular obstruction by accumulations of biliary material varying in appearance (homogeneous, granular, crystalline, lamellar, etc.) called thrombi or biliary plugs. These are probably made up of bile components and cellular debris such as fragments discharged from the pericanalicular ectoplasm and hepatocyte membranes, especially those making up the canalicular pole. At the ultrastructural level, these biliary thrombi appear in different forms: uniform, usually granular (recent thrombi, polymorphous, granular, vesicular membranous, lamellar [old thrombi]). These biliary concretions are also found in the widened intercellular spaces and the Disse space as well as the canaliculi.

– Thickening of the pericanalicular ectoplasm which sometimes shows signs of edema of the matrix which follows fragmentation.

– Widening of the intercellular spaces between adjacent hepatocytes with the development of microvilli on membranes opposite the dilated intercellular spaces.

P.M. Motta and L.J.A. DiDio (eds.), Basic and clinical hepatology, pp. 137–161. All rights reserved.

138

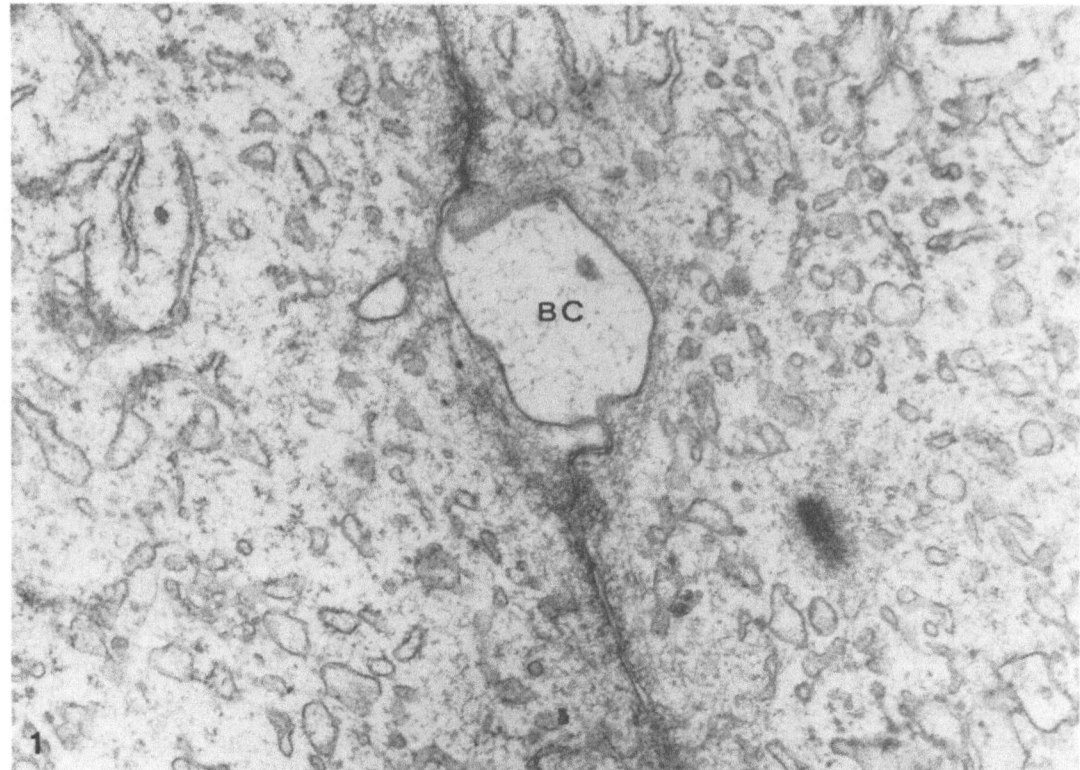

Figure 1. Cholestasis. Bile capillary (BC) dilated and without microvilli; ×16,000.

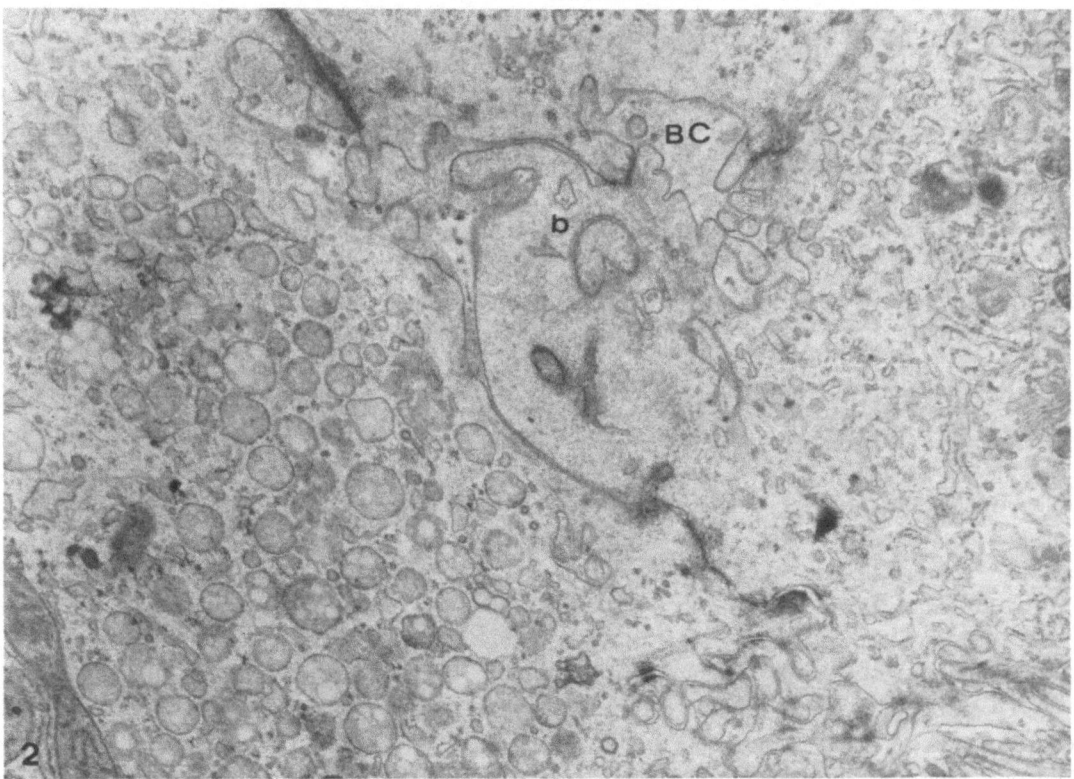

Figure 2. Cholestasis. Bile capillary (BC) showing the lumen partially occluded by a large cytoplasmic bleb (b); ×16,000.

The later secondary ultrastructural alterations include:

– Mitochondrial changes, some of which are undoubtedly aspecific (formation of myelin-like figures, better called onionoid bodies, a sign of mitochondrosis [4, 5], hyperplasia, megamitochondria, etc.), while others are considered to be more distinctive (widening and enrichment of the cristae to the formation of circular cristae).

– Dilatation, degranulation, and fragmentation of the cisternae of the rough endoplasmic reticulum which appears decreased in size with respect to normal although there seems to be an overall lipoprotein synthesis.

– Hypertrophy of the Golgi complex combined with a rearrangement of its components. In fact, the saccule membranes–vesicular membranes ratio of the hepatocytes in the periportal area becomes the equivalent of that of hepatocytes in the portal zone.

– Increase in the number of secondary lysosomes (such as lipofuscin granules), especially autophagic vacuoles. The increase in number of these organelles is found in all types of liver cell damage.

– Presence of special kinds of 'cellular inclusions', i.e., inclusions of bile pigment and pseudobiliary inclusions. In fact, as regards the former type of inclusions, it is thought that conjugated bilirubin is deposited in the cytoplasm in focal areas exposed to degenerative phenomena. Therefore there would initially be an irregular accumulation of finely granular and fibrillar material unsurrounded by membrane. In a following intermediate stage, the focal area of degeneration is thought to be sequestered and incorporated in an autophagic vacuole which later merges with lysosomal structures (including secondary ones) which discharge their enzyme content into the autophagolysosome lumen thus formed. In particular, betaglycuronidase is thought to catalyze the deconjugation of bilirubin diglucuronide. These mechanisms explain why longer-standing biliary inclusions are surrounded by a membrane and why their content reacts like unconjugated bilirubin. Pseudobiliary inclusions correspond to vacuoles surrounded by membrane containing osmiophilic material with a lamellar appearance, often arranged in a spiral and sometimes combined with variable amounts of granular material. The type of material chemically corresponding to these inclusions is not definitely known, but we do know that there is a very large number of inclusions in conditions of cellular damage optically defined as 'feathery degeneration'.

– Increase in the number of peroxysomes.

– Intracytoplasmic aggregates of microfilamentous nature in the hepatocytes of the periportal lamina, similar to the Mallory bodies of light microscopy. However, these are only found in long-standing cholestasis.

In order to understand pathogenetic mechanisms, particularly intrahepatic cholestasis, it is of fundamental importance to define which of these alterations are secondary to the pressure increase in the biliary tree and which, on the other hand, are primitive. The latter indicate the target structure on which the 'metabolic or chemical' etiologic factor acts (drugs, alcohol, virus, hereditary defects, etc.).

Experimental evidence implies an alteration in the metabolism of monohydroxylate biliary acids as the possible pathogenetic starting point. Since biliary acids are synthetized at the level of the smooth endoplasmic reticulum, particular importance has been ascribed to its ultrastructural changes as probable signs of a hydroxylation defect. Because the smooth endoplasmic reticulum appears hypertrophic in the course of cholestasis, the term 'hypoactive hypertrophic endoplasmic reticulum' was coined [6]. However, at the present time, alterations of the smooth endoplasmic reticulum are considered a result of cholestasis and not primary changes. Alterations of the rough endoplasmic reticulum, Golgi complex, mitochondria, and lysosomes are assessed in the same way.

Recent research has focused attention on the hepatocyte periphery. In fact, the canalicular membrane shows early, evident submicroscopic alterations in the course of cholestasis as well as appearing altered from the cytochemical and biochemical points of view. Alterations of the cytoskeletal components, microtubules, and microfilaments linked to integral proteins of the membrane are closely connected to changes in the plasmalemma. By acting on these proteins or on the microfilaments themselves, the pathogenic agent causes a break in the 'cytoskeleton–membrane' functional system. This lesion would be a warning sign of a reduction in tone of the canalicular plasma

140

membrane, with consequent dilatation of the canaliculus under increased biliary pressure. In relation to the pericanalicular ectoplasm, it has been demonstrated that there exists a rich population of contractile actin-like microfilaments forming a web-like structure similar to the terminal web of enterocytes, a structure which is particularly evident in canalicular microvilli [7]. Physiologically, it seems that these microfilaments play a fundamental role in the bile secretion process, and different experimental studies have shown that changes in the macromolecular structure of microfilaments can lead to an arrest in bile flow [8].

It has also been suggested that a morphofunctional alteration of contractile microfilaments lies at the basis of a considerable variety of cholestatic conditions in man [9].

However, there exist conditions of cholestasis, such as that induced by estrogens, which, due to the absence of detectable ultrastructural changes involving the biliary canaliculus, suggest that the primary lesion does not involve the cytoskeleton of the microvilli, but rather the ionic pump systems at the canalicular membrane level which regulate the secretion of fractions of biliary acids and electrolytes [10].

The hyperbilirubinemia of cholestatic jaundice can no longer be attributed to a reflux of bile into the blood through a widened junctional apparatus as was previously maintained. The current more probable hypothesis is that of so-called 'transhepatocytic regurgitation' through a retrograde diacytose process by means of vesicles through the hepatocyte cytoplasm or by inversion of the secretory polarity of hepatocytes.

3. VIRAL HEPATITIS

Electron microscopy has made a fundamental contribution to the study of the viruses responsible for hepatitis A, B and non-A non-B, enabling their morphological characterization and cellular localization to be established together with the antigens correlated to them.

3.1. Hepatitis type A virus (HAV)

This virus was observed for the first time in 1973

[11] in stools taken during the acute phase of the disease from volunteers experimentally infected with serum from patients suffering from hepatitis A. In 1974 [12], the presence of similar particles was demonstrated in the serum and liver of infected monkeys. It is a small virus (25–28 nm) with cubic symmetry and no external envelope or subunits. Both 'full' (unpenetrated by stain) and 'empty' (penetrable by stain) particles have been detected by immunoelectron microscopy. The 'empty' particles at low buoyant densities probably represent virions devoid of nucleic acid. However, these are immunologically indistinguishable from the 'full' particles. The nucleic acid contained in viral particles proved to be RNA, so that the virus should belong to the enterovirus group of picornaviruses [13]. HAV has been identified in the liver homogenate of infected marmosets by using immunoelectron microscopy [14] and later in bile, feces, and liver homogenate of experimentally infected chimpanzees [15].

Using an immunofluorescence technique, the presence of this viral antigen has been identified in the cytoplasm of hepatic cells from experimentally infected chimpanzees [15], and this finding was confirmed by an immunoperoxidase technique. The distribution of HAV was fine, granular, and 'scattered' throughout the cytoplasm, with complete negativity of the nucleus. Using immunoelectron microscopy, it has been possible to observe 27-nm particles in cytoplasmic vesicles and positive reaction at the level of vesicle membranes, rough endoplasmic reticulum, and polyribosomes [16].

The mechanism by which HAV causes hepatitis is still unknown. It remains to be established whether the virus has a cytopathic effect or whether it is the immune response to it which causes hepatocyte necrosis. Nevertheless, the majority of patients with type A viral hepatitis can expect a full recovery.

3.2. Hepatitis type B virus (HBV)

This virus corresponds morphologically to the 'Dane particle'. This is a spherical double-shelled particle with a diameter of 42 nm. It is a circular double-stranded virus composed of an inner core about 28 nm in diameter which can be immunologically and morphologically correlated with the hepatitis B core antigen (HBcAg), and a double outer shell corresponding, from an immunological point of view, to the hepatitis B surface antigen (HBsAg). The Dane particle was first identified in patients' serum by negative staining or by immunoelectron microscopy [13]. Later, it was possible to localize the particle at the ultrastructural level in the vesicles of the smooth endoplasmic reticulum [17, 18], and this finding was confirmed by immunoelectron microscopy [19]. The Dane particle has rarely been observed in the sinusoidal space [18].

This virus has at least four different types of antigen:

3.2.1. Hepatitis B core antigen (HBcAg) is the nuclear component of HBV. It has an icosahedral symmetry and measures around 27–28 nm with a 2-nm-thick envelope. HBcAg does not circulate freely, but has been identified by different authors both in the nucleus and in the cytoplasm of hepatocytes infected with HBV in the form of 'empty' or 'full' spherical particles (Figs. 3 and 4). These particles differ from those corresponding to the central part of HBV since the DNA is single-stranded and DNA polymerase is absent [20]. At high magnification it is possible to detect electron-dense subunits 2.5 nm in diameter closely connected to each other forming the envelope of the actual particle. The nucleus of the hepatocytes containing the HBcAg appears hypertrophic with marked rarefaction of the nucleoplasm and chromatin in the HBcAg-rich nuclei.

In poor HBcAg cases, these particles are evenly spread throughout the nucleoplasm without disturbing nuclear density. In some cases, HBcAg may be localized around the nuclear pores [18], and even in the perinuclear cisterna [21]. Its presence in the pars amorpha of the nucleoli has also been described [21, 22]. These particles can be found in the cytoplasm in small aggregates or as isolated particles scattered in the hyaloplasm [17], sometimes even in close proximity to the plasmalemma [23]. Similar particles with a blurred edge, hence called 'cloudy particles', have recently been observed [18], but their nature has yet to be assessed. Very rarely, aggregates of HBcAg have been localized in membrane structures, probably phagosomes.

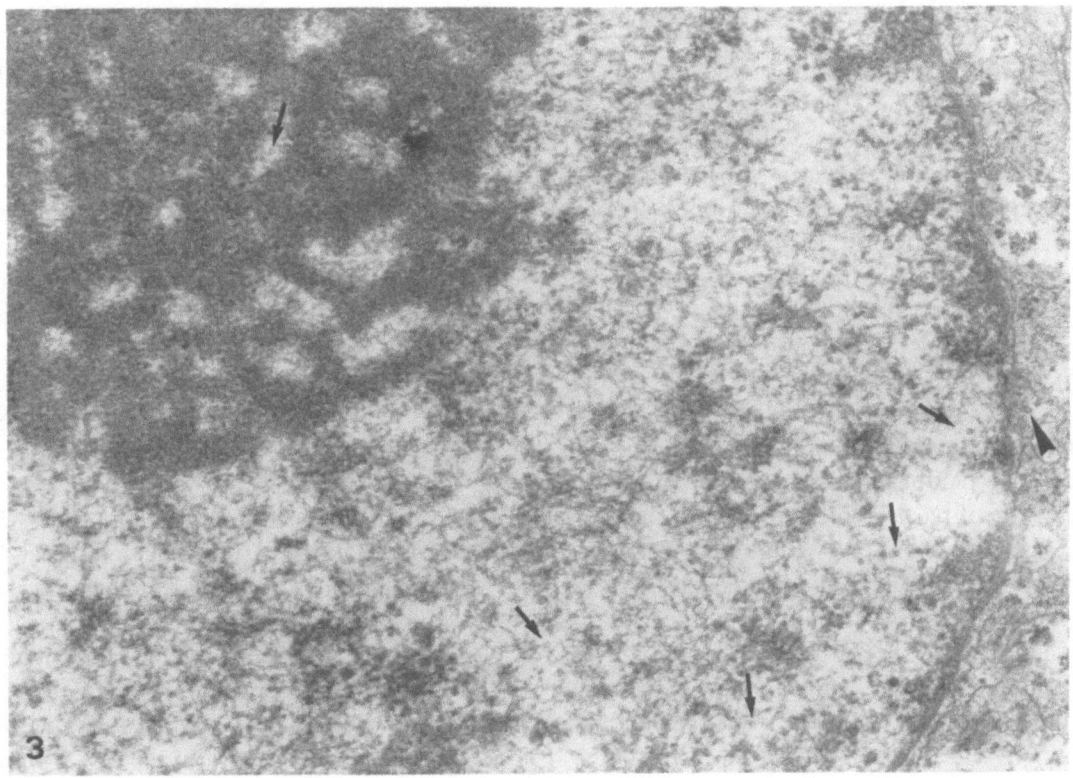

Figure 3. Hepatitis B. HBcAg in the nucleolus and nucleoplasm (arrows) and in the cytoplasm (arrowhead); × 36,000.

142

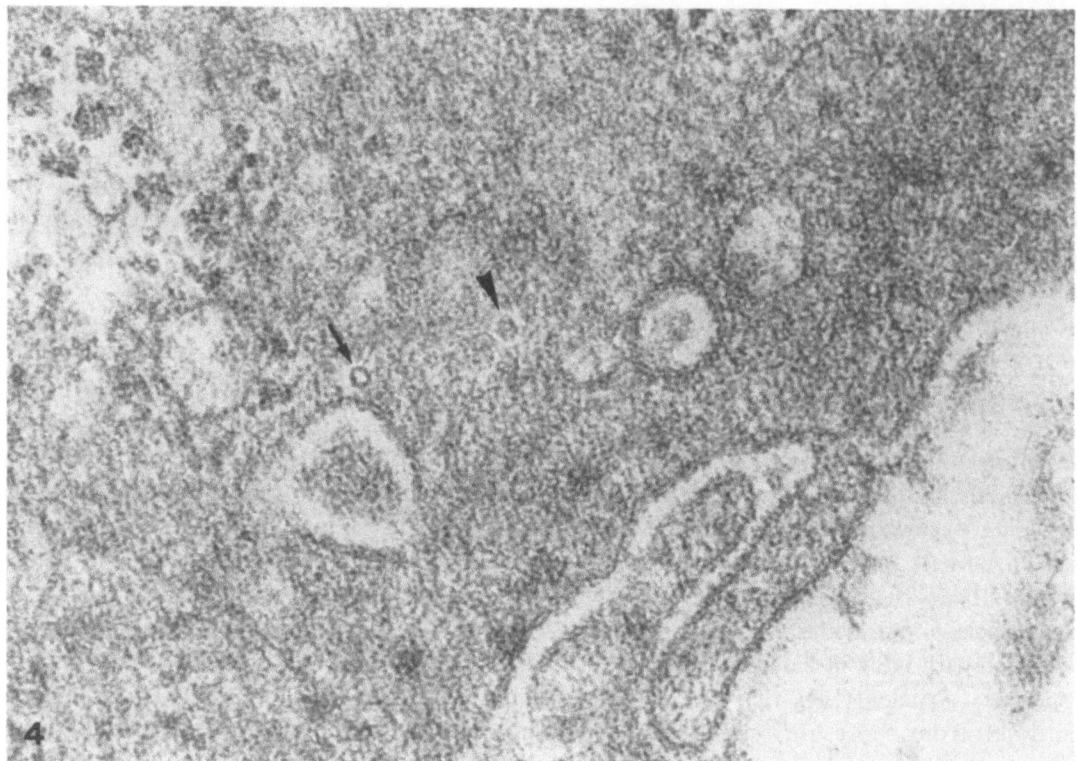

Figure 4. Hepatitis B. Empty (arrow) and full (arrowhead) HBcAg particles in the cytoplasm; ×140,000.

3.2.2. Hepatitis B surface antigen (HBsAg) can be found in the circulation by using negative staining or immunoelectron microscopy, both on the outer surface of HBV and in the form of particles 19–21 nm in diameter with a spherical or tubular shape – the latter varying in length between 50 and 230 nm [24]. Particles analogous to those observed in the serum have been identified within dilatated vesicles of the smooth and rough endoplasmic reticulum (Fig. 5) [25]. These particles made up of slightly electron-dense material may be spherical (with a diameter of around 35 nm and an electron-opaque core) or have a tubular shape variable in length. The first type of particle, often present in the same vesicle in groups of four or five, represent transverse sections of the second kind. No image ascribable to these particles has been identified in the hyaloplasm, the nucleus, or in the Golgi apparatus. Equivalent images, but with a diameter ranging 20–30 nm were later pointed out by other authors [26].

HBsAg can be found in several cytoplasmic zones of the hepatocyte or spread throughout the entire cytoplasm. With light microscopy, these hepatocytes present a cytoplasm characterized by a zone of fine, even, shiny eosinophilia and have been defined as 'ground-glass hepatocytes'. The study of this type of hepatocyte under the electron microscope has revealed a smooth, hypertrophic endoplasmic reticulum with dilatated cisternae containing the particles described above and a displacement of organelles to the periphery of the cell.

Localization of HBsAg at hepatocyte membrane level by using immunofluorescence and immunoperoxidase techniques [19, 27–29] has been interpreted as a sign of disease activity (Fig. 6). It is now accepted that HBV is not a cytopathic virus. Whatever the mechanism responsible for direct hepatocyte damage may be, viral antigens have to be found located around the plasma membrane. In this way the hepatocyte becomes a target structure for the immunocompetent reaction. Among the various antigens associated with HBV, it seems more and more probable that HBsAg is the one with a real 'target' function [23]. Nevertheless, ultrastructural research [18, 21] has not led to identification at this

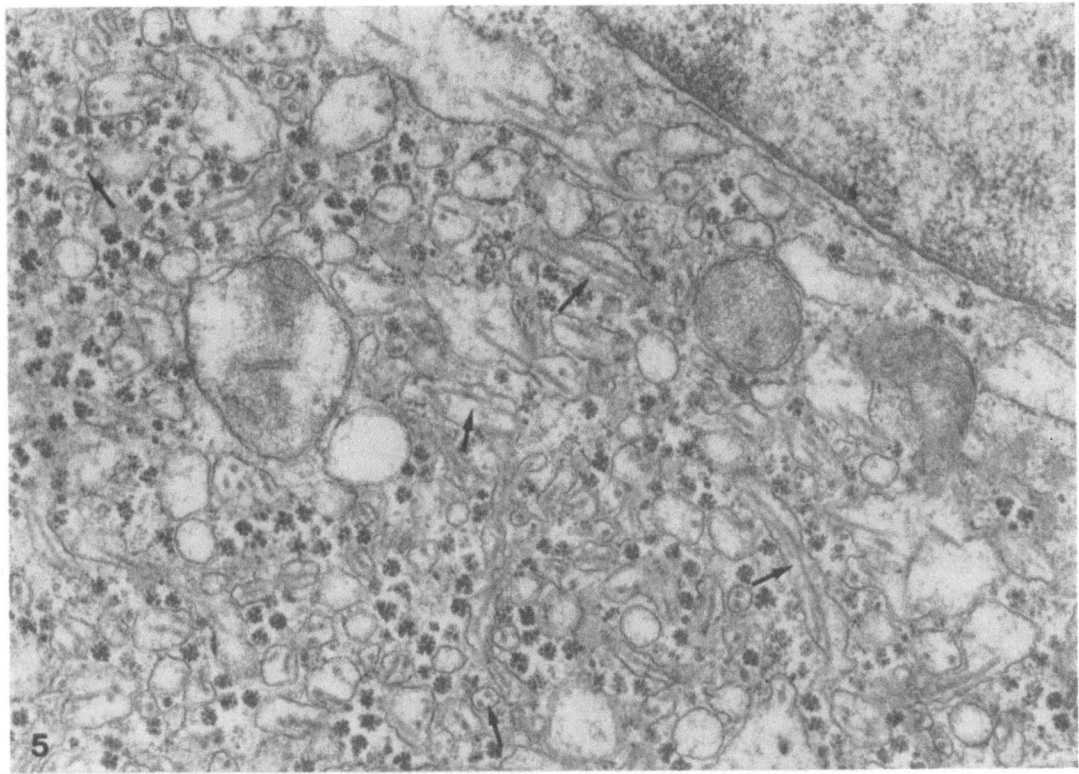

Figure 5. Hepatitis B. Clear evidence of HBsAg into the cisternae of smooth endoplasmic reticulum (arrows); × 36,000.

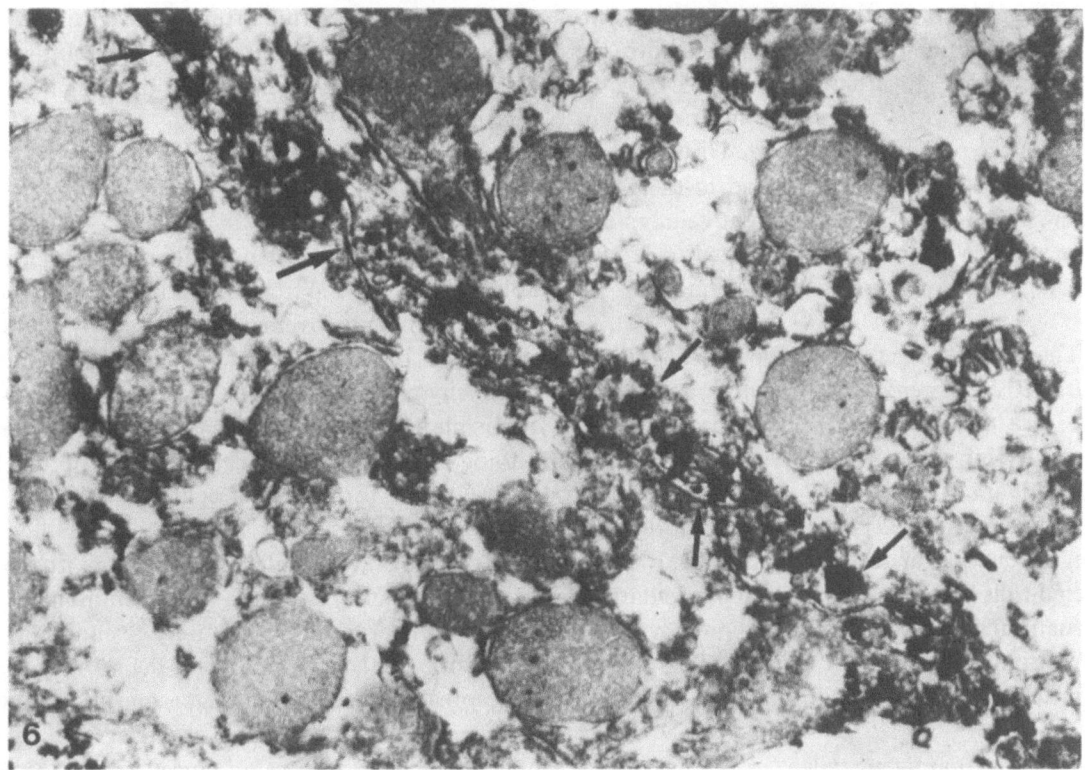

Figure 6. Hepatitis B. Immunoperoxidase technique. HBsAg localization on hepatocyte plasma membrane (arrows); × 36,000.

144

level of typical particles ascribable to HBsAg, even though a rearrangement of the plasmalemma has been detected.

Recent immunoelectron-microscopic studies [19, 30], have thoroughly characterized the two antigens, supplying further information on their exact localization, replication, and the way they are released from the hepatocyte. In some cases, the identification of HBcAg, mainly in ribosomes, free polyribosomes, and around the nuclear pores, but very rarely in the nuclei of the actual hepatocytes, has led to the hypothesis that this antigen is synthetized in the cytoplasm, migrates to the nucleus, and later returns to the cytoplasm [30] On the other hand, the localization of HBsAg in the perinuclear space in the cisternae of the endoplasmic reticulum and on its membranes, such as the hepatocyte membrane, confirms the suggestion that this antigen is produced in the endoplasmic reticulum. The fact that Dane particles have been found in the cisternae of the endoplasmic reticulum implies that once they have penetrated the nucleus from the cytoplasm, the particles corresponding to HBcAg migrate through the nuclear pores toward the cytoplasm and are coated with an HBsAg-positive membrane in the cisternae of the endoplasmic reticulum to then be released into the intercellular space together with other HBsAg-positive particles, by a process of inverse phagocytosis. This hypothesis is supported by the fact that Dane particles have been found in the Disse and intercellular spaces. The different cellular distribution of HBV antigens is recognized to have a precise diagnostic and prognostic meaning [23, 27].

3.2.3. The third antigen is the so-called *HBeAg (hepatitis B e antigen).* The fact that anti-HBe-positive sera can agglutinate Dane particles [31] implies that this antigen is present on the outer surface of Dane particles. HBeAg has been localized by some authors [31] by using immunofluorescence in the cytoplasm and by others in the nucleus of infected cells [32]. There is no evidence to date of ultrastructural identification even though various interpretations have been put forward [33, 34]. The exact nature of HBeAg is still unknown.

3.2.4. The fourth antigen, called 'δ' [35], was localized by using immunofluorescence in the nucleus of

hepatocytes from patients with HBsAg-positive chronic hepatitis, usually mutually excluding the intrahepatocyte presence of HBcAg. Using electron microscopy, electron-dense granular structures, 20–30 nm in diameter with blurred edges, have been localized at the level of these nuclei. They are frequently associated with heterochromatin and occasionally found free in the euchromatin. These observations were further confirmed by immunoelectron microscopy [36]. The nature of the 'δ' antigen is the object of current investigation.

3.3. Non-A non-B hepatitis virus (NANBV)

This virus [37] is responsible for the onset of a form of viral hepatitis that has not been correlated with any of the viruses identified to date. According to some authors, this virus is responsible for the majority of cases of posttransfusional hepatitis. Recently [38], immunoelectron microscopy has been used to detect the presence of viral-like particles, 25–30 nm in diameter, on the liver homogenate of infected chimpanzees. Electron microscopy has revealed particles 40–60 nm in size, resembling the structure of togavirus, in the urine of three patients suffering from acute viral hepatitis not ascribable to other viruses [39]. This antigen has been localized at the nuclear level by using immunofluorescence [40, 79–83].

3.4. Acute viral hepatitis

In this disease, ultrastructural alterations are detectable both in the parenchyma and in the portal tracts. Lobular subversion is caused by pleomorphism of the hepatocytes and the concomitant mesenchymal reaction. The main alterations responsible for the heterogeneity of hepatocyte morphology are acidophilic degeneration of the liver cells with the formation of acidophilic bodies, and their swelling with the formation of ballooning cells. During acidophilic degeneration, the hepatocytes, smaller in size than those commonly found in normal liver, appear extremely eosinophilic with a pycnotic nucleus. An electron-dense hyaloplasm, widespread organelle damage, and a somewhat retracted nucleus can be seen under the electron microscope. At a more advanced stage, the acidophilic body surrounded by a light halo is found displaced outside the hepatocytes or inside the Kupffer cells [41].

These roundish bodies show a strongly electron-dense hyaloplasm with a few organelles which are usually shrunken. The nucleus is wrinkled and sometimes only nuclear debris is detectable in its place. Glycogen particles and polyribosomes are no longer present. These degenerative phenomena have been ascribed to dehydration with a selective loss of potassium [41]; however, an alteration in nuclear function could also lead to early cell death.

Several hypertrophic Kupffer cells can sometimes be detected close to the acidophilic bodies, a warning sign of a phagocytosis of necrotic material.

The so-called oncocytoid cell forms part of the acidophilic degeneration. This cell is characterized by a thick cluster of mitochondria containing large granules with an electron-dense matrix and no shrinkage of the cell hyaloplasm [41].

During ballooning degeneration, the cellular volume of the hepatocyte is considerably greater than average. The cytoplasm appears studded with small, slightly eosinophilic granules mainly displaced around the nucleus. Under the electron microscope, it is possible to observe a marked proliferation and dilatation of vesicles of the smooth and rough endoplasmic reticulum which may appear degranulated. The mitochondria are swollen and take on various shapes and sizes until they look like megamitochondria or they may have a very thick matrix. Granules of bile pigment may be present in the hyaloplasm together with a reduction in the number of glycogen particles. A swelling of the sinusoidal face may also be seen with the formation of blebs which are a warning sign of a break in the plasmalemma and discharge of its content. Areas of focal lithic necrosis are sometimes detectable in the cytoplasm. The microvilli appear enlarged and distorted around the bile capillary, sometimes with an accumulation of bile matrix of granular appearance within the lumen. A complete loss of microvilli is occasionally seen together with a thickening of the pericanalicular ectoplasm, caused by an increase in contractile filamentous structures.

In acute viral hepatitis with cholestasis, the so-called lamellar bodies can be found in the hepatocyte, made up of a double chain of phospholipids produced by the interaction of bile with membrane phospholipids [41]. The nuclear membrane of the hepatocytes may be irregular and undulating with focal dilatations which may give rise to pseudoinclusions of cytoplasmic material. Real inclusions made up of fat droplets or clusters of glycogen particles can also be observed in the nucleus [41]. Nuclear chromatin appear enriched and usually displaced to the periphery of the nucleus. There is a high incidence of so-called 'nuclear bodies' [42], considered signs of a state of hyperactivity on the part of the hepatocyte. Several cells are bi- or multinucleate and nucleoli are often increased in number. These aspects can be ascribed to the hepatocyte's regenerative processes.

Alongside hepatocyte pleomorphism, the intralobular mesenchymal response contributes to subversion of the lobular structure. Kupffer and endothelial cells increase in number and appear hypertrophic. The former show an intense phagocytic activity, incorporating cellular debris and necrotic material. They are densely packed with granules of yellowish-brown pigment, known as 'ceroid pigment.' Under the electron microscope, the structure of the Kupffer cells is characterized by a marked increase in the rough endoplasmic reticulum and the presence of various dense bodies, probably lysosomes, amorphous debris, hemosiderin, lipofuscin, and biliary material.

Polymorphonuclear leucocytes and lymphocytes are also found in the Disse space, sometimes invading the intercellular space. The appearance of a thin basal membrane around the sinusoidal face of the hepatocyte, together with an increase in collagen fibers in the Disse and intercellular spaces, may be responsible for disorders in microcirculation and hence a reduction in the hepatocyte's average life. This alteration has been called 'sinusoidal capillarization' [43].

A marked infiltration of mononuclear cells, mainly lymphocytes mixed with histiocytes, plasma cells, and sometimes neutrophil granulocytes can be seen around the portal space and, in some cases which often develop toward the chronic stage of the disease, around the periportal space as well. The bile ductules present alterations soon after the onset of jaundice. In most cases, the lumen is dilated with a reduction or disappearance of the microvilli of epithelial cells which reveal different hyaloplasmic densities. Cytoplasmic 'blebs' or cellular debris may appear within the lumen. The ductules and the ducts are constantly infiltrated by lymphocytes and neutrophil granulocytes [44].

3.5. Chronic hepatitis

Portal and periportal alterations predominate over intralobular ones in chronic hepatitis. Persistent chronic hepatitis is characterized by a marked portal inflammation composed mainly of lymphocytes and histiocytes and, to a lesser extent, fibroblasts, plasma cells, and eosinophil and neutrophil leucocytes. A slight increase also occurs in the number of ductules and ducts, which always have a lumen. The boundary line between the portal tract and the lobular periphery parenchyma is clearly marked. The periportal hepatocytes show a slight dilatation of the cisternae of the endoplasmic reticulum, an increase in glycogen granules and fat droplets, with no alteration of other organelles. The lobular structure is retained. At the lobular level, a very slight pleomorphism of the hepatocytes and their nuclei can be detected, accompanied by a negligible mesenchymal reaction. The size and shape of the mitochondria is often above average with paracrystalline inclusions in their matrix. At the nuclear level, various nuclear bodies can be identified.

3.6. Chronic aggressive hepatitis

A more serious involvement of the portal and periportal spaces occurs in chronic aggressive hepatitis, with a spread of the inflammatory infiltrate beyond the limits of the portal tract and consequent piecemeal necrosis of the hepatocytes in zone 1 of the Rappaport acinus. In some cases, lymphocytes can be observed closely adhered to the hepatocyte membrane, causing lysis of the latter [45]. In the periportal region, ballooning cells and acidophilic bodies are easily recognizable, surrounded by lymphocytes, macrophages, and fibroblasts. Subcellular changes in the hepatocytes found in the Rappaport zones 2–3 are characterized by a decrease in the rough endoplasmic reticulum, proliferation of the smooth endoplasmic reticulum, and vesicular transformation of both. Mitochondrial alterations, autophagosomes, and accumulations of hemosiderin and lipofuscin can be found together with areas of cytoplasmic focal necrosis [41].

Collagen fibrils are packed into the Disse and intercellular spaces, isolating the hepatocytes from the rest of the parenchyma and producing a rearrangement in the lobular structure. Lipocytes are present in large numbers and, as the precursors of fibroblasts, they take an active part in the process of hepatic fibrosis [46]. Cellular debris, hypertrophic Kupffer cells, lymphocytes, and plasma cells are found in the sinusoidal spaces. A dilatation of the intercellular space between the hepatocytes is frequently observed with a proliferation of microvillous formations. An increase in the number of ductule structures, sometimes devoid of a lumen and placed directly in contact with the hepatocytes, is visible in the portal space dilated due to intense fibrosis and inflammatory infiltration [45].

As the lymphoplasma cell infiltration process continues, accompanied by the simultaneous necrosis of individual hepatocytes, septa of connective tissue spread within the parenchyma. These septa are considered active in that they are formed by inflammatory infiltration, fibroblastic proliferation, and neoformation of connective tissue fibers. The septa disturb the lobular structure, but do not cause nodular regeneration at this stage. In cases of chronic active hepatitis with cholestasis, the typical modifications of cholestasis are added. More than half the patients with the above alterations develop cirrhosis.

An important ultrastructural study of the livers of chimpanzees infected with HAV and HBV has revealed several significant differences. In HAV infection, the most conspicuous alterations have been detected at the cytoplasmic level in the mitochondria, which are roundish with a thickened matrix and irregular-shaped cristae while the smooth endoplasmic reticulum appears vacuolized. In HBV infection, on the other hand, the mitochondria show no particular alterations and the smooth endoplasmic reticulum reveals tubular hypertrophy [43]. Evidence of two different pathogenetic mechanisms has therefore been suggested. At the present time, there are no comparative ultrastructural studies on HBV and non-A non-B viral hepatitis.

4. ALCOHOLIC LIVER DISEASE

There are basically three morphologic types of liver

damage from alcohol: hepatic steatosis, alcoholic hepatitis, and cirrhosis.

Alhough an excessive intake of alcohol is almost always associated with liver steatosis, it does not necessarily lead to alcoholic hepatitis or cirrhosis since sex and genetic factors are also involved in this progression [48]. These three morphological pictures can be observed separately or together. The accumulation of lipids detectable in a morphological examination is preceded by small collections of fat which can be revealed only with chemicals. Liver steatosis is characterized by the intracytoplasmic presence of lipids (mostly triglycerides and, to a lesser extent, phospholipids and cholesterol) in the form of fine droplets or large vacuoles which stretch the cytoplasm to the point of displacing the nucleus to the periphery. Fatty deposits may be spread throughout the lobule or be preferentially displaced in the centrolobular zone. Parenchymal inflammation is absent or slight at this stage and the portal spaces are normal or slightly infiltrated by mononuclear cells with a slight amount of newly formed fibrous tissue.

Under ultrastructural observation, the fat vacuoles have a diameter varying from 30 to over 200 nm. Initially, the smallest lipid droplets are displaced around the sinusoidal face. Later, the largest ones may be displaced anywhere in the hyaloplasm. Sometimes these vacuoles are surrounded by a membrane. Hepatocytes called lipogranulomes, whose cytoplasm is almost completely replaced by a large fat vacuole and appears surrounded by mononuclear cells and histiocytes, can also be seen in most cases of alcoholic hepatitis. Mitochondrial changes of various types are already observed at this stage. Mitochondria of normal size are noted with disorientated cristae, increase in size of the dense granules of the matrix, and the presence of vacuoles with fibrillar and lamellar inclusions and paracrystalline structures. Some mitochondria appear larger, with a considerably polymorphous appearance [49]:

– Spherical megamitochondria with a maximum diameter of 10–12 μm and a matrix density the same as normal mtochondria.
– Elongated megamitochondria (up to 15 μm), usually containing protracted crystalline inclusions with the major axis parallel to the longest part of the organelle.
– Irregular megamitochondria with a large number of cristae and variously displaced crystalline inclusions.

Nevertheless, megamitochondria should not be considered specific alterations of alcohol liver damage since they are found in other liver diseases.

There is a proliferation of the vesicles of the smooth endoplasmic reticulum which may appear dilated.

When hepatic steatosis is complicated by the onset of alcoholic hepatitis, the histological diagnosis is based on the presence of alcoholic hyaline Mallory bodies surrounded by neutrophil polynucleates in the liver cells, especially the centrolobular ones, and on a process of necrosis and fibrosis which occludes the centrolobular veins, so-called 'acute hyaline sclerosing necrosis.' The portal spaces appear enlarged with an increase in mononuclear cells and a proliferation of bile ductules. A slight interstitial fibrosis is associated with portal fibrosis. In some cases, intercellular biliary thrombi and hepatocellular bile pigment can be observed. Cholestasis has been related to the formation of Mallory bodies [50].

Mallory bodies are highly indicative of alcohol liver damage, even though they are seen in other liver diseases [50]. As well as in hepatocytes, these bodies have been reported in bile duct cells [51] and ductule cells [52]. Their massive presence may signify a probable evolution toward cirrhosis [53]. They are composed of cytoplasmic accumulations of filamentous material of a lipoprotein nature due to synthesis increase. These filaments seem to contain an actin-like protein [54], and some authors are inclined to consider them similar to the intermediate filaments of the liver cell [55] and that their aggregation derives from an antimicrotubulin action of ethanol [48]. In fact, Mallory bodies appear to interfere with normal hepatocyte functions, reducing them to those of transport and secretion. It is thought that they may represent neoantigens able to evoke T-lymphocyte hyperreactivity [56].

There also is an association between Mallory bodies and lymphocytic infiltrates, even though the latter are not necessarily found in the same zone as the Mallory bodies [48]. The presence of these lymphocytic infiltrates implies that they have a cytotoxic effect equivalent, though to a lesser degree, to that detectable in chronic active hepatitis. Furthermore, an in vivo chemotactic activity of Mallory bodies for polymorphonuclear leucocytes has been identified [57]. In fact, polymorphonuclear leucocytes attack the cells containing Mallory bodies, destroying their plasmalemma and coming into direct contact with cellular organelles.

Three morphological variants of Mallory bodies are known at the ultrastructural level [38]:

- type 1, made up of fibrils in a parallel arrangement with a diameter of 14.1 nm;
- type 2, the most frequent, composed of filaments orientated at random, with an average diameter of 15.2 nm;
- type 3, characterized by the almost complete disappearance of fibrillar structures composed of granular or homogeneous electron-dense material.

There are also other hepatocellular alterations correlated with this disease, even though they are nonspecific. The nuclei are large with prominent nucleoli [58]. There is a reduction in the number of profiles of the rough endoplasmic reticulum, which is recognized by aspects of dilatation, degranulation, fragmentation, and vesiculation. The Golgi complex appears hypertrophic and dilated, and a considerable increase in small electron-dense droplets, 30–40 nm in diameter, are noted within its membranous structures. There is an increase in autophagic vacuoles containing lamellar and osmiophilic amorphous material. The onset of the phenomenon called 'sinusoid capillarization' occurs in the Disse space, with subsequent interference in nutritive exchanges between the hepatocyte and the sinusoidal blood. This event may be an important factor in the pathogenesis of alcoholic liver disease [59].

The Kupffer cells are increased in number and are hypertrophic, and are rich in vacuoles of pinocytosis and phagocytosis.

Fibrosis and/or cirrhosis occur in 10%–30% of patients with a history of chronic alcoholism. It has been proved that alcoholic hepatitis is associated with an exasperated turnover of collagen tissue [60]. In fact, when the alcoholic disease becomes chronic, the presence of an increased number of fibroblasts

in close apposition to bands of collagen fibers is noted between hepatocytes and sinusoids and in the portal space. This leads to a neoformation and deposition of collagen fibers with the consequent formation of septa followed by cirrhotic nodules. Alongside the fibroblasts, numerous myofibroblasts are noted, probably involved in the retraction of fibrous septa given their contractile capacity. Furthermore, there is a considerable increase in lipocytes [61], considered the precursors of fibroblasts, which are also in close contact with small bands of fibrils packed on the extracellular wall of the plasma membrane.

5. PRIMARY BILIARY CIRRHOSIS

Primary biliary cirrhosis is a chronic liver disease, probably of immunological pathogenesis, characterized by a significant reduction in interlobular and septal ducts with a consequent progressive alteration in bile flow [62]. The disease is divided into four different histological patterns which may occur separately or together. Stage I: destructive nonsuppurative cholangitis or florid duct lesions; stage II: ductular proliferation; stage III: scarring phase; stage IV: fully developed cirrhosis. However, florid duct lesions are detectable in 38% of cases in stage I, 45% in stage II, 19% in stage III, and 15% in stage IV [62].

Bile duct lesions seem to be mediated by the formation of immune complexes [63] and are the most characteristic lesions of stages I and II, together with the accumulation of inflammatory cells (mainly lymphocytes, macrophages, and plasma cells) in the portal spaces and the presence of lymphatic follicles with germinative centers, epithelial granulomes with giant cells, and the swelling of the ductal epithelial cells.

Under ultrastructural observation, the bile ducts present a dilated lumen with a reduction in the number of microvilli, which appear shortened and edematous to the point of disappearing completely. Numerous cytophagosomes and lysosomes containing myelinic figures can be observed in the cytoplasm of duct cells. At this stage, a few scattered filamentous structures can already be seen in the hyaloplasm, arranged separately, or grouped in bands. Numerous cytophagosomes and mitochondria showing curling of the cristae and crystalline inclusions in their matrix are present in the liver cells. 'Glycogen bodies' and peroxysomes increased in volume have also been described [52]. The bile canaliculi appear normal even though edematous microvilli are sometimes seen.

As the bile ducts are gradually destroyed and replaced by fibrous tissue, there is a proliferation of bile ductules (stage II) displaced to the marginal zone of the periportal space, surrounded in turn by an abundant lymphoplasma cellular exudate.

Near the periportal space, the hepatocytes show signs of irregularly spread cholestasis and cytoplasmic agglomerates which have the staining and ultrastructural characteristics of Mallory hyaline substance [64]. Periportal fibrosis is also present.

Under the electron microscope, the lumen of bile ductules devoid of microvilli is often dilated and the surface of the ductule cells facing the lumen contain electron-lucent vesicles which may rise from the luminal surface, completely filling the lumen. In the epithelial cells of the bile ductules, a marked increase in filamentous structures can be seen grouped in thick bands, displaced close to the cellular membrane or grouped around the mitochondria and other organelles (Fig. 7). A reduction in the number of cytophagosomes and lysosomes occurs while a vacuolization of the rough endoplasmic reticulum appears with degranulation. The basal membrane may still be intact [52] or doubled with many collagen fibers wrapped around the ductule. The number of cytophagosomes in the hepatocytes is clearly below that of stage I, and intramitochondrial crystals can still be observed. The periphery bile canaliculi, especially those situated between three or more cells, are dilated with a loss of microvilli which appear shortened and edematous.

As the disease gradually develops, the bile ductules are destroyed as well, the inflammatory process declines, and an irregular often star-shaped scar is formed (stage III). Connective septa then spread out of the portal space, followed by the formation of regenerative nodules (stage IV).

During these stages, the most characteristic sign is that of a large number of hepatocytes in the periportal region or at the periphery of the regenerative nodules, which become heavily stained due to the copper [62]. The typical ultrastructural alterations of stages III and IV consist of thickening

and doubling, followed by breakage of the basal membrane of residual bile ductules, while the plasma membrane of the ductule cells remains intact. A reduction in the ductule lumen with an absence of microvilli also occurs [52, 65]. A further increase in filamentous structures is detectable in the cytoplasm of the epithelial cells of the bile ductules [66], which also reveal hypertrophy of the Golgi complex and rarefaction of the rough endoplasmic reticulum, which appears vesiculated or vacuolized [65]. A reduction in the ribosomal component also occurs. Some authors have also observed a significant presence of cytophagosomes and lysosomes increased in volume during these stages [65].

The cells of the biliary epithelium usually present an increased volume with an electron-lucent cytoplasm, alternated with other cells with a thickened cytoplasm tightly packed with organelles. The bile ducts are often surrounded by macrophages and sometimes infiltrated by polymorphonuclear leucocytes [52].

Hepatocytes may reveal the characteristic alterations of cholestasis, with extensive rearrangement at the biliary pole level. They have lysosomes increased in volume, cytophagosomes [65] and megamitochondria with crystalline inclusions in extremely complicated shapes [52]. The phenomenon of sinusoid capillarization is a fairly common finding.

It is well known that the antimitochondrial antibody can be found in circulation in most cases of primary biliary cirrhosis: by using immunoelectron microscopy, the antigen can be localized on the internal face of the membrane and on the mitochondrial cristae [67].

6. CONSTITUTIONAL HYPERBILIRUBINEMIA

Disorders of bilirubin metabolism in hepatocytes are the cause of nonhemolytic constitutional hyperbilirubinemia (NHCH). It is possible to recognize characteristics of familiarity with genetic transmission which is not always fully established. The pathogenesis of this disease probably lies in an hereditary enzymatic defect connected to carrier systems of the vascular pole, metabolic conjugation systems of the smooth endoplasmic reticulum, and enzymatic systems of canalicular excretion. Two main groups of NHCH have been identified:

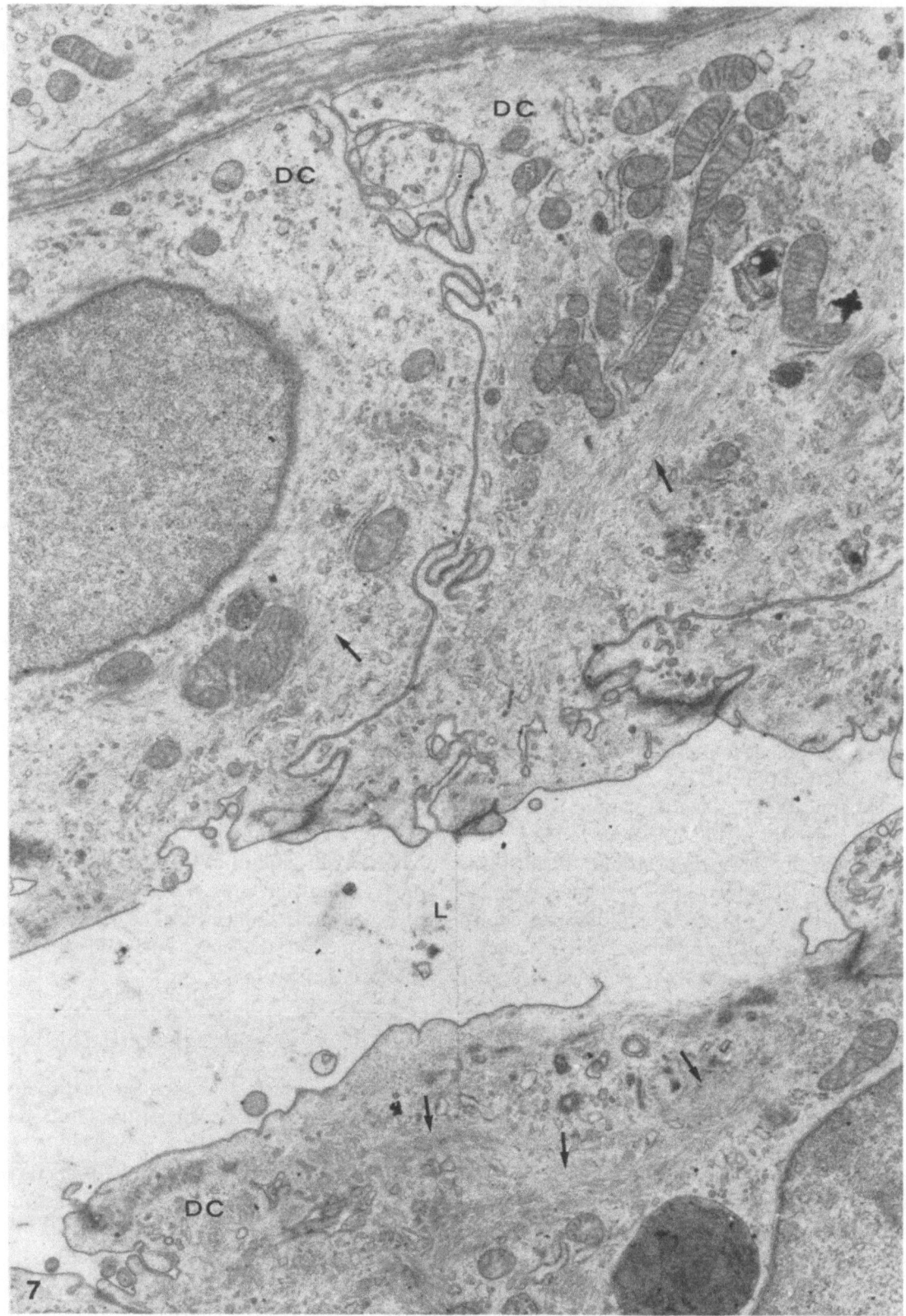

Figure 7. Primary biliary cirrhosis. Bundles of microfilaments (arrows) in the cytoplasm of ductular epithelial cells (DC). L, lumen; ×12,000.

– Nonconjugated bilirubin hyperbilirubinemia due to purification and conjugation deficiencies such as Gilbert syndrome and Crigler-Najjar syndrome.

– Conjugated bilirubin hyperbilirubinemia due to purification, accumulation and excretion deficiencies such as Rotor syndrome and Dubin-Johnson syndrome.

Light-microscopic analysis of liver biopsies from such patients produces findings which are usually normal and only reveal the pathognomonic sign of an accumulation of pigment in a few cases. Therefore, the submission of biopsies from suspect patients to electron-microscopic analysis has long been advised for NHCH.

Nevertheless, even though NHCH is theoretically an excellent model of submicroscopic research (study of samples which are already known 'a priori' to be deficient or lacking a specific functional activity), considerable difficulties still exist in making an etiopathogenetic connection between ultrastructural observations and functional data relative to disorders of bilirubin metabolism. In fact, at the current stage of interpretation, the ultrastructural characteristics of bioptic samples from these patients do not seem to help either a better understanding of pathogenetic mechanisms or the differential diagnosis of the disease.

The alterations most commonly observed and reported in the literature which have gradually been assessed or reconsidered concern [68, 69]:

– The hepatocyte vascular pole. Aspects of 'sinusoidal fragility' are seen (to variable degrees), i.e., a reduction and distortion of hepatocyte microvillous expansions together with the presence of amorphous material, mainly fragments of organelles or hepatocyte hyaloplasmic inclusions, in the Disse space (sometimes dilated) or in the sinusoidal lumen, aspecific changes in the endothelial cells and bands of collagen fibers in the Disse space. According to some authors, these aspects constitute a defect of the vascular pole of the hepatocyte and of the sinusoidal endothelium (endothelial-hepatocyte meiopragia). This finding is considered to be of some pathogenetic interest especially in unconjugated bilirubin congenital jaundice (Gilbert syndrome) and in an acquired from (Kalk posthepatitic hyper-

bilirubinemia) probably caused by a purification deficiency which is thought to be produced by a structural defect of the cellular membrane and/or the Disse space.

– Hepatic pigmentation. In particular, those forms of pigment inclusions, commonly called 'specific inclusions', should be taken into account. Ultrastructural findings show them surrounded by a membrane and made up of two basic morphologically separate components present in variable amounts, depending on the type of syndrome in question (Gilbert syndrome, Rotor syndrome, Dubin-Johnson syndrome). In fact, a granulofilamentous component of medium to low density (of protein nature) is found together with a component of globular–amorphous aspect (which can probably be ascribed to unsaturated fatty acids). It seems that these inclusions are in some way correlated with lysosomal structures (secondary lysosomes) and at least one of them (which accumulated in Gilbert syndrome and is made up of a small amount of granulofilamentous material which surrounds prominent lipid globules) cannot really be distinguished from lipofuscin granules.

– Mitochondria which reveal aspecific alterations such as variable shapes and sizes and frequently the presence of paracrystalline inclusions in the matrix.

– Smooth endoplasmic reticulum which sometimes appears hypertrophic and dilated.

6.1. Gilbert syndrome

From a pathogenetic point of view, Gilbert syndrome is considered the result of low hepatocyte bilirubin–UDP–glycuroniltransferase activity. Nevertheless, it seems that alongside this primary enzymatic deficiency, other enzyme systems ought to be involved. The alteration of these systems can also be primary or secondary: enzyme chains responsible for the formation of diglycuronide–bilirubin, but also membrane enzyme systems with a carrier function carrying out the purification and transport of molecules of free bilirubin [70].

A light-microscopic examination of the hepatic specimen generally reveals a substantially preserved lobular structure. According to several recent observations [71], electron-microscopic study enables Gilbert patients to be divided into two subpopulations, one showing marked hypertrophy of the

152

smooth endoplasmic reticulum (so-called Gilbert EM +) (Fig. 8), and the other characterized by hepatocytes with a submicroscopic aspect very similar to that of normal subjects (so-called Gilbert EM —). This morphological distinction also seems to be retained in the evaluation of results of calorie restriction and nicotinic acid stimulation tests. In fact, the EM + subpopulation shows a significant increase in free bilirubin compared with EM — patients and controls in response to calorie restriction, while the response to nicotinic acid stimulation does not produce statistically significant values, even though the difference between the subpopulations persist. Nevertheless, in our opinion, hypertrophy of the smooth endoplasmic reticulum is too aspecific a submicroscopic finding.

6.2. Crigler-Najjar syndrome

Crigler-Najjar syndrome is an extremely rare condition of serious unconjugated bilirubin hyperbilirubinemia of very early onset and chronic evolution. According to the most recent interpretations, the Crigler-Najjar syndrome presents important

similarities with a situation of fetal liver persistence with no glycuronyl transferase activity. In fact, this syndrome appears to be the result of a serious deficiency in the hepatocytes' ability to conjugate bilirubin [70, 72].

Ultrastructural observations [73] of biopsies from carriers of the Crigler-Najjar syndrome have produced wholly aspecific findings.

6.3. Dubin-Johnson syndrome

In this disease, hyperbilirubinemia is mainly of the conjugated type, but there may also be an increase in the amount of unconjugated bilirubin [70]. Macroscopically, the bioptic specimen is black or dark brown. Under light-microscopic analysis, the lobular structure appears normal without inflammatory alterations or significant changes in silver impegnation. Pigment, much darker than lipofuscin, is deposited in the hepatocytes and may even be very widespread. If the hepatocyte is not packed, the pigment collects in the pericanalicular ectoplasm, especially in the centrolobular hepatocytes. Pigment is also present in the Kupffer cells. His-

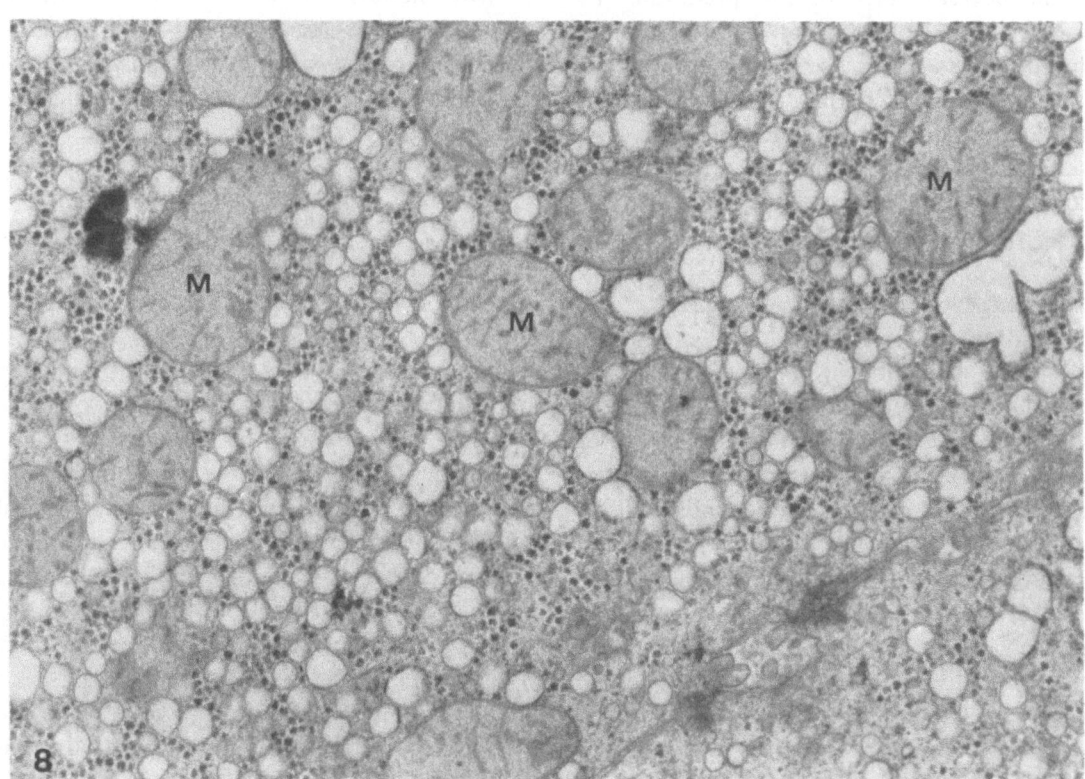

Figure 8. Gilbert syndrome. Smooth endoplasmic reticulum hypertrophy. M, mitochondria; ×16,000.

tological signs of cholestasis are not present. Under submicroscopic analysis, changes in the plasma membrane at the sinusoidal pole are slight as are those of the rough (fragmentation, vesiculation) and smooth (hypertrophy) endoplasmic reticulum, mitochondria (paracrystalline inclusions in the matrix), and the Golgi complex. A particular ultrastructural finding is that of oval-shaped pigment granules, 0.5–2.5 μm in diameter, bound by a membrane, especially concentrated around the pericanalicular ectoplasm (Fig. 9). Each granule is made up of two subunits: a filamentous one, probably of protein nature, which constitutes the main fraction of the pigment; and a globular one of probable lipid nature (unsaturated fatty acids) present in smaller amounts. In the Dubin-Johnson syndrome, the granulofilamentous component of protein nature predominates over the globular lipid one in the pigment granules [68].

The overall chemical nature of the pigment is not very clear. Some authors consider it to be of the lipofuscin type while others think that it is composed of melanin, or at least an anomalous melanin variant. Recent studies based on data obtained from the ESR spectra of Dubin-Johnson pigment [74] exclude the normal or anomalous melanin component. The exact molecular characterization of the pigment has not yet been achieved, but it is almost certainly not uroporphyrin or coproporphyrin. Ultrastructural studies carried out by numerous authors on bile canaliculi in the course of the Dubin-Johnson syndrome have not revealed significant abnormalities, apart from the limited dilatation of the canalicular lumen with a slight decrease in the number of microvillous evaginations of the canalicular plasma membrane and the variable presence of pigment granules within the actual lumen.

6.4. Rotor syndrome

For a number of years, Rotor syndrome was considered a variant of the Dubin-Johnson syndrome and hence the result of an altered canalicular excretion of conjugated bilirubin. Later, the demonstration of patients showing symptoms consistent with Rotor syndrome, but with kinetic tests of cholephylic stains indicating a deficiency in the

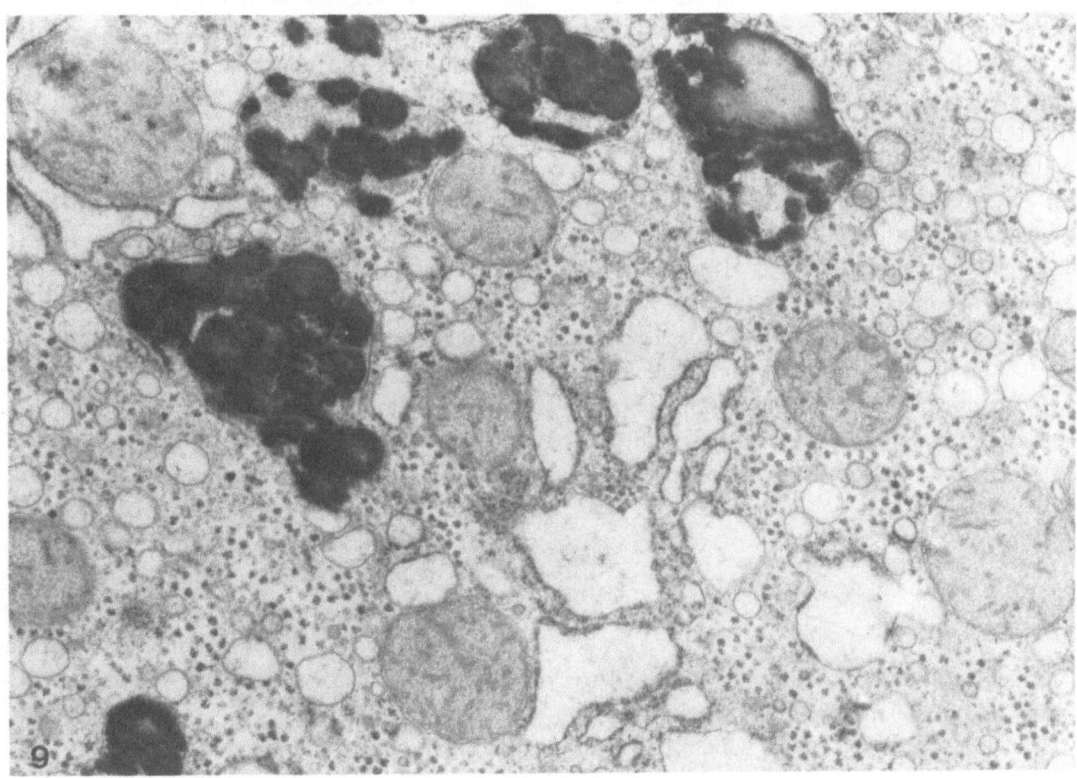

Figure 9. Dubin-Johnson syndrome. Pigment deposits into pericanalicular dense bodies; × 18,000.

uptake and storage phases of the organic anions, led this form of NHCH to be reassessed from a new pathogenetic perspective. Most patients suffering from Rotor syndrome are carriers of a primary deficiency in hepatocyte uptake and storage of bilirubin [70].

From a morphological point of view, according to traditional descriptions, the absence of pigmentation constitutes the distinctive sign of Rotor syndrome compared with the Dubin-Johnson syndrome. However, according to some authors, there are cases of liver cell accumulation of pigment. Ultrastructural findings offer a very limited contribution to the explanation of the pathogenetic mechanism underlying Rotor syndrome. Sporadic, aspecific alterations have been described at the level of the sinusoidal pole, such as a reduction in the microvilli of the hepatocyte plasmalemma. The perisinusoidal recesses and interhepatic spaces appear dilated. Data on mitochondrial changes are highly conflicting: according to some authors, these alterations are usual and include the size, shape, and matrix density of these organelles, up to the appearance of frequent megamitochondria [75]. According to others [69], the abnormalities consist solely of the appearance of paracrystalline structures in the matrix of the mitochondria. There have been some reports of hypertrophy of the smooth endoplasmic reticulum and many vesicles and vacuoles in the Golgi complex. At the canalicular pole level, a dilatation of the biliary canaliculi has been described with a reduction in the number of microvilli [69]. This extreme variability is also detectable at the submicroscopic level, both as regards the amount of pigment stored and its aspect, i.e., the relation between the two protein and lipid components. According to some authors [68], the pigment characteristic of Rotor syndrome is made up of equal parts of the two components, at least in the majority of cases.

7. STORAGE DISEASES

Several congenital metabolic disorders can lead to intracellular storage of metabolites. Schematically, there are at least four ways in which this can happen:

– Synthesis of molecules with an anomalous structure which can no longer be recognized by the cell's catabolic systems (as in two forms of glycogenosis, dextrinosis and amylopectinosis).

– Reduction (congenital or acquired) in the ability of some substrates to bind particular metabolites (for example, in Wilson's disease or hepatolenticular degeneration in which ceruloplasmin is deficient or in some forms of atransferrinemia).

– Congenital anomaly of the synthesis control mechanism of some macromolecules, followed by their hyperproduction, as in some forms of cholesterosis.

– Storage of metabolites within the cell due to their reduced catabolism.

All the peculiar clinical metabolic disorders produced by these four pathogenetic mechanisms are called storage diseases [76].

In recent years, growing importance has been given to the now extensive group of storage diseases which forms part of 'congenital lysosomal diseases' caused by the intracellular degradation deficiency of some macromolecules produced or penetrated within the diseased cell [77]. Electron microscopy has made a decisive contribution to pathogenetic investigation of this particular group of diseases and today it is also a very useful diagnostic tool [78]. In fact, in recent years, it has been possible to identify not only the type of organelle in which storage occurs, i.e., lysosomes, but also the exact morphological aspect of the stored substrate (Figs. 10–12).

There is no satisfactory classification of congenital lysosomal diseases. The traditional subdivision into mucopolysaccharidosis, glycolipidosis, and glycogenosis, which referred to the stored substance, now seems inadequate because a large number of forms with mixed storage have been noted due to the frequency of the phenomenon of genetic heterogeneity. These diseases regard single, multiple, or as yet unidentified enzyme defects which cause the simultaneous storage of several macromolecules. There also exist congenital lysosomal diseases with anatomoclinical characteristics which do not fall within the groups already defined.

Table 1 lists the main congenital lysosomal diseases in which visceromegaly is a prominent early symptom and which therefore involve liver disease.

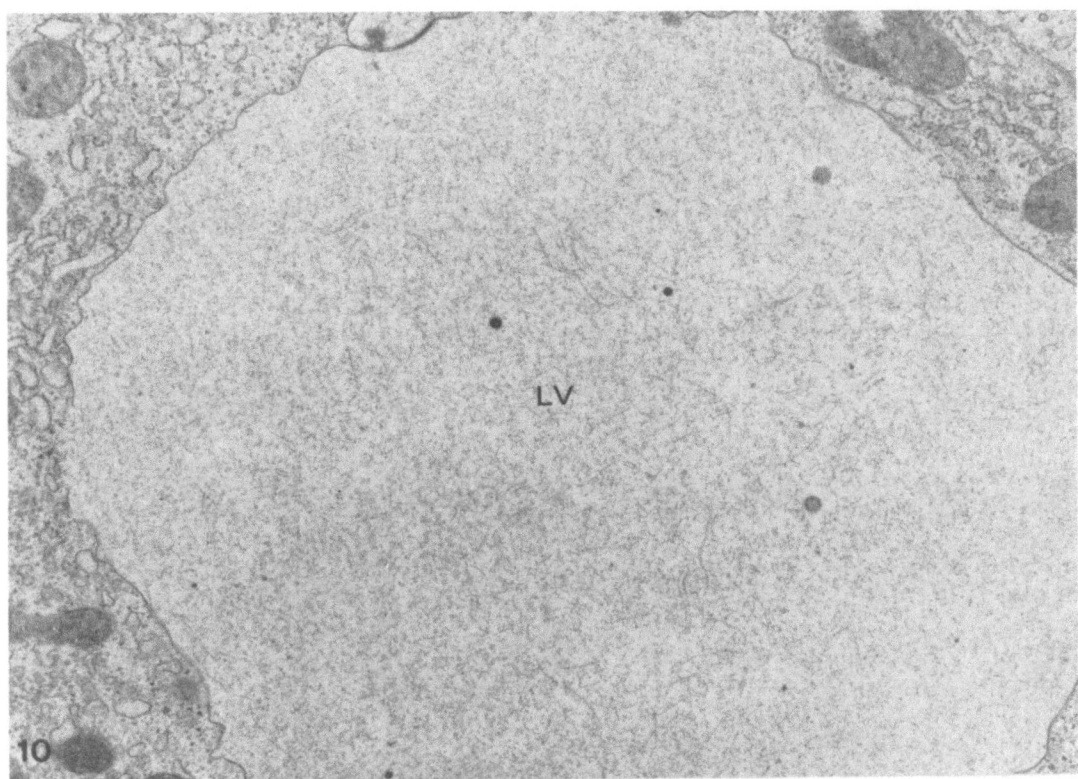

Figure 10. Mucopolysaccharidosis. Great lysosomal vacuole (LV) filled with granulofilamentous material; ×14,000.

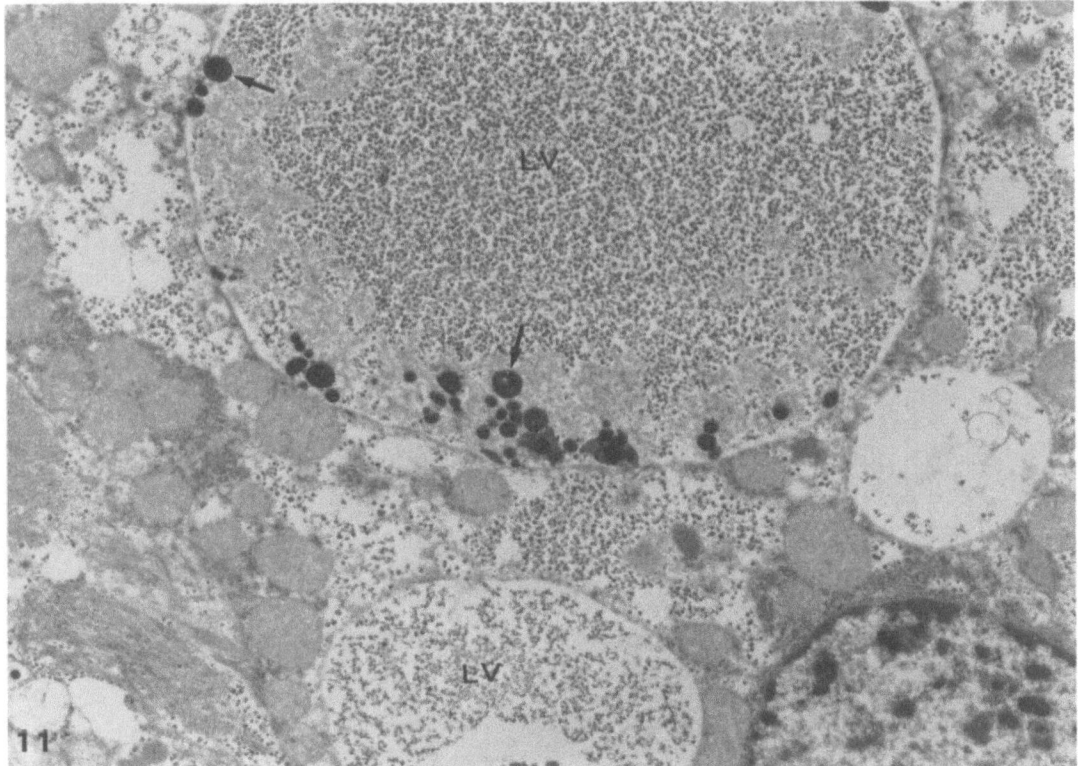

Figure 11. Mucolipidosis. Lysosomal vacuoles (LV) filled with glycogen particles, granulofilamentous material, and dense lipid droplets (arrows); ×8600.

156

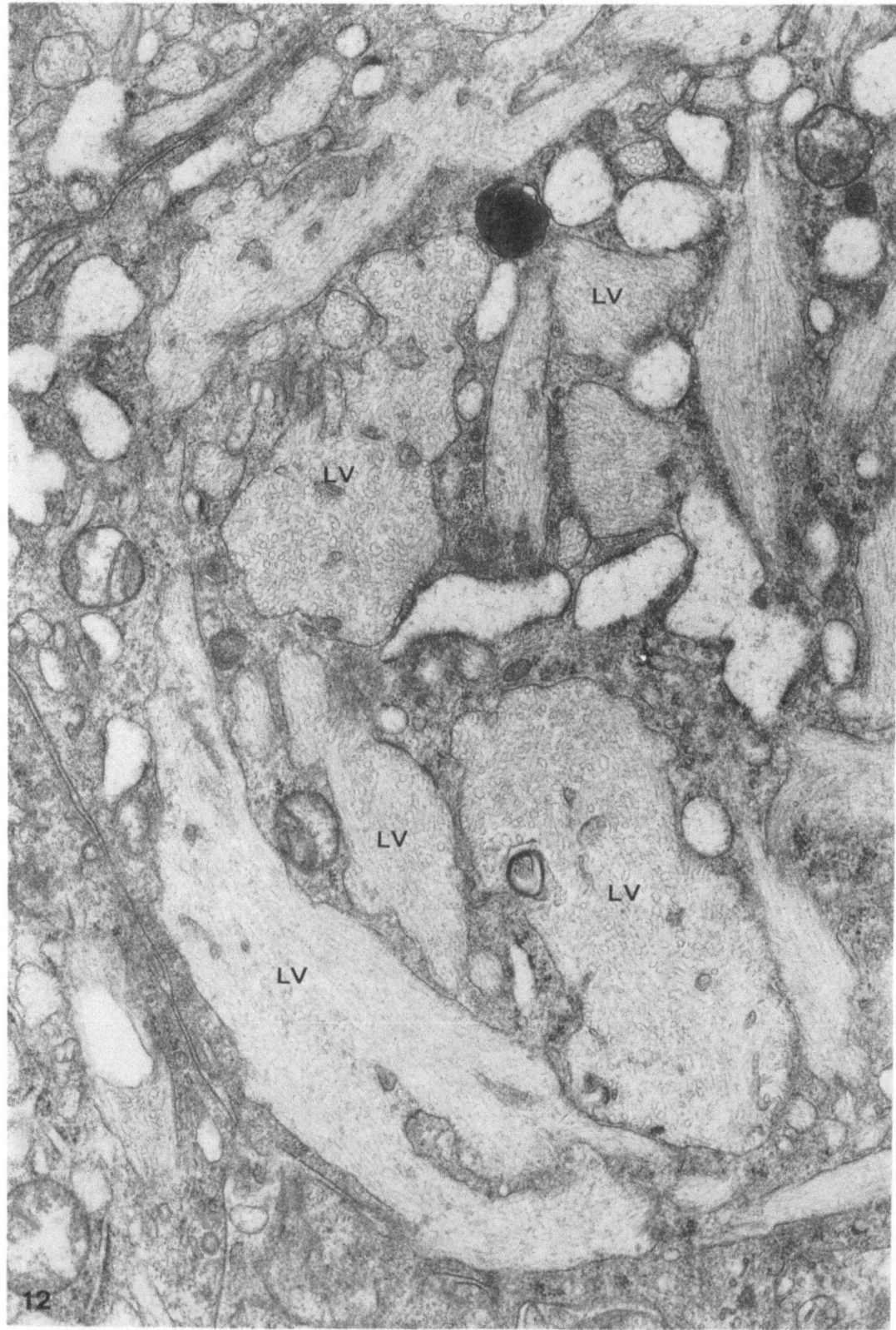

Figure 12. Gaucher disease. Kupffer cell. Numerous large, irregular lysosomal vacuoles (LV) filled with characteristic tubular material; × 34,200.

Table 1. Main congenital lysosomal diseases with visceromegaly

---

Mucopolysaccharidosis
    IH
    IH/S
    II
    III
    IV
    VI
    VII (neonatal hepatitis)

Glycolipidosis
    Niemann-Pick disease types A, B, C
    Gaucher disease: acute, juvenile, adult
    Fabry disease

Oligosaccharidosis
    Aspartilglycosaminuria
    Mannosidosis
    Fucosidosis

Mixed storage diseases
    Known deficiency: Gangliosidosis
                       Austin disease
    Unknown deficiency: mucolipidosis II
                        mucolipidosis III

Known deficiency disease not covered by the preceding forms
    Pompe disease
    Wolman disease
    Cholesterol storage of esters disease (CSED)

7.1. Mucopolysaccharidosis

Light microscopy reveals the presence of vacuoles highly variable in size and number within the hepatocytes. The ultrastructural equivalent is made up of numerous roundish cytoplasmic vacuoles, 5–15 μm in diameter, bound by a membrane. These vacuoles are not located at any particular site within the cytoplasm and only seem to prefer areas of the pericanalicular ectoplasm in some cases. Their content is scattered in flocculent-like formations which ultrastructural cytochemical techniques have shown to be of mucopolysaccharide nature (Fig. 10). Other vacuolar inclusions may contain polymorphous formations, such as more or less electron-dense spherules or clusters of finely granular material. The content sometimes appears arranged in filamentous formations, while inclusions containing lamellar membranous structures are rare. Acid phosphatase activity is constantly high at the level of all these vacuoles. Kupffer cells sometimes seem to contain 'zebra bodies' as well as a large number of lysosomes with a clear matrix. In these cells, the lysosomal vacuoles

are smaller than those of hepatocytes and are rarely over 5 μm in diameter.

7.2. Niemann-Pick disease

Three main forms can be identified on the basis of clinical signs and the degree of enzyme deficiency (acute infantile form, subacute form, and adult form) which all share the same hepatosplenomegaly.

Prior to the development of electron microscopy, the morphological diagnosis of Niemann-Pick disease was formed on the basis of the presence of Pick cells, large elements with a diameter over 40 μm sometimes with two nuclei and often pycnotic. After treatment with lipid solvents, these cells reveal a fine areolar reticulum which gives them a characteristic vacuolated honeycomb appearance or that of foam cells. Using the May-Grunwald-Giemsa method, sphingomyelin storage can be demonstrated by revealing blue (lipidic) granules which also prove positive to Sudan Black B and PAS staining. Characteristic 'Maltese crosses' sometimes appear under the polarizing microscope. At ultrastructural examination, lysosomal vacuolar inclusions can be observed in the hepatocyte cytoplasm with a matrix containing membranous structures. This storage product is often arranged in alternate dark and light lamellae with the characteristic periodicity of complex lipids and a tendency to settle concentrically or one parallel to the other. Acid phosphatase tests are always positive at the level of these lysosomal inclusions. Normal peribiliary lysosomes are very scarce and sometimes absent. The typical Niemann-Pick elements also present lysosomal cytoplasmic inclusions containing electron-dense material sometimes alternated with transparent lamellae, each at a distance of 4–5 nm. Kupffer cells appear larger than normal and their cytoplasm is often packed with roundish lysosomal formations containing granular or granulofilamentous material, rarely lamellar in appearance.

7.3. Gaucher disease

Three main clinical forms of Gaucher disease have been identified on the basis of the period of onset and evolution (acute or infantile form, subacute or

158

juvenile form, and adult form), all of which are characterized by splenomegaly. A cerebrosidic thesaurosis lies at the basis of this disease, i.e., intracellular storage of glucosilcerebrosides. Conspicuous storage of these lipids at the level of the reticulohistiocyte cells is explained by the fact that they are found in enormous quantities in erythrocytes and leucocytes. In light microscopy, the diagnosis of Gaucher disease is formulated on the basis of the finding of characteristic Gaucher cells, histiocytes containing glucosilcerebrosides, in bone marrow, the splenic red pulp and in lymphonodular bioptic material. These cells appear large (20–80 μm in diameter), round or oval, and are usually mononucleate. At high magnification, their cytoplasm presents typical, often parallel streaks. Ultrastructural analysis of Gaucher cells reveals how their cytoplasm contains roundish or fusiform inclusions, 0.6–4.0 μm in size, bound by a membrane and detectable as lysosomes overloaded by constant positivity to acid phosphatase. The structure of the material stored within these inclusions appears characteristic. They are tubular structures between 13 and 75 nm thick, tightly packed, and usually parallel to the main axis of the lysosomal vacuole (Fig. 12). They are separated by a thin line of clear transparent matrix and are not penetrated by electron staining methods. Erythrophagosomes are also present in Gaucher cells and this explains their rich ferritin content detectable by using suitable analytic ultrastructural methods. The hepatocytes appear exempt from storage. From an ultrastructural point of view, apart from the storage site, Gaucher disease can be distinguished from other forms of lipidosis by the peculiar submicroscopic characteristics of the glucocerebrosides within dilated lysosomes, practically the only complex lipids never to produce pseudomyelinic lamellar figures.

7.4. Gangliosidosis GM 1 (Norman-Landing disease)

Ultrastructural analysis of material from the liver biopsies of patients with Norman-Landing disease reveals the presence of vacuolar formations in the hepatocytes. These formations are 0.3–11.0 μm in diameter, bound by a membrane, and acid phosphatase positive with a matrix which has a basically flocculent or medium-granular appearance and a

marked storage of disordered filamentous material as well as rare amorphous-homogeneous spherules. Each filament is 10–20 nm thick and 1.0–1.5 μm in length; rarely the microfilaments are stacked in groups of four to five. A more limited number of hypertrophic secondary lysosomes contains lamellar lipidic formations with a circular development. The remaining organelle population of the hepatocytes seems undamaged, and hypertrophy of the smooth endoplasmic reticulum is noted only in some cases while there is a certain decrease in the rough reticulum. Vacuolar inclusions of lysosomal nature, wholly similar to those of the hepatocytes, are found in the sinusoid endothelial cells and Kupffer cells.

7.5. Glycogenosis type II or Pompe disease

In Pompe disease, glycogen storage occurs within the lysosomes of numerous parenchymal cells due to the deficient action of acid maltase (acid alpha-1,4-glucosidase). Light-microscopic analysis of the hepatocytes of patients with Pompe disease produces findings which can be added to those detectable in other forms of glycogenosis, such as Von Gierke disease. Under the electron microscope, a considerable increase in the amount of hyaloplasmic glycogen can be seen in the hepatocyte, mainly in the form of rosettes. At the same time, the glycogen appears enclosed in vacuoles containing acid phosphatase, called 'glycogen residual bodies.' The glycogen contained in them may appear both in the form of rosettes and as single particles and is called 'lysosomal glycogen.' It is therefore clear that submicroscopic analysis is the only morphological test able to distinguish between this and other forms of glycogenosis. Most of the lysosomes overloaded with glycogen are found in the hepatocytes, but hypertrophic lysosomes of the 'glycogen residual bodies' type can also be found in the endothelial cells, Kupffer cells, and the epithelial cells of the bile ductules.

In conclusion, as can be seen from this concise chapter, electron microscopy has contributed a great deal of new, important information to the study of human liver pathology, together with a better understanding of the data supplied by the use of light microscopy. Further progress, particularly as regards the more detailed morphological identification of the different etiological agents of hepatitis, shall result from the development and routine use of more and more sophisticated techniques, and from growing collaboration between pathologists practicing electron microscopy and clinicians.

REFERENCES

1. Laschi R (1978) Diagnostic ultrastructural du foie. Arch Anat Cytol Pathol 26: 267–270
2. Desmet VJ (1972) Morphologic and histochemical aspects of cholestasis. In: Popper H, Schaffner F (eds) Progress in liver diseases, vol 4. New York: Grune and Stratton, pp 97–132
3. Schaff Z, Lapis K (1979) Cholestasis. In: Johannessen JV (ed) Electron microscopy in human medicine, vol 8. London: McGraw-Hill International, pp 80–88
4. DiDio LJA (1971) Myocardial mitochondrosis or mitochondritis: an electron microscopic study. Ateneo Parmense [Acta Biomed] 4:359–399
5. Faller A (1977) Gibt es eine Mitochondriose? Acta Anat (Basel) 99:263–264
6. Schaffner F, Popper H (1969) Cholestasis is the result of hypoactive hypertrophic smooth endoplasmic reticulum in the hepatocyte. Lancet 2:355–359
7. Holborow EJ, Trencher PS, Dorling J, Webb J (1975) Demonstration of smooth muscle contractile protein antigens and epithelial cells. Ann NY Acad Sci 254:489–504
8. Phillips MJ, Oda M, Mak E, Fisher MM, Jeejeeboy KN (1975) Microfilament disfuncton as a possible cause of intrahepatic cholestasis. Gastroenterology 69:48–58
9. French SW (1976) Is cholestasis due to microfilament failure? Hum Pathol 7:243–244
10. Erlinger S (1978) Cholestasis: pump failure, microvilli defect, or both? Lancet 1:533–534
11. Feinstone SM, Kapikian AZ, Purcell RH (1973) Detection by immune electron microscopy of a virus-like antigen associated with acute illness. Science 182:1026–1028
12. Hilleman MR, Provost PJ, Wolanski BS (1974) Characterization of CR 326 human hepatitis A virus, a probable enterovirus. Presented at the International Association of Biological Standardization Symposium on Viral Hepatitis, Milan, Italy, December 1974
13. Report of the WHO Expert Committee on Viral Hepatitis (1977) Advances in viral hepatitis. WHO Tech Rep Ser 602:1–62
14. Provost PJ, Wolanski BS, Miller WJ, Ittensohn OL, McAleer WJ, Hilleman MR (1975) Physical, chemical and morphologic dimension of human hepatitis A virus strain CR 326 (38578). Proc Soc Exp Biol Med 148:532–539
15. Mathiesen RL, Feinstone SM, Purcell RH, Wagner J (1977) Detection of hepatitis A antigen by immunofluorescence. Infect Immun 18:524–530
16. Shimizu YK, Mathiesen LR, Lorenz D, Drucker J, Feinstone SM, Wagner JA, Purcell RH (1978) Localization of hepatitis A antigen in liver tissue by peroxidase-conjugated antibody method: light and electron microscopic studies. 121:1671–1679
17. Gudat F, Bianchi L, Sonnabend W, Thiel G, Aenishaenslin W, Stalder GA (1975) Patterns of core and surface expression in liver tissue reflects state of specific immune response in hepatitis B. Lab Invest 31:1–9
18. De Vos R, Ray MB, Desmet VJ (1979) Electron microscopy of hepatitis B virus components in chronic active liver disease. J Clin Pathol 32:590–600
19. Huang SH, Neurath AR (1979) Immunohistologic demonstration of hepatitis B viral antigens in liver with reference to its significance in liver injury. Lab Invest 40:1–17
20. Hirschan SZ, Gerber M, Garfinkel E (1975) Observations on the core particles of hepatitis B virus and the DNA polymerase associated with hepatitis B antigen. Am J Med Sci 270:141–149
21. Busachi CA, Badiali De Giorgi L, Gardelli T, Bianchi FB, Pisi E, Laschi R (1980) Studio immunoistochimico ed ultrastrutturale degli antigeni del virus della epatite B (HBsAg–HBcAg) nelle epatopatie croniche. In: Gasbarrini G, Miglio F, Bernardi M (eds) Attualità in epatologia. Bologna: Editrice Compositori, pp 23–25
22. Michalak Y, Nowoslawski A (1977) Hepatitis B virus in nucleoli of liver cells. N Engl J Med 297:787–788
23. Bianchi L, Gudat F (1979) Immunopathology of hepatitis B. In: Popper H, Schaffner F (ed) Progress in liver diseases, vol 6. New York: Grune and Stratton, pp 371–392
24. Bayer ME, Blumberg BS, Werner B (1968) Particles associated with Australia antigen in the sera of patients with leukaemia, Down's syndrome and hepatitis. Nature (Lond) 218:1057–1059
25. Stein O, Fainaru M, Stein Y (1972) Visualization of virus-like particles in endoplasmic reticulum of hepatocytes of Australia antigen carriers. Lab Invest 26:262–269
26. Gerber MA, Hadziyannis S, Vissoulis C, Schaffner F, Paronetto F, Popper H (1974) Hepatitis B antigen: nature and distribution of cytoplasmic antigen in hepatocytes of carriers. Proc Soc Exp Biol Med 145:863–867
27. Ray MB, Desmet VJ, Bradburne AF, Desmyter J, Fevery J, De Groote J (1976) Differential distribution of hepatitis B surface antigen and hepatitis B core antigen in the liver of hepatitis B patients. Gastroenterology 71:462–469
28. Gudat F, Bianchi L (1977) HBsAg: a target antigen on the liver cell? In: Popper H, Bianchi L, Reutter W (eds) Membrane alterations as basis of liver injury. Lancaster: MTP, pp 171–178
29. Busachi CA, Ray MB, Desmet VJ (1978) An immunoperoxidase technique for demonstrating membrane localized HBsAg in paraffin sections of liver biopsies. J Immunol Methods 19:95–99
30. Yamada G, Nakane PK (1979) Hepatitis B core and surface antigens in liver tissue. Lab Invest 36:649–659
31. Trepo C, Vitvitski L, Neurath R, Hashimoto N, Schaefer R, Nemoz G, Prince AM (1976) Detection of e antigen by immunofluorescence in cytoplasm of hepatocytes of HBsAg carriers. Lancet 1:486
32. Arnold W, Niesen JO, Hardt F, Meyer Zum Buschenfeld KH (1977) Localisation of HBe antigen in nuclei of hepatocytes in HBsAg-positive liver disease. Gut 18:994–996
33. Neurath AR, Strick M (1977) Host specificity of a serum marker for hepatitis B: evidence that 'e antigen' has the properties of an immunoglobulin. Proc Natl Acad Sci USA 74:1702–1706

34. Vyas GN, Peterson DL, Townsend RM, Damle SR, Magnuisho W (1977) Hepatitis B 'e' antigen an association with lactate dehydrogenase isozyme-S. Science 198:1068–1070

35. Rizzetto M, Canese MG, Aricò S, Crivelli O, Trepo C, Bonino F, Verme G (1977) Immunofluorescence detection of new antigen-antibody system (δ/anti δ) associated to hepatitis B virus in liver and serum of HBsAg carriers. Gut 18:997–1003

36. Canese MG, Rizzetto M, Aricò S, Crivelli O, Zanetti AR, Macchiorlatti E, Ponzetto A, Leone L, Mollo F, Verme G (1979) An ultrastructural and immunohistochemical study on the δ antigen associated with the hepatitis B virus. J Pathol 128:169–175

37. Prince AM, Brotman B, Grady GJ, Kuhns WJ, Harri C, Levine RW, Millian SJ (1974) Long-incubation post-transfusion hepatitis without serological evidence of exposure to hepatitis-B virus. Lancet 2:241–246

38. Bradley DW, Cook EH, Maynard JE, McCaustland KA, Ebert JW, Dolana GH, Petzel RA, Kantor RJ, Heilbrunn A, Fields HA, Murphy BL (1979) Experimental infection of chimpanzees with antihemophilic (factor VIII) materials: recovery of virus like particles associated with non-A, non-B hepatitis. J Med Virol 3:253–269

39. Coursaget P, Maupas P, Levin P, Barin F (1979) Virus-like particles associated with non-A, non-B hepatitis. Lancet 2:92

40. Vitvitski L, Trepo C, Prince AM, Brotman B (1979) Detection of virus-associated antigen in serum and liver of patients with non-A, non-B hepatitis. Lancet 2:1263–1267

41. Trump BF, Kim KM, Iseri OA (1976) Cellular pathophysiology of hepatitis. Am J Clin Pathol [Suppl] 65:828–847

42. Scotto JM, Stralin HG (1976) Relationship between nuclear bodies and intranuclear invaginations in parenchymal liver cells of patients with viral hepatitis. J Microsc Biol Cell 25:233–235

43. Schaffner F, Popper H (1963) Capillarization of hepatic sinusoids in man. Gastroenterology 44:239–242

44. Cavalli G, Bianchi FB, Bacci G, Casali AM (1971) Ultrastructural studies of bile ductules in the course of acute hepatitis. Acta Hepatosplenologica 18:355–363

45. Lapis K, Schaff Z (1979) Chronic hepatitis. In: Johannessen JV (ed) Electron microscopy in human medicine, vol 8. London: McGraw-Hill International, pp 137–157

46. Hopwood D, Nyfors A (1976) Effect of methotrexate therapy in psoriatics on the Ito cells in liver biopsies, assessed by point-counting. J Clin Pathol 29:698–703

47. Schaffner F, Dienstag JL, Purcell RH, Popper H (1977) Chimpanzee livers after infection with human hepatitis viruses A and B. Arch Pathol Lab Med 101:113–117

48. French SW, Burbige EJ (1979) Alcoholic hepatitis: clinical, morphologic, pathogenic, and therapeutic aspects. In: Popper H, Schaffner F (eds) Progress in liver diseases, vol 6. New York: Grune and Stratton, pp 557–579

49. Iseri OA, Gottlieb LS (1971) Alcoholic hyalin and megamitochondria as separate and distinct entities in liver disease associated with alcoholism. Gostroenterology 60:1027–1035

50. Gerber MA, Orr W, Deuk H, Schaffner F, Popper H (1973) Hepatocellular hyalin in cholestasis and cirrhosis: its diagnostic significance. Gastroenterology 64:89–98

51. Fortin R (1973) Dégénérescence hyaline de Mallory à localisation inhabituelle. Ann Anat Pathol (Paris) 18:459–462

52. Chedid A, Spellberg MA, De Beer RA (1974) Ultrastructural aspects of primary biliary cirrhosis and other types of cholestatic liver disease. Gastroenterology 67:858–869

53. Popper H, Schaffner F (1974) Steatosis. Mallory's hyalin-cirrhosis: can their relationships be resolved by an experiment of nature? Gastroenterology 67:185–188

54. Nenci I (1975) Brief communication: identification of actin-like proteins in alcoholic hyalin by immunofluorescence. Lab Invest 32:257–260

55. French SW, Sim JS, Caldwell MG (1977) Thick microfilaments (intermediate filaments) and chronic alcohol ingestion. In: Popper H, Bianchi L, Reutter W (eds) Membrane alterations as basis of liver injury. Lancaster: MTP, pp 311–325

56. Zetterman RK, Leevy CM (1975) Immunologic reactivity and alcoholic liver disease. Bull NY Acad Med 51:533–544

57. Schaffner F (1971) Electron microscopy of acute alcoholic hepatitis. In: Gerok W, Sickinger K, Hennekeuser HH (eds) Alcohol and the liver. New York: FK Schattauer, pp 273–279

58. Yokoo H, Minick O, Batti F, Kent G (1972) Morphologic variants of alcoholic hyalin. Am J Pathol 69:25–32

59. Orrego H, Medline A, Blendis LM, Rankin JG, Kreaden DA (1979) Collagenisation of the Disse space in alcohol liver disease. Gut 20:673–679

60. Mezey E, Potter JJ, Maddrey WC (1975) Hepatic fibrogenesis in alcoholism. In: Khanna JM, Israel Y, Kalant H (eds) Alcoholic liver pathology. Ontario: Addiction Research Foundation, pp 145–156

61. Tanikawa K (1975) Fine structural alterations and biochemical changes of the liver in acute alcohol intoxication. In: Popper H, Becher K (eds) Collagen metabolism in the liver. New York: Stratton Intercontinental Medical, pp 93–99

62. Dickson ER, Fleming CR, Ludwig J (1979) Primary biliary cirrhosis. In: Popper H, Schaffner F (eds) Progress in liver diseases, vol 6. New York: Grune and Stratton, pp 487–502

63. Thomas HC, Potter BJ, Sherlock S (1977) Is primary biliary cirrhosis an immune complex disease? Lancet 2:1261–1263

64. Monroe S, French SW, Zamboni L (1972) Mallory bodies in a case of primary biliary cirrhosis: an ultrastructural and morphogenetic study. Am J Clin Pathol 59:254–262

65. Lapis K, Schaff Z (1979) Cirrhosis. In: Johannessen JV (ed) Electron microscopy in human medicine, vol 8. London: McGraw-Hill International, pp. 158–187

66. Busachi CA, Badiali De Giorgi L, Bianchi FB (1979) Increased ductular microfilaments in primary biliary cirrhosis. J Submicrosc Cytol 11:409–412

67. Bianchi FB, Penforld PL, Roitt IM (1973) Mitochondrial antibodies in primary biliary cirrhosis. V. Ultrastructural localization of the antigen to the inner mitochondrial membrane using a direct peroxidase conjugate. Br J Exp Pathol 54:652–657

68. Gautier A, Okolicsànyi L, Gardiol D (1968) Constitutional non hemolytic hyperbilirubinemia and the passage of bilirubin through the hepatocyte. A critical and experimental contribution to ultrastructural investigation of the liver. In: Sherlock S, Dioguardi N (eds) Liver reactivity. Milano: Fondazione Carlo Erba, pp 17–42

69. Lapis K (1979) Metabolic disorders. In: Johannessen JV (ed) Electron microscopy in human medicine, vol 8. London: McGraw-Hill International, pp 20–79

70. Berthelot P, Dhumeaux D (1978) New insights into the classification and mechanisms of hereditary, chronic, non haemolytic hyperbilirubinaemias. Gut 19:474–480

71. Dawson J, Carr-Locke DL, Talbot JC. Rosenthal FD (1979) Gilbert's syndrome: evidence of morphological heterogeneity. Gut 20:848–853

72. Arias IM, Gartner LM, Cohen M, Ben-Ezzer J, Levi AJ

(1969) Chronic non hemolytic unconjugated hyperbilirubinemia with glucuronyl transferase deficiency. Clinical, biochemical pharmacologic and genetic evidence for heterogeneity. Am J Med 47:395–409

73. Minio-Paluello F, Gautier A, Magnenat P (1968) L'ultrastructure du foie humaine dans un cas de Crigler-Najjar. Acta Hepatosplenologica 15:65–71

74. Swartz HM, Sarna T, Varna RR (1979) On the nature and excretion of the hepatic pigment in the Dubin-Johnson syndrome. Gastroenterology 76:958–964

75. Tanikawa K (1979) Liver pathology. In: Trump BF, Jones RT (eds) Diagnostic electron microscopy, vol 2. New York: John Wiley, pp 15–46

76. Resibois A, Tondeur M, Mockel S, Dustin P (1970) Lysosomes and storage diseases. Int Rev Exp Pathol 9:93–149.

77. Hers HG, Van Hoof F (1979) Lysosomes and storage diseases. New York: Academic

78. Dustin P, Tondeur M, Libert J (1979) Metabolic and storage diseases. In: Johannessen JV (ed) Electron microscopy in human medicine, vol 2. London: McGraw-Hill International, pp 151–221

79. Shimizu YK, Feinstone SM, Purcell RH, Alter HJ, London WT (1979) Non-A, non-B hepatitis: ultrastructural evidence for two agents in experimentally infected chimpanzees. Science 205:197–200

80. Bradley DW, Maynard JE, Cook EH, Ebert JW, Gravelle CR, Tsiquaye KN, Kessler H, Zuckerman AJ, Miller MF, Ling C, Overby LR (1980) Non-A/non-B hepatitis in experimentally infected chimpanzees: cross-challenge and electron microscopic studies. J Med Virol 6:185–201

81. Busachi CA, Realdi G, Badiali De Giorgi L, Alberti A (1980) Hepatocellular ultrastructural changes in patients with acute and chronic non-A, non-B hepatitis. J Submicrosc Cytol 12:681–686

82. Tsiquaye KN, Bird RG, Tovery G, Wyke RJ, Williams R, Zuckerman AJ (1980) Further evidence of cellular changes associated with non-A, non-B hepatitis. J Med Virol 5:63–71

83. De Woolf-Peeters C, De Vos R, Desmet V, Ray MB, Desmyter J, De Groote G, Fevery J, Broeckaert L, De Groote J (1981) Human non-A, non-B hepatitis: ultrastructural alterations in hepatocytes. Liver 1:50–55

10. RADIOLOGY OF THE LIVER

A.J. CHRISTOFORIDIS

1. INTRODUCTION

The advent of computed tomography (CT) opened new horizons in the study of the gross radiologic morphology of the liver and its pathological manifestations in vivo [1–5]. The use of ultrasound and radionuclide imaging plays an active role in the daily routine of clinical radiology. CT scanning, however, with the now achieved short times of exposure, from one to ten seconds, and the availability of thin layers down to one millimeter thickness, together with the reconstruction capabilities of the newer CT units, gives a distinct advantage in many cases over the other noninvasive modalities. The cost of the examination and the absence of the CT scanner even today from many hospitals, of course, remains a serious obstacle in the utilization of this most important modality as a routine procedure in the daily clinical praxis. Invasive procedures, such as arteriography, splenoportography, transhepatic cholangiography, biliary drainage procedures, needle aspiration biopsies of the liver, and retrograde pancreaticocholangiography, remain important radiologic interventional procedures used commonly in medical centers in the last several years. The scope of this edition with its limitation of space prevents us from describing these important invasive radiological modalities in the examination of the liver. Reference, however, to these will be made in the discussion primarily of computed tomographic examination of the liver, which is considered to the most important development in diagnostic radiology of the abdominal organs in reent years. It is not within the objectives of this chapter to discuss useful and time-honored examinations such as oral cholecystography and intravenous cholangiography, which will be mentioned only in the discussion of more recent developments. Important diagnostic modalities such as radionuclide imaging and ultrasound will be discussed and their merits and important applications will be illustrated and compared with computed tomography.

The use of CT in the evaluation of hepatic diseases did not decrease the significance of the use of radionuclide scanning or the valuable and, many times, unique contributions offered by ultrasonography or angiography. This becomes evident in the discussion of the merits of each of these modalities in solving individual clinical problems. However, the specific advantages of computed tomography, particularly the accuracy of the morphologic findings and the importance of the attenuation characteristics of different disease entities, resulted in reassessment of the indications and the proper sequence in the utilization of the other imaging modalities. While in some instances the CT examination can satisfactorily establish a diagnosis without further need to resort to the utilization of other procedures, in many cases and particularly in the most problematic ones, the other methods should be applied in combination and in a logical sequence so that the diagnostic accuracy can be potentiated resulting often in the exact diagnosis for the patient's benefit. It should be emphasized that in order to obtain the best results, each clinical problem should be studied individually and with the full knowledge of the advantages as well as the limitations of each examination. With this background information, the proper sequence of these modalities can be meaningfully selected. We recognize the fact that some differences in approaching individual clinical situations do exist, and that there may be differences from one medical center to another. These are dictated sometimes by the previous experience of the radiologic team and the available equipment.

2. COMPUTED TOMOGRAPHY OF THE LIVER

The technique for examining the liver by computed tomography might not be a uniform one in all medical centers as indicated above. In our department we use the following steps. We administer to the patient approximately 300–400 cc of a 2% solution of Gastrogafin approximately 30–35 min prior to the patient's CT examination. The objective of this, of course, is to have the small bowel and possibly the right colon outlined by the contrast medium in order to avoid any interference of fluid-filled bowel loops which might resemble soft tissue densities while the opacified small bowel loops serve as a reference point to facilitate the demonstration of other intraabdominal organs [6]. Subsequently, and in approximately 3–5 min before the beginning of the CT scanning, another 200–300 cc of 2% solution of Gastrogafin is administered in order to secure the visualization of the stomach and the duodenal C-loop. The examination is performed using as a reference point the xyphoid process and at 1-cm intervals from the dome of the liver to the most caudal part of the organ. As expected, other adjacent organs such as the pancreas, spleen, kidneys, adrenals, aorta, and inferior vena cava, to mention some of the more important ones, are included in these sections and frequently render valuable and occasionally unexpected findings contributing to the better understanding of the patient's diagnostic problem.

A scout view of the abdomen is obtained to facilitate and expedite the sectioning at the desired levels, as these differ from patient to patient (Fig. 1). Subsequently follows the routine of administration of intravenous contrast medium in the form of a bolus of approximately 60 cc Conray 400 or in the form of an infusion of 150–200 cc of contrast

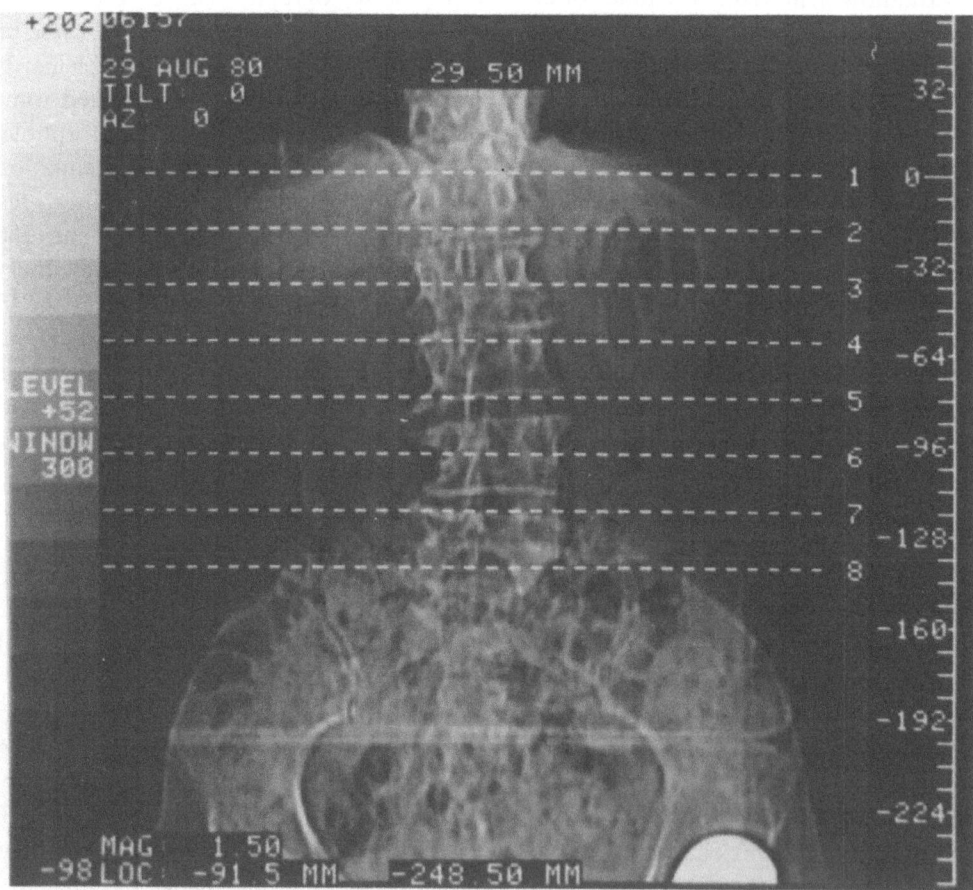

Figure 1. The broken lines from 1 to 8 in this scout view indicate the levels selected for the sectioning. The sections which are made subsequently correspond exactly to the predetermined levels. This feature of the CT scanner not only expedites the examination but also precludes any error regarding the accuracy of the examination at the desired levels.

medium with half the concentration of the contrast used in the bolus injection. The use of cholangiographic contrast, although theoretically attractive for opacifying the biliary system, did not prove in our experience to be very productive because of the associated side effects such as nausea, vomiting, and discomfort of the patient during the examination. These side effects might actually result in undesirable movement of the patient, and misleading partial volume effect detrimental particularly in the definition of smaller lesions. Although a lesion such as a cyst, an abscess, or a mass can be demonstrated adequately without the intravenous administration of contrast medium, the increase in the difference of the attenuation coefficient following the intravenous injection makes the diagnosis more accurate and improves the definition of the lesion. The significance of the contrast enhancement becomes more vital in cases of primary or metastatic lesions which, although usually of smaller attenuation number than the hepatic parenchyma, occasionally are almost or actually isodense. In this case, the administration of contrast medium becomes very important for the diagnosis.

The most common artifacts detrimental to the examination are those related to motion and specifically to the patient's respiration which can be avoided in many cases with the proper instruction to the patient. This is easier now with the newer scanners and their shorter exposure times. Cardiac motion transmitted to the upper part of the adjacent liver presents a lesser source of potential artifacts to be kept in mind, however, during the interpretation. The supine position is the one we use routinely for the examination of the liver. The scanning of the patient is monitored by the radiologist during the progress of the examination. He can, therefore, decide for possible modifications of the examination, if additional sections should be made depending on the available information, if additional contrast should be given, or if the examination should be terminated.

3. HEPATIC PARENCHYMAL DISEASE

Computed tomography can accurately demonstrate the size of the liver and its shape. It has a distinct advantage over other modalities in diffuse diseases when these result in the decrease or increase of the attenuation value of the hepatic parenchyma. A classic example is the fatty infiltration manifested by generalized diminished density of the parenchyma in which case the blood vessels within the liver are strikingly seen as areas of arborizing structures of increased attenuation surrounded by the diminished density of the liver parenchyma (Fig. 2). On the other side of the spectrum are the idiopathic hemosideroses or secondary hemosideroses manifested as generalized increased density of the liver while the vessels are easily detected as less dense branching structures.

In other diffuse diseases, specifically in hepatitis and cirrhosis, the CT findings are variable depending on the degree and extension of the disease. In early cases, the CT findings might give the appearance of a normal liver while, in advanced stages of atrophy, one can see areas of regenerated nodules which have the appearance of lobulations on the surface of the liver and which are more evident when they are profiled along the contour of the liver. Large intrahepatic vessels and particularly the hepatic veins can be easily demonstrated. Radionuclide scans are of significant diagnostic value here, enhancing the accuracy of the computed tomographic examination particularly in the early cases where the CT findings are not yet clearly detectable [7, 8].

On the other hand, it should be mentioned that in patients with cirrhosis where the radionuclide examination demonstrates focal difference in uptake, raising the question of metastatic disease, abscess or possibly hepatoma, the CT examination, following intravenous administration of contrast medium, will demonstrate that the attenuation of the regenerated nodules in cirrhosis will blend imperceptably with the surrounding hepatic parenchyma, thus pointing to the correct diagnosis. The presence of ascites (Fig. 3) can be detected easier and with greater accuracy with computed tomography than with any of the other available modalities, including radionuclide scanning or ultrasound [9–12]. The CT sections of the liver, besides demonstrating the size and contour of the hepatic parenchyma, include also an adequate outline of adjacent organs in general and of the spleen in particular, the condition of which is of specific interest in cases of cirrhosis. Enlargement of the

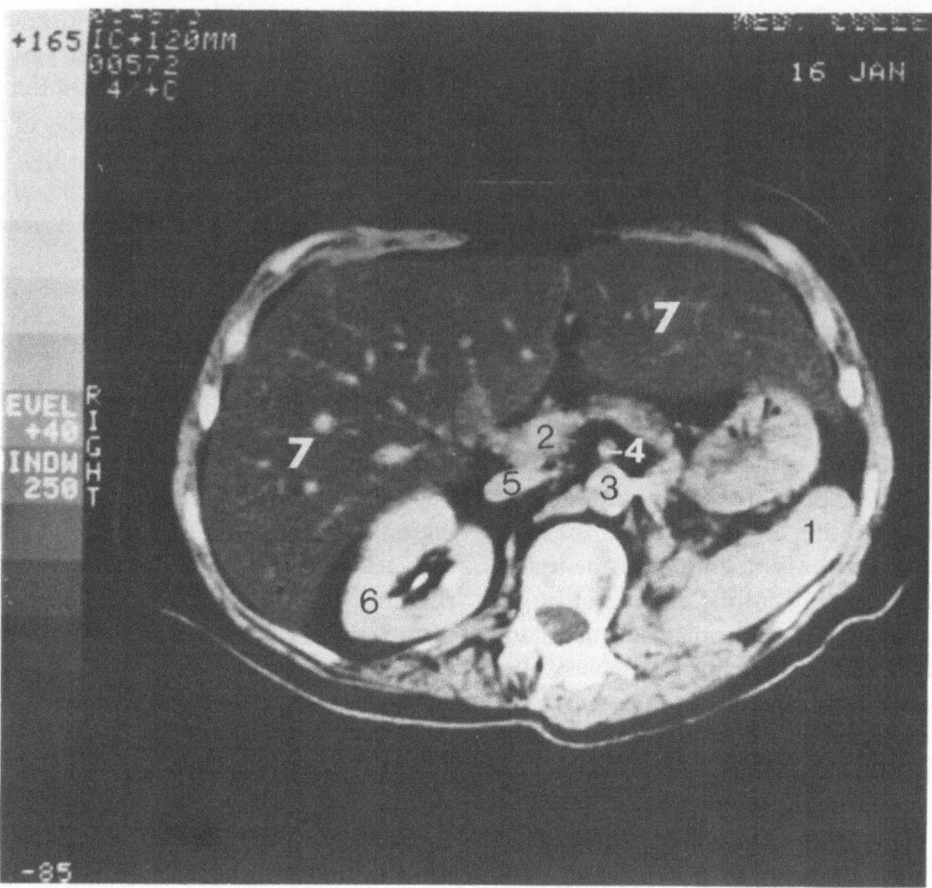

Figure 2. Fatty infiltration of the liver. Notice the decreased attenuation of the liver (7) and the relative increased density of the intrahepatic vessels; spleen (1), pancreas (2), aorta (3), superior mesenteric artery (4), inferior vena cava (5), right kidney (6).

spleen with associated splenic vein enlargement, and lobulations of the liver which might be small or of normal size, in addition of the presence of small amounts of ascites detected by computed tomography, will help in establishing the diagnosis of cirrhosis.

4. HEPATIC TRAUMA

The question of hepatic trauma is a relatively common one particularly in emergency rooms where victims of car accidents are frequently seen. Most of the patients are young, below the age of forty. Blunt abdominal trauma may be associated with multiple other injuries. The mortality rate is rather high. Computed tomography, representing a noninvasive and expeditious technique, has become the radiologic examination of choice. Intrahepatic as well as subcapsular haematomas are detectable

due to the high attenuation number of the fresh blood. The exact location and extension of the hematoma can be ascertained accurately. Older hematomas, however, have a lower attenuation number; therefore, differential diagnosis from other conditions such as abscess or cyst might be more difficult (Fig. 4a and b). Other radiologic modalities such as ultrasound, demonstrating a radiolucent area, radionuclide study, or hepatic artery angiogram might be of value although they will include the same differential diagnostic problems. The correlation with the clinical history might be important although it is not always as contributory as in the cases of recent acute trauma. Complications of previous hepatic trauma such as hepatic or subhepatic abscess, liver necrosis, or vascular injuries will make the diagnosis of an old trauma more difficult and, in this case, additional radiologic examinations including radionuclide study (i.e., gallium 67) for the detection of abscess [13] and

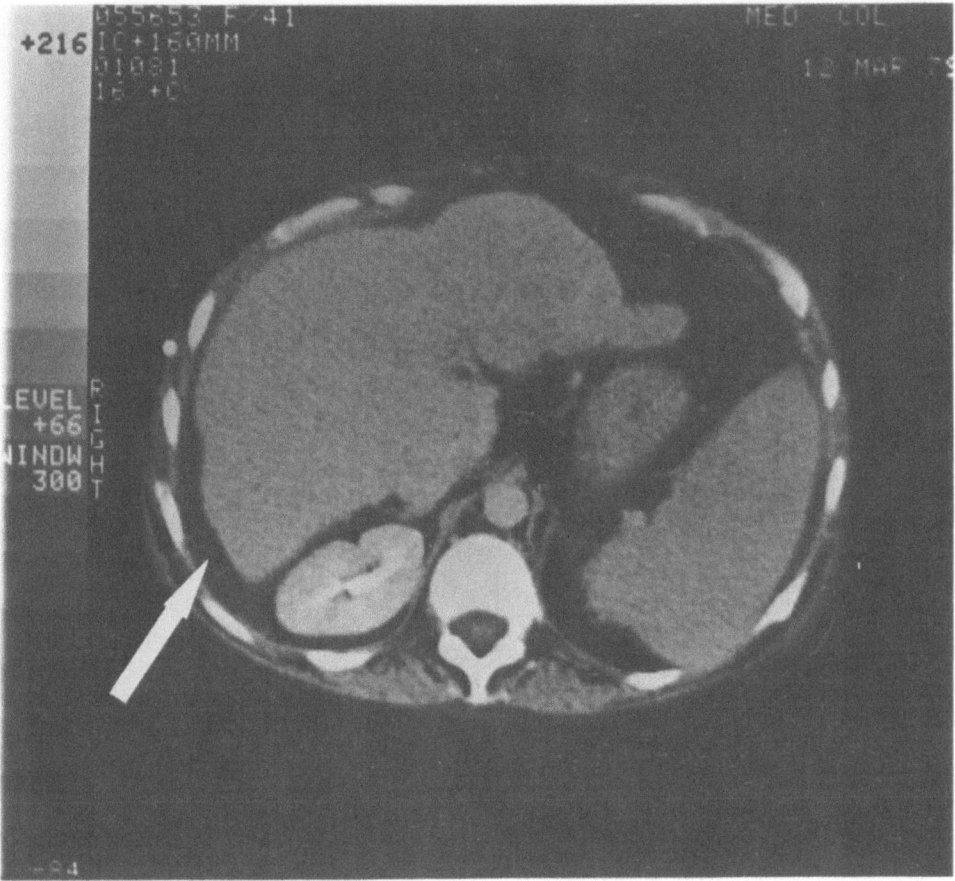

Figure 3. Patient with cirrhosis. Notice the nodular liver, enlarged spleen and the presence of ascites (arrow).

hepatic angiography for vascular lesions will be necessary for a more definitive diagnosis.

5. MASS LESIONS OF THE LIVER

The recognition of a mass lesion within the liver with CT is primarily dependent on the difference of the attenuation number of the tumor from that of the normal hepatic parenchyma [14, 15]. Generally speaking, the majority of lesions detected by computed tomography have a lower attenuation number than the surrounding normal liver tissue. Exceptions to this rule, such as an occasional metastatic lesion from the gastrointestinal tract where the lesion might be isodense, are rare. The difference in attenuation numbers could be very small or could be as high as 50 or 60 numbers (on a scale from −1000 to +1000), depending on the nature of the mass lesion. As a rule, when the difference is

significant, no enhancement by means of injection of intravenous contrast media is necessary; however, when the outline of a mass lesion is barely detectable or uncertain, it becomes mandatory to further evaluate the questionable mass by enhancement via the injection of intravenous contrast medium. As a rule, the normal hepatic parenchyma is accentuated more than a tumor mass. In a cystic lesion, the increase will be practically zero while in a malignant neoplasm it will differ depending on the nature and vascularity of the neoplasm. The information provided by the degree of the change in the attenuation number in the postcontrast examination becomes very important. In addition to rendering the lesion more visible by virtue of the increased difference between the normal liver parenchyma and the neoplasm, it might also contribute to the characterization of the lesion [16, 17]. The vascularity of the mass as a whole, of the periphery of the lesion, or of certain areas only of the mass

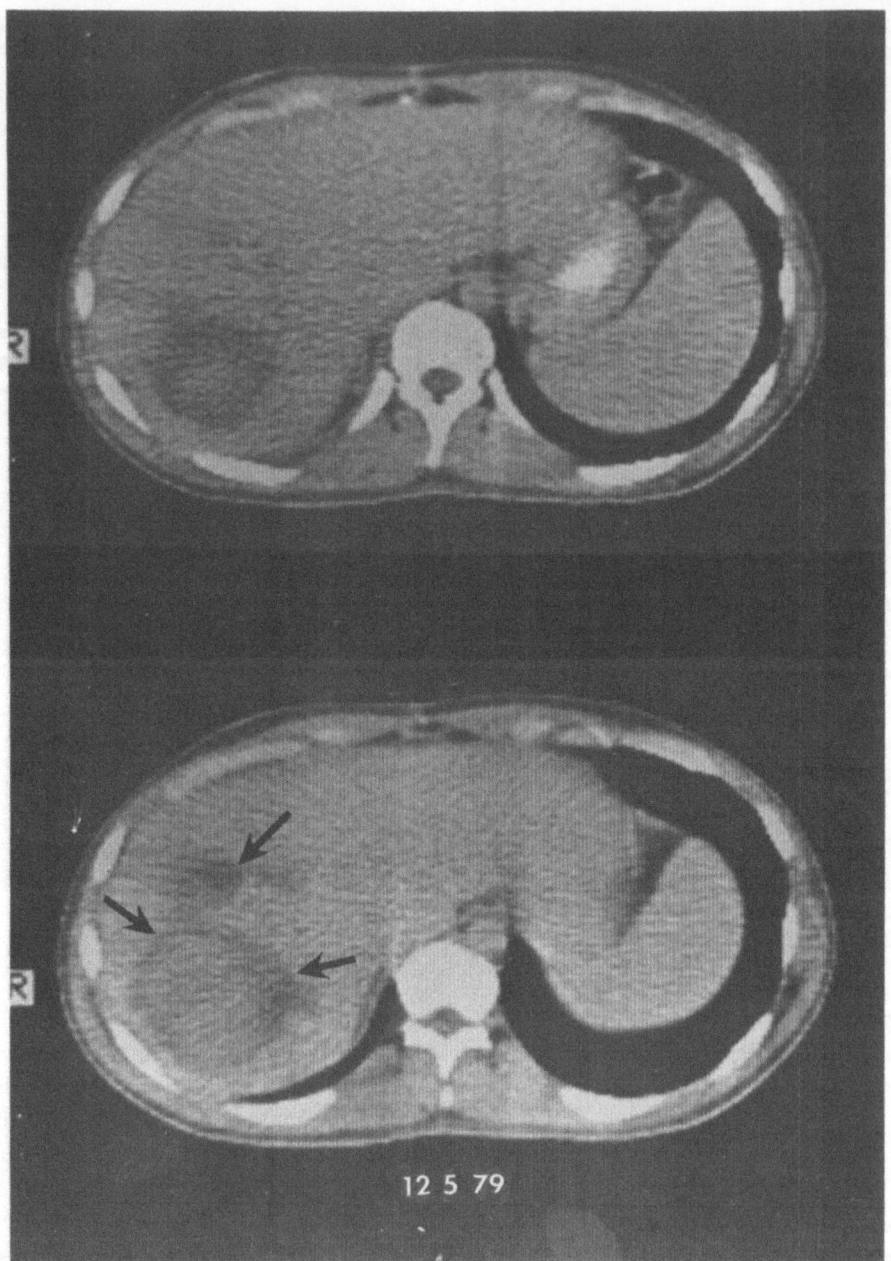

Figure 4a. Recent intrahepatic hematoma following trauma (5 Dec 1979).

constitutes important information. This is an advantage of computed tomography over other modalities, and we expect that this information will become even more accurate with the utilization of thinner sections and of the computed reconstruction in coronal and sagittal planes. Mass lesions can be further classified into benign and malignant.

In this respect we should briefly mention the more common masses:

5.1. Cysts. Hepatic cysts may be single or multiple. They are sharply defined and their shape might be round or oval and of water density, i.e., they have a smaller attenuation number than the surrounding normal hepatic tissue.

As in the case of renal cysts, the solitary hepatic cysts are many times asymptomatic and usually represent incidental findings. On the other hand, a polycystic disease of the liver, easily demonstrated

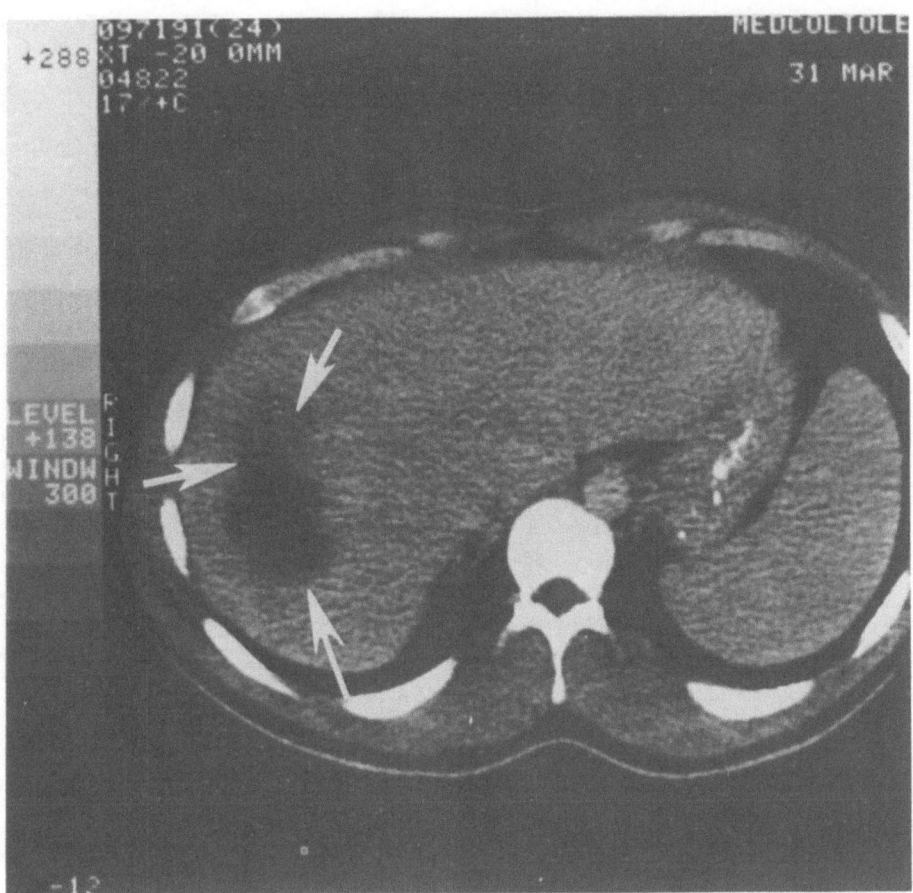

Figure 4b. Old intrahepatic hematoma four months later (31 Mar 1980). Notice the decreased attenuation (density) of the old hematoma.

by computed tomography, frequently is associated with polycystic disease of the kidneys. The exact dimensions of the cyst can be quickly demonstrated by the computer, and the thickness and uniformity of the wall can be appreciated. A cyst 1 cm in diameter can be easily demonstrated with the now available CT scanners. Enhancement with contrast medium of thin sections of 3–5 mm can assist in avoiding partial-volume averaging, thus making accurate determination of the attenuation number and rendering a clear outline of the cystic lesion. No other radiologic method can so accurately localize a small cystic lesion of 1 cm or less in size.

5.2. Hepatic abscess. A liver abscess might, at first glance, resemble a cyst; however, the two basic differences from the morphologic point of view, which should be looked for, are the outline of the abscess and the attenuation density. The definition of the abscess wall is not as sharply demarcated as in the case with cysts, while the wall is somewhat thicker. With contrast enhancement, the wall of the abscess usually shows some increase in density and occasionally a contour irregularity [18]. An increase in density of the parenchyma immediately adjacent to the wall of the abscess may be observed due to the associated inflammatory reaction in contradistinction to the contents of the abscess which, as expected, remain unchanged. Occasionally a cavitating tumor with an enhancement of its wall might imitate the presence of an abscess; however, besides the morphologic changes, the clinical history and the follow-up examination should not make difficult the differentiation of the two entities. As a matter of fact, computed tomography serves admirably in the follow-up of an abscess during the medical management. The decrease in the size of the abscess and also the reaction of the surrounding liver tissue can be well demonstrated in comparative follow-up studies (Fig. 5a–d).

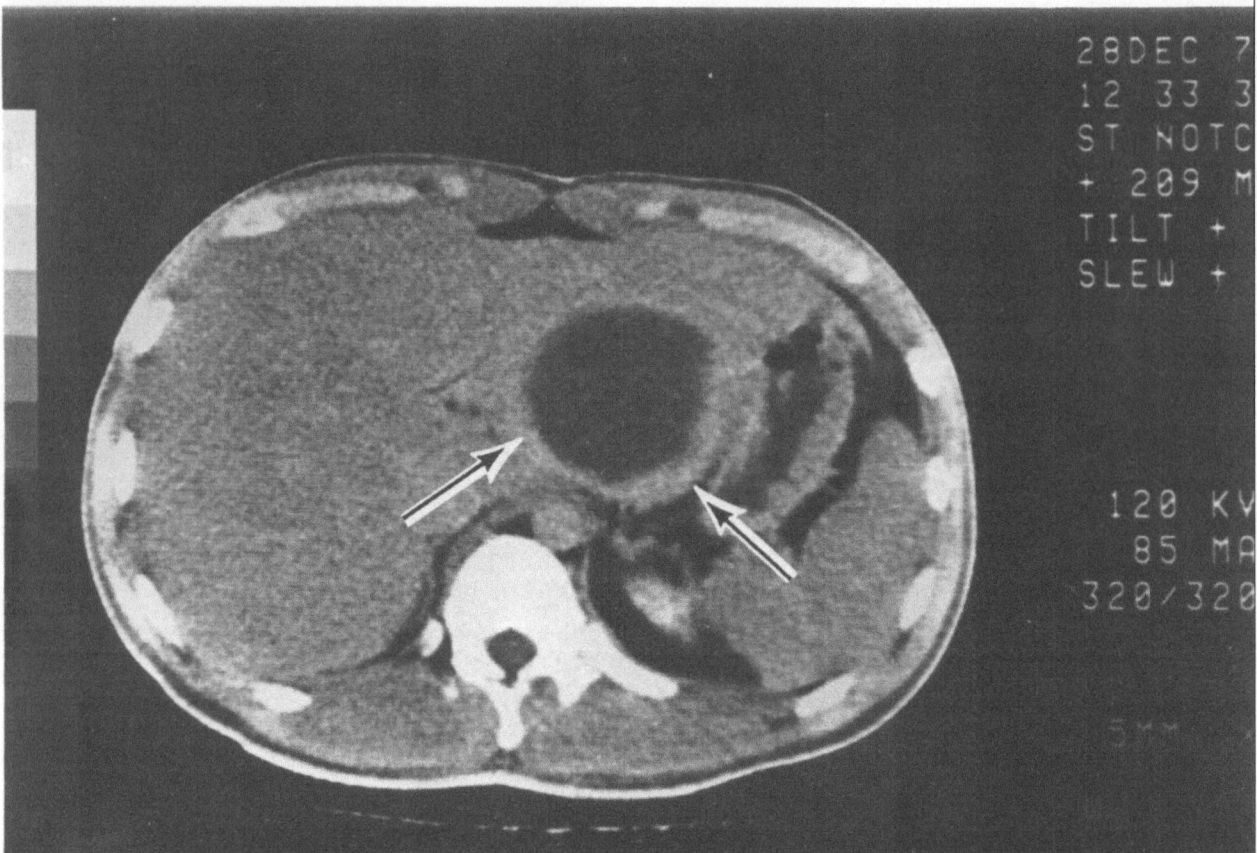

Figure 5a. Liver abscess. Notice the relatively thick and irregular wall with the increased attenuation number of the wall of the abscess and the adjacent inflammatory reaction of the hepatic parenchyma.

5.3 Malignant hepatic tumors. As mentioned above, almost all of the tumors of the liver, benign and malignant, exhibit a density which is lower to some degree from that of the normal hepatic parenchyma and varies from the almost isodense to that which might be necrotic, thus raising the question of differential diagnosis of an abscess formation (Fig. 6).

These neoplasms, if needed, can be further evaluated by enhancement with the use of intravenous contrast media, in which case it is expected that the difference with the attenuation of the surrounding liver parenchyma will increase and therefore outline even more clearly the presence of the neoplastic tissue. Occasionally some neoplasms are sharply outlined and round in shape, in which case they may raise the question of being cysts or old encapsulated hematomas (Fig. 7). In both cases, the attenuation number will be lower than that of a neoplastic lesion and, even more, their number will

remain unchanged following the intravenous injection of iodinated medium for enhancement purposes.

Differentiation between primary and metastatic lesions or between different histologic types of neoplasms has been attempted. There is indication that while some tumors are enhanced in a homogeneous way, other neoplasms such as those originating from the gastrointestinal tract show foci of increased density within the metastases. This as well as other suggested signs has not been as yet adequately tested and therefore should not be considered as reliable at this time. Attention should be paid to the fact that not infrequently sections of the liver include small radiolucent areas representing intrahepatic vessels which an unexperienced observer might consider as being due to small metastases, particularly in a patient with a known primary neoplasm. Two observations, in this regard, might solve the problem: (a) the fact that these small

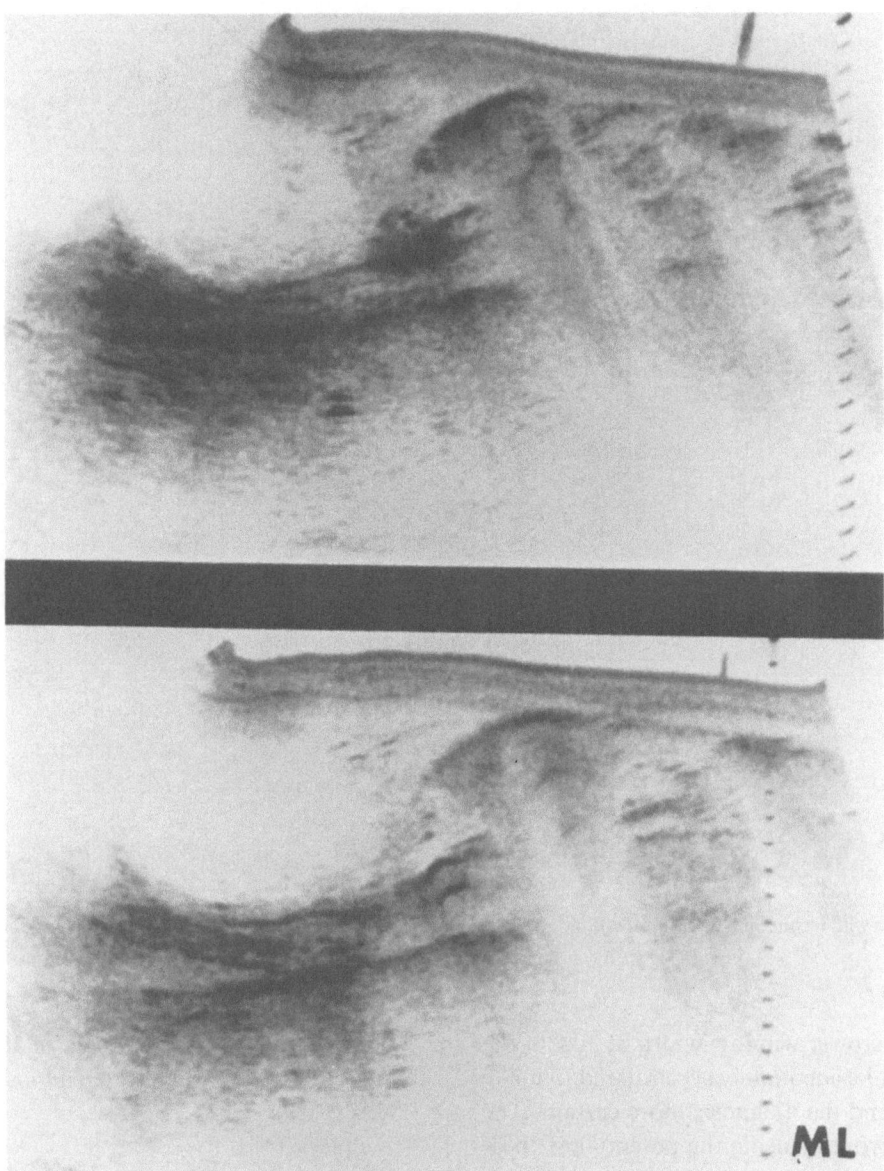

Figure 5b. Ultrasound study – midline longitudinal section. Notice the sonolucent area with some increased echoes which are not present in simple (noninfected) cystic lesions.

roundish filling defects become smaller when closer to the peripheral parts of the hepatic parenchyma, and (b) the observation that, following the injection of contrast medium, these round areas show a higher attenuation number comparable to the density of the adjacent inferior vena cava or aorta. The neoplastic tissue might also be enhanced, but not to the same degree as the vascular structures.

In discussing small metastatic lesions, a very common daily problem, we should again emphasize the use of thin sections in the range of 3–5 mm, easily obtainable with the present-day equipment, in order to demonstrate accurately these lesions which otherwise (with thicker slides of 1–2 cm) might not be demonstrated due to volume averaging. Another important factor of which we should be acutely aware is the proper utilization of the window setting. This is actually critical when the density of a neoplasm is barely discernible from the adjacent hepatic parenchyma. With a standard window setting, i.e., of 200, a tumor density might be barely perceptible, while with the use of a

172

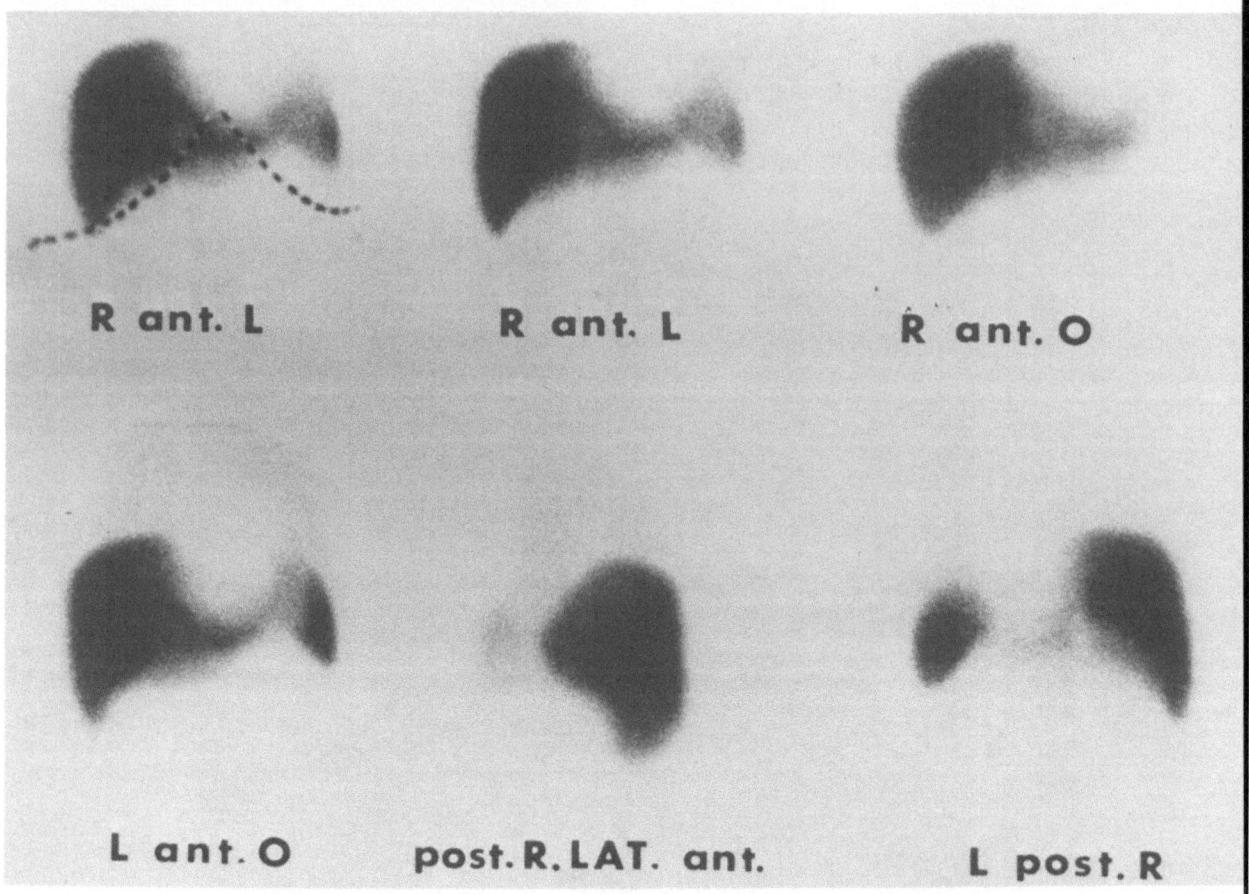

R ant. L   R ant. L   Ṙ ant. O

L ant. O   post. R. LAT. ant.   L post. R

Figure 5c. Liver scan with technetium 99m sulfur colloid. Nonspecific, large, rounded filling defect involving parts of the right and left lobes of the liver.

considerably narrower window width of 20–30, the difference might be adequately accentuated to make the distinction and the diagnosis more certain. The importance of properly using the potential of these versatile characteristics of computed tomographic units by adjusting the window setting and level cannot be overemphasized.

Gross tumor characterization based on the CT findings and with proper evaluation of the pre- and postcontrast enhancement studies can be made in cases of cavernous hemangiomas where in the pre-enhancement study the density is lower than that of the hepatic parenchyma and higher than that of a cyst or old hematoma. Following enhancement, the tumor and particularly its most peripheral part, due to rich vascular channels, exhibits an attenuation number higher than that expected in cases of an ordinary tumor and at the same time shows areas of considerably less opacification attributed to the presence of obliterated channels of the cavernous hemangioma due to the clotted blood.

6. EVALUATION OF THE BILIARY TREE

Under normal conditions, the larger ducts of the right and left lobe can be visualized following the administration of the cholangiographic contrast medium. The normal intrahepatic duct system and in particular the hepatic radicals are not visualized on CT scans, even following the intravenous administration of a contrast medium such as Cholografin. However, the attenuation number of the dilated and, therefore, visualized biliary duct system is almost similar to that of water density and can be differentiated from the vascular structures of the liver which have a density similar to that of the inferior vena cava. In case of doubt and for further

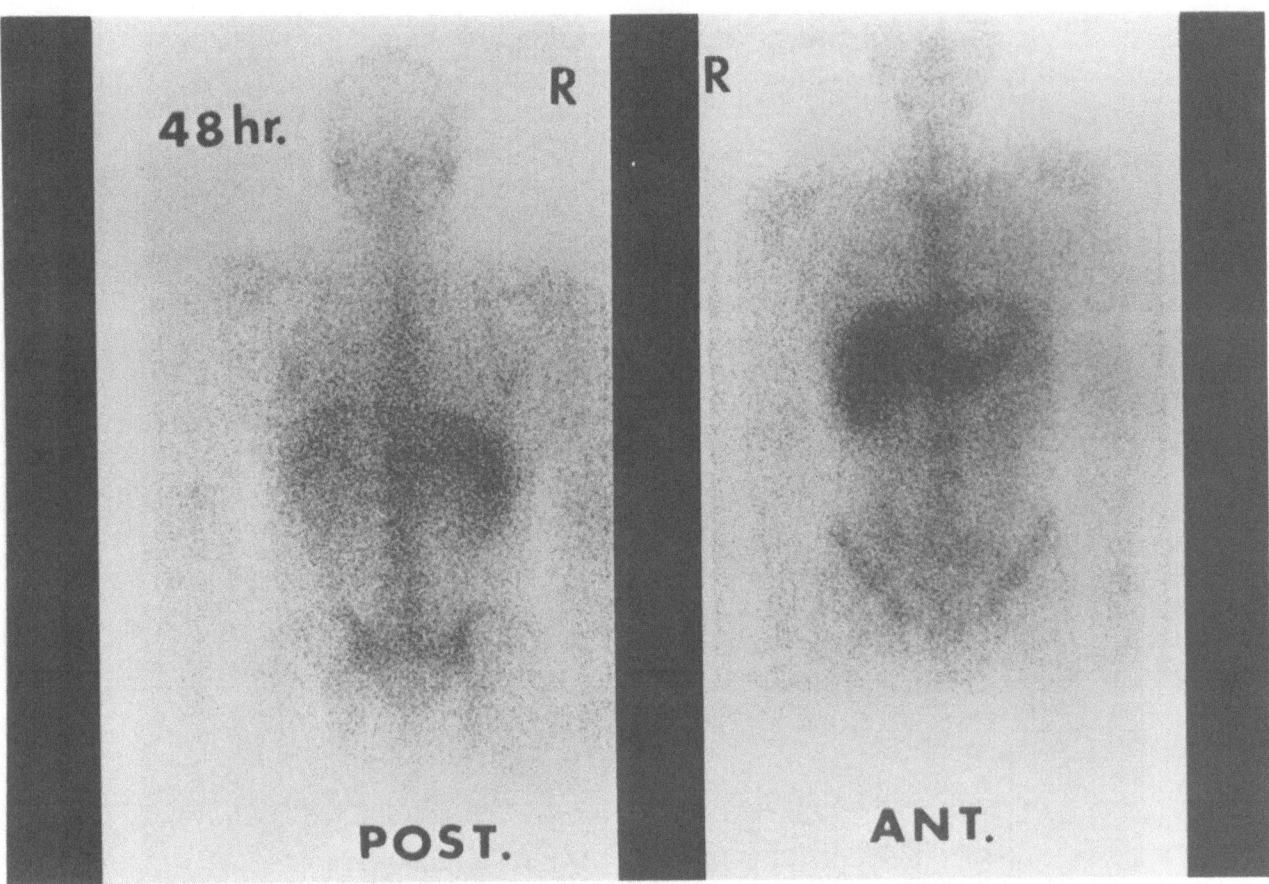

Figure 5d. Gallium-67 study. Follow-up at 48 h.

clarification, an intravenous injection of contrast medium will accentuate the vascular system, making in this way the differentiation from the biliary ducts rather obvious.

As a matter of fact, following the injection of intravenous iodinated medium, the increase in the parenchymal density of the liver accentuates even further the difference of the density of the biliary system, the detection of which should not present a problem. One may follow the pathway of the common bile duct and the intrahepatic bile system, when dilated, as they are branching from the region of the porta hepatis. Occasionally these are visualized as elongated, oval in shape, or even round structures. The extrahepatic duct system projects slightly laterally and anteriorly to the portal vein while the common bile duct during its course is located just medially to the duodenal C-loop and posteriorly to the pancreatic head where it is partially embedded. The diameter of the common bile duct normally varies from 5 to 8 mm. The low attenuation density of the common bile duct can be accentuated by means of intravenous injection of contrast medium which, while it leaves the bile duct unaffected, enhances the surrounding pancreatic parenchyma and also the adjacent vascular structures, thus making the bile duct more visible by virtue of a relatively lower attenuation number and the measurement of its dimensions more accurate.

The gallbladder is practically always demonstrated while sectioning the lower part of the liver, provided that the patient has had no previous cholecystectomy, information which, surprisingly, might not always be available to the radiologist at the time of the examination [19]. Of course, CT is not the routine nor the suggested modality for the examination of this structure, which belongs to the territory of cholecystography and ultrasonography through which one can obtain a thorough examination [20]; however, while the patient is referred

174

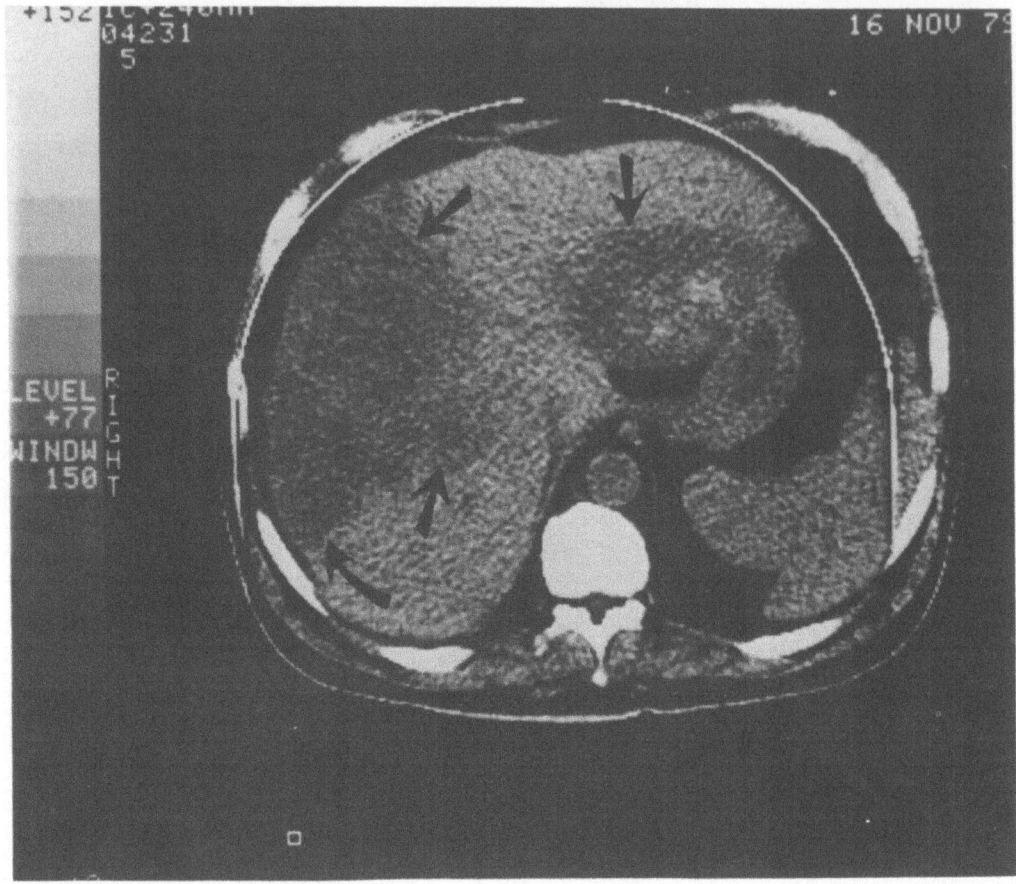

Figure 6. Multiple large metastases. Notice the decreased attenuation of the metastases in relation to the higher attenuation number of the remaining normal hepatic parenchyma.

for the examination of an abdominal problem in general or specifically of the liver, the gallbladder which has not been previously examined but which is, necessarily, also included in the CT sections might demonstrate the presence of a thickened wall due to cholecystitis or might show the presence of gallstones, information which should be taken into consideration in the patient's clinical evaluation.

7. THE JAUNDICED PATIENT

The jaundiced patient represents a rather common entity in the hospital population. The determination of the presence or absence of a dilated biliary duct system is of obvious importance for the study of the jaundiced patient. Differentiation of surgical and medical jaundice is a prerequisite for correct patient management. This does not always repre-

sent a diagnostic problem, particularly following biochemical studies and the appropriate correlation with the patient's clinical history and physical examination. In a number of cases, however, the differentiation is not certain and, therefore, the radiologist is called for consultation and for the performance of the appropriate radiologic diagnostic modality.

The radiologist today has at his disposal a number of procedures with which the exact nature of the jaundice can be accurately established. Cholecystography and intravenous cholangiography are not informative in view of the fact that the serum bilirubin of these patients usually is significantly elevated, rendering the studies useless. Radionuclide imaging is of relatively small value although the recently introduced utilization of radioactive hepatobiliary compounds (PIPIDA, HIDA) can give useful information [21–24]. Per-

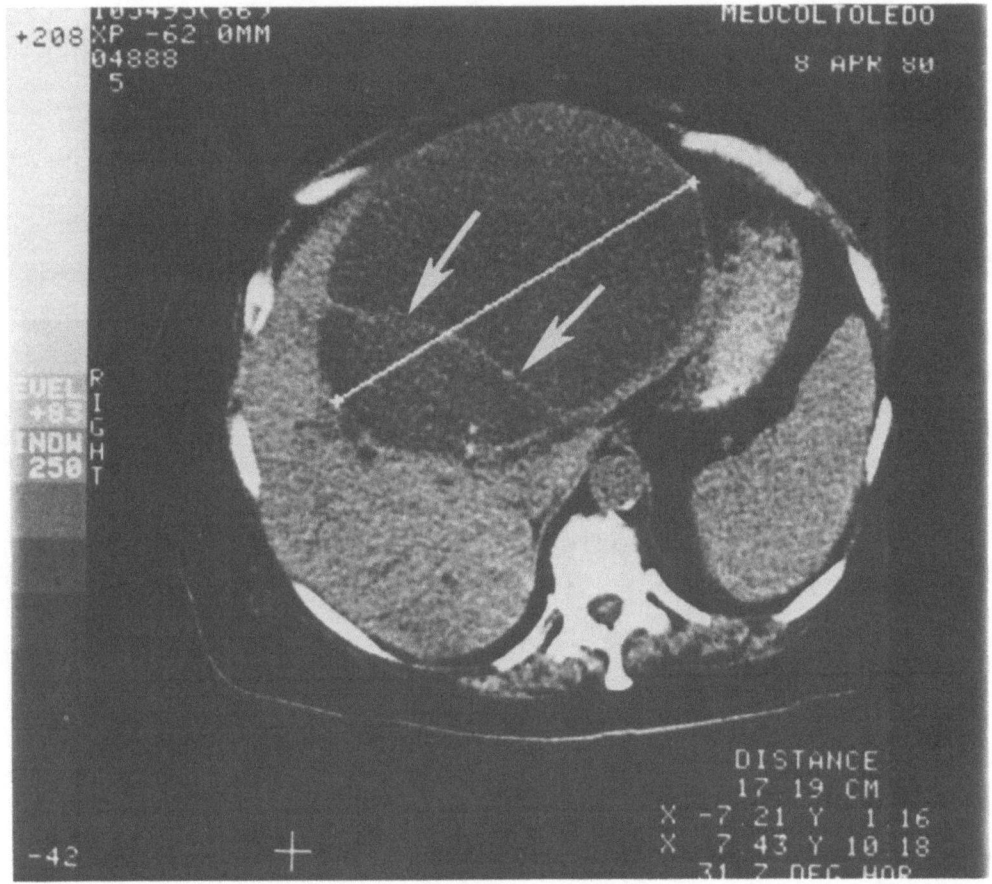

Figure 7a. Cystadenocarcinoma. Notice the cystic, septated appearance of this very large tumor, measuring 17.19 cm as indicated in this section. The attenuation (density) is distinctly lower than that of the remaining normal hepatic parenchyma.

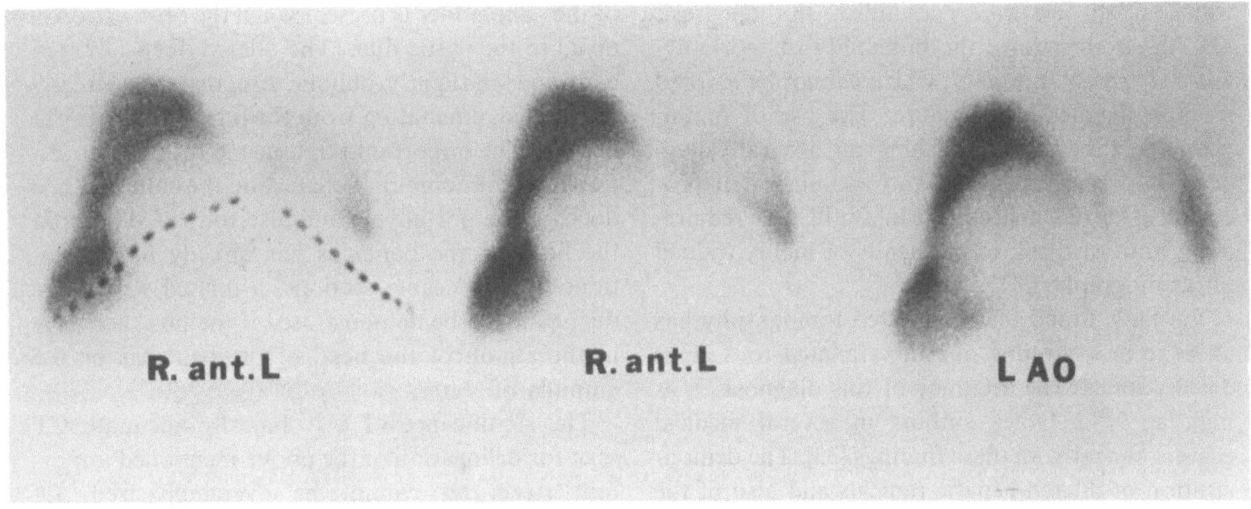

Figure 7b. Technetium 99m sulfur colloid scan shows the large, nonspecific sharply demarcated defect.

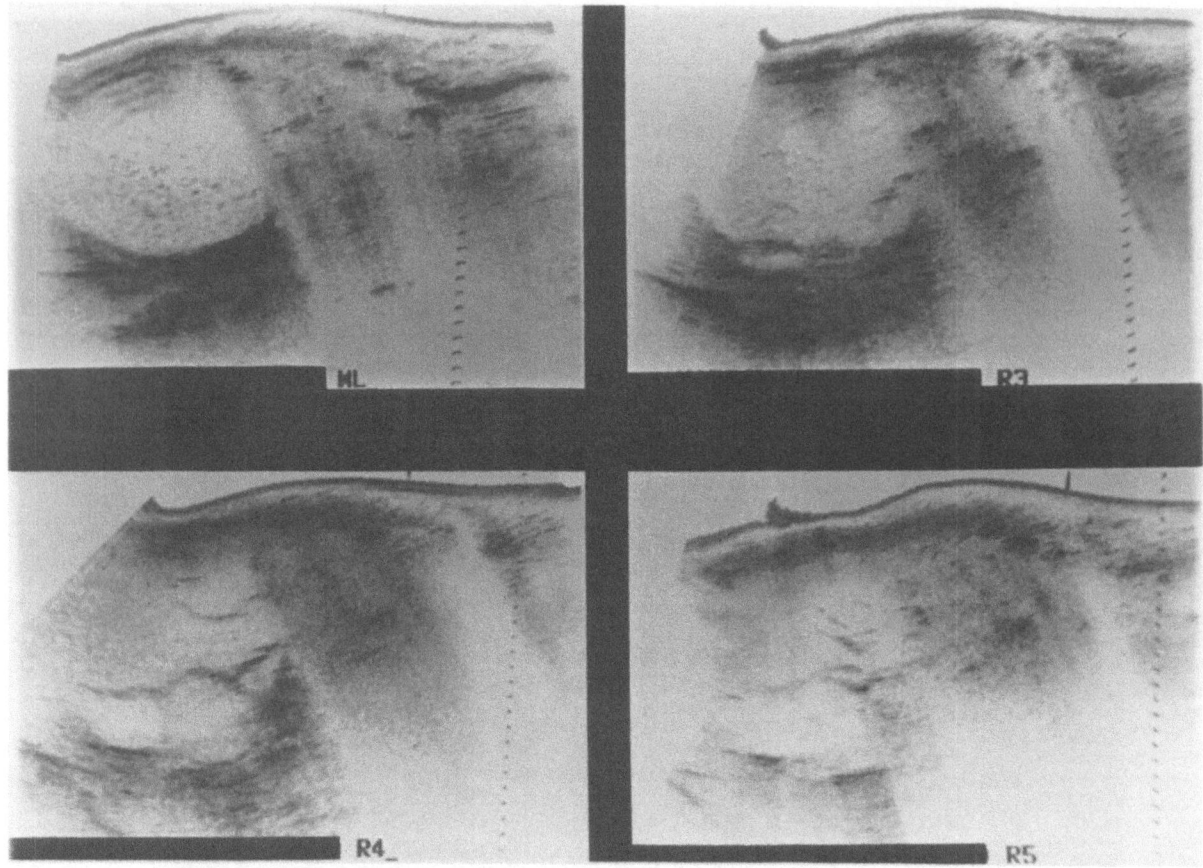

Figure 7c. Ultrasound study – longitudinal section at midline (ML) and at 3, 4, and 5 cm to the right of the midline, demonstrating internal echoes and septations (R4, R5).

cutaneous transhepatic cholangiography and endoscopic retrograde pancreaticocholangiography represent two useful, although invasive, procedures which might accurately establish the diagnosis [25–30]. Both involve the possibility of morbidity and very rarely mortality, which cannot be ignored for any diagnostic procedure. The use of noninvasive methods in establishing an accurate diagnosis is preferable to the above-enumerated procedures. Ultrasonography can fulfill this requirement in most cases, in the hands of highly trained ultrasonographers [31, 32].

We have found that computed tomography has an edge in answering questions related to a jaundiced patient. The accuracy of this diagnosis is as high as 97%. Other authors in several medical centers concur with these findings [33]. The demonstration of dilated hepatic radicals and also of the common hepatic and common bile ducts indicates the presence of obstructive (surgical) jaundice; however, the exact localization of the site of obstruction represents useful information for the surgeon before the patient's laparotomy. Associated dilatation of the gallbladder is present when the obstruction is distal to the cystic duct. The dilated ducts are seen as round or slightly oblique structures, as already mentioned, emanating from the region of the porta hepatis. The important relationship for the identification of the common hepatic and the common bile ducts to the portal vein and also to the C-loop and the head of the pancreas has already been mentioned. In the same sections, a dilated pancreatic duct can also be demonstrated if the obstruction is in the region of the head of the pancreas or the ampulla of Vater.

The significance of a technically adequate CT scan for delineation of the above-mentioned important structures cannot be overemphasized. Of course, suspension of the respiratory movement during the exposure, the use of intravenous contrast medium, short x-ray exposures, and the use of proper technical factors will render excellent morphological details with one of the third- or fourth-generation CT scanners. Under these conditions, the identification of the dilated biliary system containing the low attenuation bile is accurate and dependable. Although the extrahepatic duct system is easily recognized, the intrahepatic radicals can be better demonstrated following the intravenous injection of iodinated contrast medium enhancing the liver parenchyma and the vascular structures and delineating more clearly the dilated and nonopacified biliary duct system. In this way, even slightly dilated ducts can be visualized while otherwise these might not be recognized.

The use of Cholografin or other media intended to opacify the biliary tree is unnecessary, as the opacification will be minimal, if any, in patients with jaundice. The minimal enhancement might not exceed the density of the hepatic parenchyma or

may even become isodense. This will make the identification of the biliary tree practically impossible. Therefore, the administration of the cholangiographic contrast media is not only unnecessary but also counterproductive. The low attenuation number of the dilated biliary ducts when sectioned in a transverse plane may raise the question of intrahepatic metastases; however, in cases of metastases, the lack of any branching pattern as well as the nonorderly distribution and size should make the differential diagnosis of the metastatic disease from the dilated biliary radicals not a difficult one.

On rare occasions we have found that the exact nature and site of the obstruction might not be definite and therefore other invasive radiologic procedures such as the percutaneous cholangiography or the endoscopic retrograde pancreaticocholangiography might render further more-definitive and specific information [34–36] (Fig. 8).

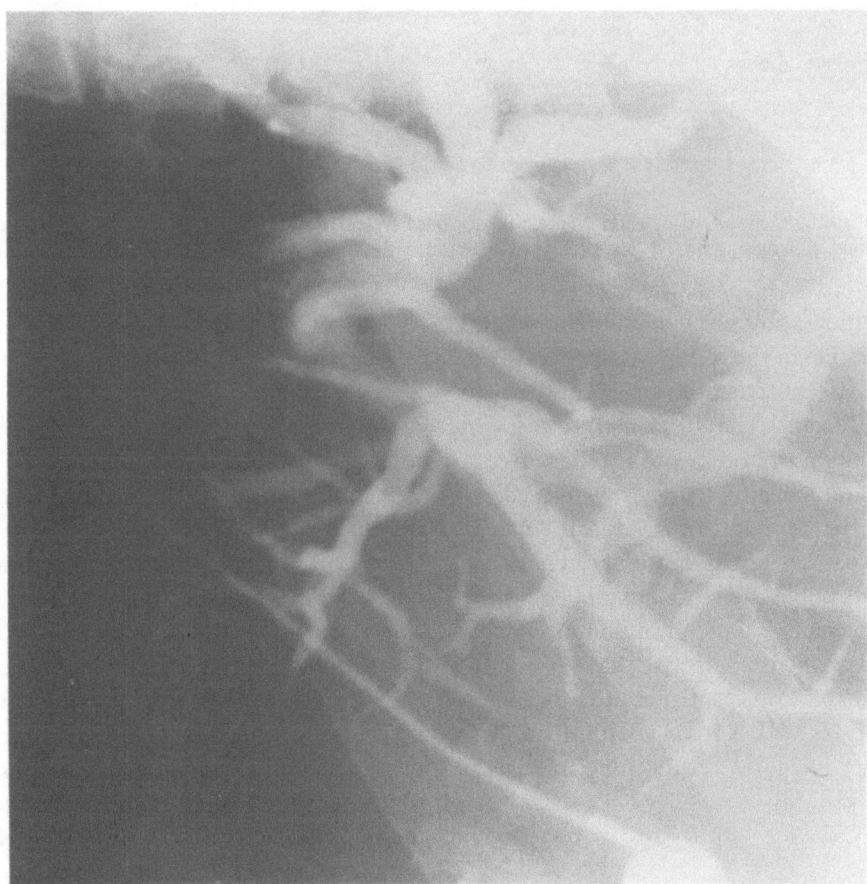

Figure 8a. Percutaneous cholangiography shows marked dilatation of the hepatic biliary system, including the common hepatic and common biliary ducts.

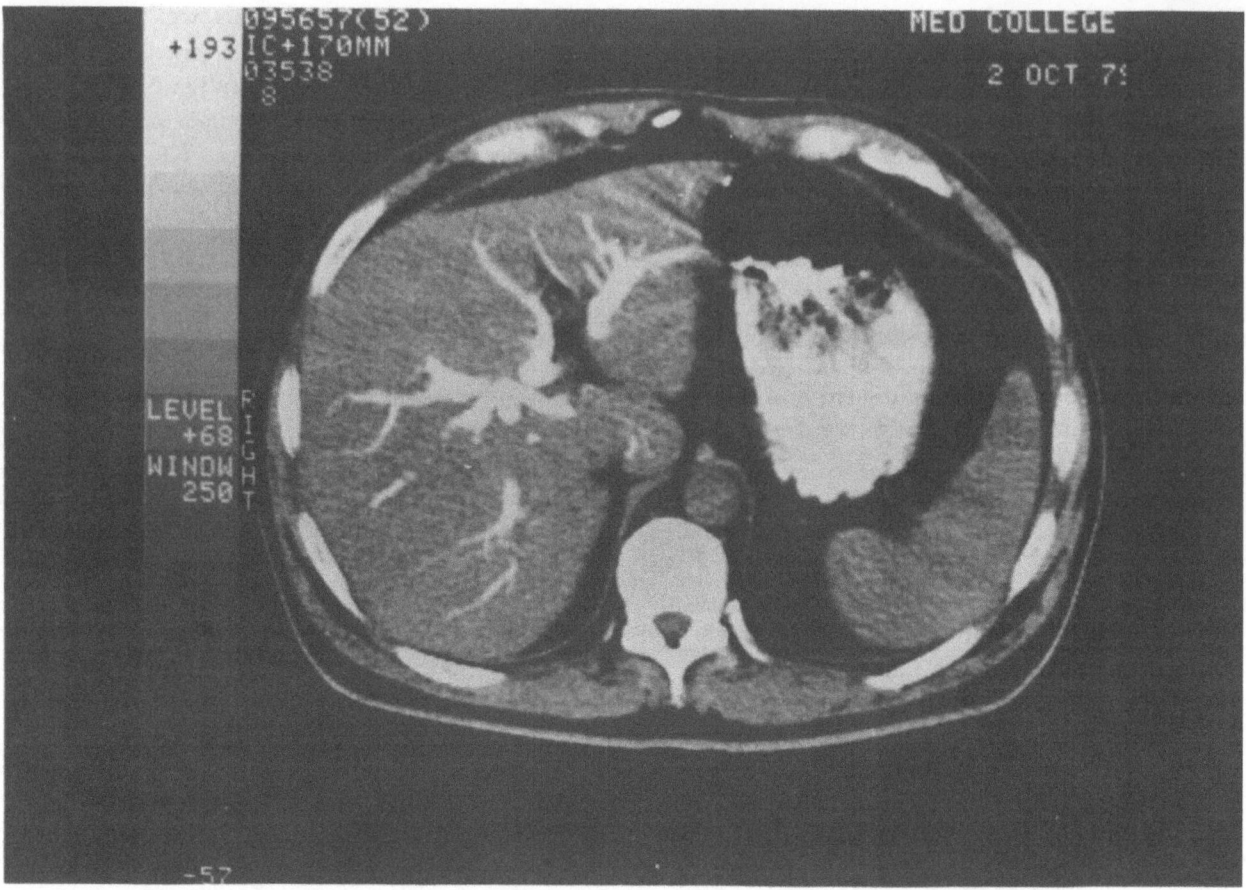

Figure 8b. Notice the dilated and opacified intrahepatic biliary duct system. The opacification is due to remaining contrast from previous percutaneous cholangiogram. The stomach is opacified due to administration of 2% Gastrogafin.

Computed tomography gives highly reliable and accurate information in the differential diagnosis of cholestasis due to obstruction or secondary to hepatocellular disease. The demonstration of a normal caliber and morphology of the biliary tree is a prerequisite in establishing a diagnosis of medical jaundice which, of course, can be due to one of several hepatic diseases, including biliary cirrhosis, viral hepatitis, alcoholic hepatitis, complication of pharmacologic agents, and granulomatous diseases. It should be mentioned here that CT is now used successfully for biopsies. Computed-tomography-guided biopsies with special 'cutting needles' have been used with good results now in several medical centers [37, 38].

8. EVALUATION OF OTHER DIAGNOSTIC PROCEDURES

As we mentioned above, we consider computed tomography the newest modality in the armamentarium for the evaluation of diagnostic problems of the liver when the routine and time-honored procedures such as cholecystography and GI study do not solve the diagnostic problem of a patient [39]. There is, however, a distinct place for the application of other diagnostic methods such as *ultrasonography* and *radionuclide scanning*, two important, noninvasive imaging modalities which we consider many times as complimentary to computed tomography. Hepatic angiography, on the other hand, used extensively in the last 30 years, has been replaced to a great extent by the above-mentioned modalities except when the information desired is related to the exact nature of the blood supply of

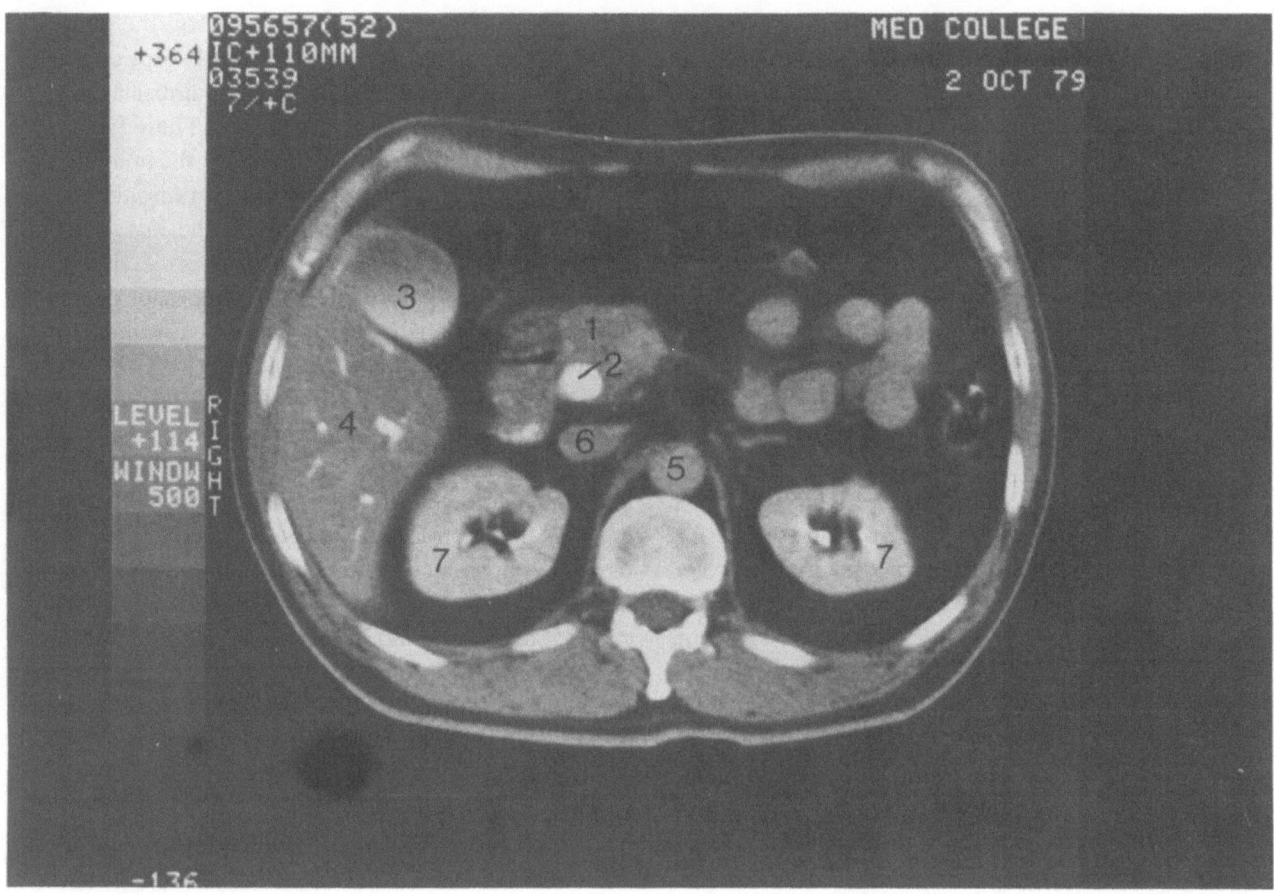

Figure 8c. Section of the liver 6 cm lower than Figure 8b. Notice the markedly dilated common biliary duct embedded in the posterior part of the enlarged and nodular head of the pancreas just before the level of obstruction of the common duct due to carcinoma of the head of the pancreas (2); dilated gallbladder (3), liver (4), aorta (5), inferior vena cava (6), kidneys (7).

the liver. It should be stated at this point that the latest of the diagnostic modalities in the examination of the liver, i.e., computed tomography, resulted in the reevaluation of the other methods, particularly the radionuclide and ultrasonic studies, eliminating some of the indication or altering and rearranging the order of their use.

Before discussing other modalities in the investigation of hepatic diseases, attention should be focused on some of the potential sources of interpretative difficulties in computed tomographic studies. We consider that awareness of the potential pitfalls will lead to a better understanding of this extraordinarily accurate and still evolving procedure. This awareness will also indicate those cases in which the proper use of other modalities should be made in order to clarify diagnostic problems by recognizing the limitations of the modality under certain conditions. The unusual case of an isodense tumor, for example, not being detected in the scan before or even after the enhancement with the contrast medium, should be further evaluated, particularly where a strong clinical suspicion of such a lesions persists, with a radionuclide or ultrasonographic examination.

The use of enhancement with the intravenous injection of iodinated contrast media should be used judiciously. It should be acknowledged that there is a tendency for overutilization, either for the demonstration of a suspected lesion not seen in the unenhanced scan as mentioned above, or in order to better demonstrate a lesion, thus improving the level of confidence of the radiologist and demonstrating the disease process more convincingly for the referring physician charged with the patient's treatment. This additional factor of increased confidence for the diagnosis is often of great significance in daily medical practice.

180

Not uncommonly, motion artifacts may present a problem, particularly in infants or very sick patients with tachypnea. One should also be aware of the possibility of an artifact in the upper part of the liver adjacent to the dome of the diaphragm, due to the transmission of the cardiac motion. Rapid movement of intestinal loops and also of gas within the gastrointestinal tract might produce linear artifacts altering somewhat the contour and the density, particularly of the left lobe of the liver. Familiarity with this type of artifact will simplify this problem.

In evaluating the CT numbers, especially when detecting small lesions, one should be aware of the so-called 'partial volume effect' where the CT number might be misleading in that the lesion occupies only part of the thickness of the CT slice. If the lesion, for example, measures 1 cm while the thickness of the slice used is 2 cm, then the CT number will be approximately the average of the number of the lesion and of the surrounding hepatic parenchyma. Therefore, if the actual difference in CT numbers is relatively small, i.e., ten attenuation numbers, then a false reading of only five numbers difference will be given, which might be barely perceptible. A thinner slice in this case or a possible enhancement with contrast medium might solve the problem and result in a more accurate diagnosis. At this point, one should also be reminded of the appropriate use of the window width and height in studying questionable lesions.

The differentiation between the biliary duct system and the vascular structures can be accomplished, as mentioned above, by intravenous injection of contrast medium which will opacify the the vascular structures but not the biliary duct system. Remember that small metastatic lesions might also be misinterpreted as axial sections of vessels or biliary ducts. Again, the administration of contrast medium in such problematic cases will improve the accuracy of the diagnosis.

9. COMPUTED TOMOGRAPHY VERSUS RADIONUCLIDE STUDIES

The imaging of the liver, and for that matter of any organ by computed tomography, is a function of the differential absorption of the x-ray beam by the tissues through which the photons of the x-ray beam are passing. The degree of absorption, as known, is dependent on the atomic number as well as on the overall mass of the tissues. These factors eventually will influence the quality of the image. In the case of the most commonly used radionuclide, the technetium 99m sulfur colloid, the image will depend on the physiologic properties of the reticuloendothelial cells, which are, for practical purposes, evenly distributed throughout the mass of the liver, and comprise approximately 14%–16% of the liver cell population.

By understanding the different mechanisms of the modalities, one can appreciate the advantages and disadvantages of the two methods of examination. In general, it is accepted that the anatomy of the organ and the presence of lesions, particularly small ones, can be more distinctly and accurately demonstrated by means of computed tomography, which practically demonstrates the real cross-sectional anatomy of the organ itself. The image, on the other hand, produced by the radionuclide study using technetium 99m sulfur colloid is the reflection of the function of the displaced or damaged reticuloendothelial cells. While a lesion of 1 cm or even less can be demonstrated by means of computed tomography, for practical purposes, it is impossible to demonstrate such a small lesion with the radionuclide study. The resolution with the computed tomography is, of course, superior. This becomes also significant for even larger lesions when these are present deeply within the mass of the liver where the attenuation factor and also the greater amount of scattered radiation compromises the quality of the image produced. Under these conditions, lesions of up to 2 cm or even larger might not be detected by using the radionuclide study. To some extent, the resolution of small lesions is also compromised by the motion of the liver, which moves approximately 2–3 cm during quiet respiration. The time of exposure, therefore, is more important in the case of radionuclide studies than in the shorter time exposures by the now available CT equipment. The net result is that the examination of the same patient who has small lesions, such as metastases, can be demonstrated in a patient undergoing CT examination but not detected in a technetium 99m sulfur colloid study done on the same day. This has been our experience as well as that of many others [7, 40] (Fig. 9).

Anatomic variations and also lesions adjacent to the liver or encroaching on the liver from the surrounding organs are better and more accurately demonstrated by using the CT examinations, while the radionuclide study might result in false-positive results. This is a common experience, particularly with thin left lobes of the liver or with unusual locations of the gallbladder. These structures do not present any problem with the CT, which demonstrates the exact anatomy of the axial section of the liver or, by reconstruction, the coronal or sagittal planes.

Due to the nature of the radionuclide examination, which depends on the function of the reticuloendothelial cells, in cases of lack or compromised function of these cells in certain areas, as a result of different pathologic processes such as fibrosis, previous radiation, and the use of toxic

drugs including chemotherapeutic agents, the area of impaired function might be presented as a defect. In a search for metastatic disease, these defects due to impaired function will be represented as false-positive results for metastases. In other words, the demonstration of a mass in the CT examination represents a direct anatomic visualization of the lesion while in the radionuclide study this is dependent upon the function of the reticuloendothelial cell population, which might be impaired not only as a result of metastatic desease, but also due to other nonneoplastic diseases.

While this dependence of the radionuclide image on the function of reticuloendothelial cells results in inadequacies and false-positive images, it might in some cases become a distinct advantage over the CT examination and particularly in nonneoplastic diseases such as hepatitis, cholangitis, and cirrhosis of the liver, where the compromised function is reflected in the radionuclide examination but not in

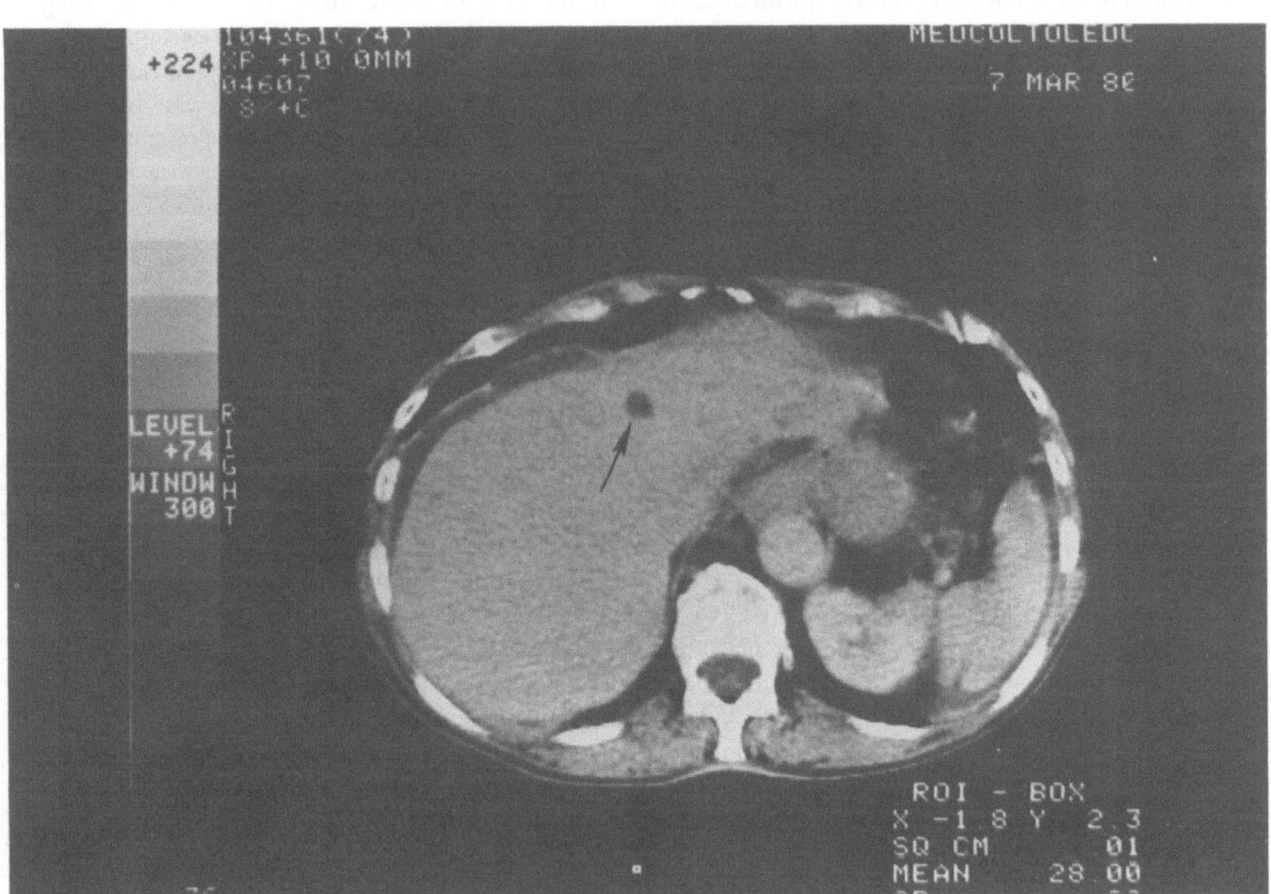

Figure 9. Small metastasis in the liver. This lesion was not demonstrated by radionuclide study nor by the ultrasound examination.

182

the CT, which primarily demonstrates accurately the anatomy of the organ particularly when the examination is done with slices of a few millimeters. Incidentally, the compromise of the function of the reticuloendothelial cells of the liver is reflected in a radionuclide study with sulfur colloid with the increased uptake by the reticuloendothelial cells of other organs, mainly the spleen and bone marrow.

Gallium-67 citrate is used primarily for demonstration of abscesses, with serial studies at different time intervals, including 24, 48, and 72 h following the administration of the radionuclide. Gallium 67 is also concentrated in hepatomas and in approximately 50% of metastatic lesions of the liver. It is not taken up, usually, by the fibrotic nodules in cases of liver cirrhosis or in areas of regeneration of hepatic tissue [13].

This brief comparison indicates the superiority in the detailed examination of the morphologic changes of the liver by computed tomography. The two examinations, however, can complement each other particularly when the radionuclide study is used as a screening method. The CT then can more accurately determine the nature of the lesion in cases where the radionuclide study is equivocable or where the clinical suspicion persists in spite of the negative radioisotopic examination [41].

10. ULTRASONOGRAPHY

With the significant breakthrough and the technical advances of the gray-scale ultrasonography and its high resolution since the early 1970s, this modality represents a significant and useful contribution to the evaluation of the liver and biliary system [42]. The contribution of the digital gray scale and the real-time equipment has markedly improved the resolution and the signal-to-noise ratio.

Gray-scale ultrasonography has a particular ability to demonstrate adequately the hepatic radicals and the duct system [43, 44]. The common bile duct caliber, as well as the size of the hepatic and intrahepatic ducts, can be accurately seen. The advantage, initially, of ultrasound over computed tomography, due to the shorter scan time in patients unable to suspend respiratory movement, however, is no longer true with the introduction of the fast, 1- to 10-s CT scanners. It is possible for

ultrasonography to detect hepatic metastases of more than 2 cm in size due to the disruption of normal acoustic characteristics of the liver parenchyma [45]. Sonolucent lesions, particularly cysts, are easily detectable with ultrasound and almost as accurately as with computed tomography. Ultrasonography can further clarify suspicious or questionable areas detected by radionuclide study, especially in the region of the liver hilum, where the percentage of false-positive nuclear images is relatively high. Another area where there has been increased application of ultrasonic studies is in the detection of gallbladder abnormalities and particularly following a nonvisualizing gallbladder after oral cholecystogram [46].

It is a common experience that gallstones can easily be detected with ultrasound and their identification becomes reliable with the strong acoustic shadow which the gallstones produce (Fig. 10). The size of the gallbladder can be measured accurately. An increase of more than 10 cm in the long diameter in the fasting patient will certainly raise the question of possible hydrops. The thickening of the wall of the gallbladder, which can be fairly accurately shown, will suggest the presence of an inflammatory process. It is the practice in most medical centers to routinely examine a nonvisualized gallbladder after oral cholecystography by using ultrasonography [47, 48]. Of course, the presence of gas in the intestinal tract and particularly a distended transverse colon might severely compromise the quality of the results. The overlapping of the liver by the rib cage, as in hypersthenic individuals, will render the examination more difficult, and while the presence of fat, and in general the examination of an obese individual, is advantageous for the CT examination, the image definition in these patients, by means of ultrasound, might be compromised. Postsurgical patients with dressings, sutures, or postsurgical scars, tubes, or other changes related to surgery or trauma will interfere with the examination. The spatial resolution, although improved markedly with the introduction of the gray-scale ultrasonography, is not as adequate as the one obtained with the CT scanners of today. The accurate detection, therefore, of small lesions such as metastases can be more accurately achieved by means of computed tomography. The significance of this becomes evident when we consider that

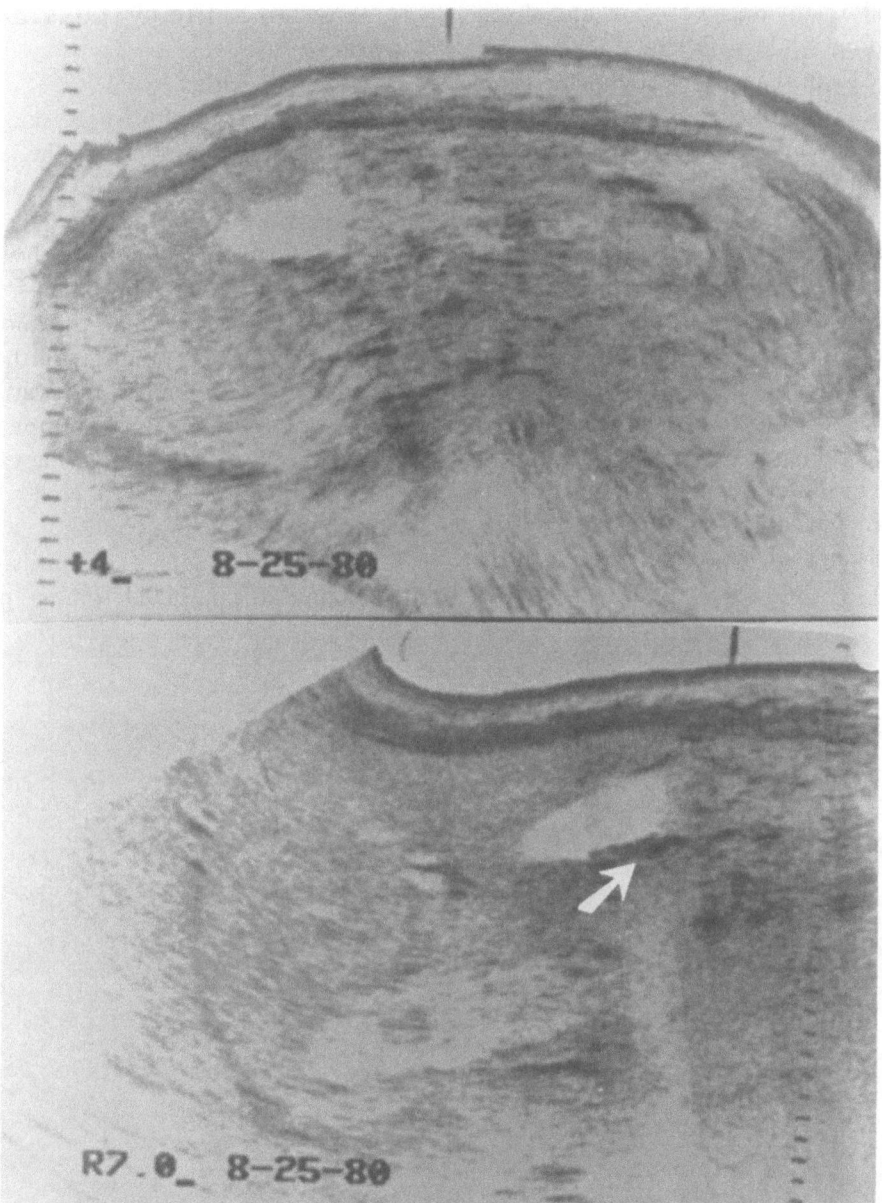

Figure 10. Ultrasound. Multiple gallstones. Notice the strong acoustic shadows (arrow). Transverse and longitudinal sections.

one of the most common considerations for which the liver is examined radiologically is for the detection of possible metastatic disease, in view of the fact that the liver represents one of the most frequent targets of metastatic involvement. Due to the fact that ultrasonography is a considerably more operator-dependent study than the other modalities (radionuclide and CT), it should be kept in mind that the reproduction of the examination in a patient for follow-up studies in the same or in other institutions might create problems of ac-

curacy and dependability.

Detection of multiple or isolated cysts of the liver, most of which are congenital in nature, are easily detectable by ultrasound when their size is larger than the width of the ultrasonic beam. In smaller cystic lesions, however, these can be mistaken as small, necrotic lesions or small abscesses.

In diffuse disease of the liver parenchyma such as in fatty infiltration and cirrhosis, the diagnosis can be suspected by using ultrasound. Fatty infiltration, as known, is diagnosed very accurately be means of

CT. Ultrasound usually does not show any change in the attenuation while with the CT there is a significant increase in the attenuation of the beam, due to fibrosis, in cases of cirrhosis. The increase in the attenuation depends on the degree of fibrosis and the extension of the cirrhotic process in the liver [49].

Among the advantages of ultrasonic examination, particularly in cases where there is comparable accuracy with the other modalities, we should mention the nonionizing nature of ultrasound and, in comparison with the CT examination, that it represents a more economical test. Obviously, when only one of the two modalities is available in an institution, and this happens to be the ultrasonographic equipment, then the question of choice or selection of modality, by necessity, is 'simplified.'

11. ANGIOGRAPHIC EVALUATION OF THE LIVER

The use of angiography in the diagnosis of liver diseases is not as common as in the 1960s and early 1970s. At the present time, this modality is utilized for diagnostic purposes on patients suspected of having vascular lesions such as hemangiomas or aneurysms (Fig. 11) or on patients anticipated to undergo liver surgery, where the knowledge of the details of the vascular anatomy of the organ might be significant. Anomalies and variations in the vascular supply of the liver are not as unusual as once was thought. In addition, the vascular supply of the tumor to be excised could be significant information for the surgeon.

Before the routine use of ultrasound and the introduction of computed tomography, the mor-

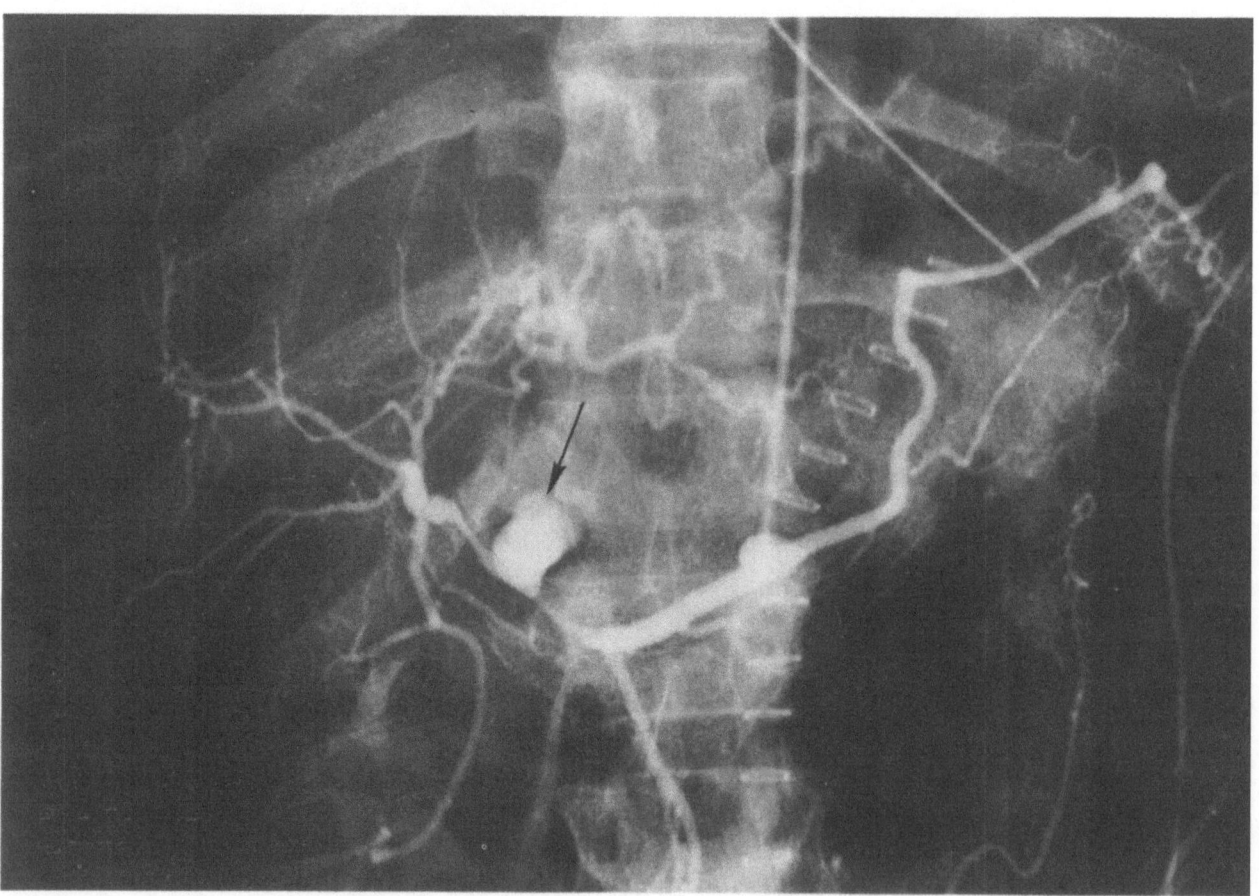

Figure 11. Posttraumatic pseudoaneurysm of the hepatic artery. The selective arteriogram shows a 2-cm aneurysm (arrow). Notice the spasticity of the hepatic artery proximal and distal to the site of the aneurysm.

pphologic evaluation of the liver was mainly obtained by means of radionuclide studies. The relatively high number of false-negative and false-positive results of the radionuclide studies and the lack of specificity of defects made the arteriographic examination in many cases of vital importance. Such an arteriographic study could have demonstrated that a filling defect was due to a normal variation, an intrahepatic gallbladder, or a benign lesion such as a cyst, and, therefore, arteriography could have saved the patient an unnecessary operation. Cases of very thin or even absent left lobe of the liver submitted to abdominal exploration were not extremely rare. With the introduction, however, of ultrasound studies and mainly after the availability of the computed tomography, the indications for arteriography of the liver have been substantially decreased. Even cases of a suspected cavernous hemangioma, which is not a very common lesion, can be characterized and diagnosed by means of computed tomography and, therefore, the patient might be operated on without the necessity of hepatic arteriography.

For the above reasons, the number of patients undergoing hepatic arteriography had been restricted primarily to those who, as a result of an accurate diagnostic workup, are going to the submitted to surgery and where the accurate knowledge of the blood supply to the liver is significant. In these patients, arteriography will more precisely guide the surgical treatment with the needed information as related to the exact size, location, and the vascular supply of the lesion and the liver in general. This may be particularly useful information, as the blood supply to the area might be of specific significance to the surgeon.

12. NEW RADIOLOGIC MODALITIES: EVALUATION

The radiologic study and investigation of patients with hepatic disorders should follow a rational approach [50]. The factors involved are several and in many cases depend on the background, experience and expertise of the examiners. Of course, the availability of all modern modalities in a hospital or diagnostic center is taken for granted when one is faced with the best choice

for the method to be used in a special clinical problem. Other factors might also include economic considerations and radiation exposure. Most medical centers have established guidelines for the logical sequence of the diagnostic methods to be used in different categories of clinical situations (Table 1). While there are differences from one medical center to another, the same philosophy and rationale in general is used as a common denominator.

The majority of diagnostic examinations of the liver requested from a radiology department have as their objective the investigation for metastatic disease in patients who are known the have a primary neoplasm. Another less frequent, although very important, reason for requesting the use of imaging radiologic procedures is the investigation of patients with hepatomegaly, suspected diffuse parenchymal disease, or abnormal laboratory tests. Finally, one should include the patients who are admitted on an emergency basis due to abdominal trauma in whom this large and not so well protected organ might be involved.

In cases of question of metastatic disease and differentiation between a benign lesion, such as a hepatic cyst, from solitary or multiple metastatic lesions, the radionuclide examination is the least specific with a relatively high false-positive rate of approximately 20% and with a false-negative rate of almost 25% [51]. It is understandable, therefore, that this study should not be considered as highly reliable in such cases and that it should be used mainly as a screening test. Ultrasound represents a more accurate and more specific diagnostic test, while the accuracy of the CT due to spatial resolution can detect smaller lesions in comparison with the other modalities. It should be mentioned at this point that on many occasions these modalities might be complementary and, therefore, it is not superfluous, in nonconclusive cases, to use two of these or even all three of these noninvasive imaging modalities, if necessary, in a logical sequence [11] (Table 1).

The significance of using contrast media for better evaluation of suspected space-occupying lesions during the computed tomographic examination has been discussed already. In the majority of cases, hepatic neoplasms, most of which are metastatic, exhibit a lower attenuation number, i.e.,

186

Table 1. Guidelines for utilization of imaging modalities

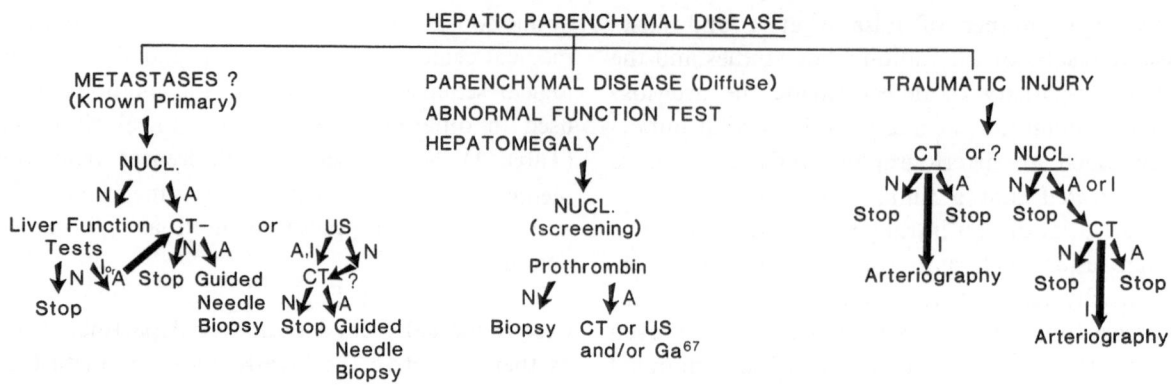

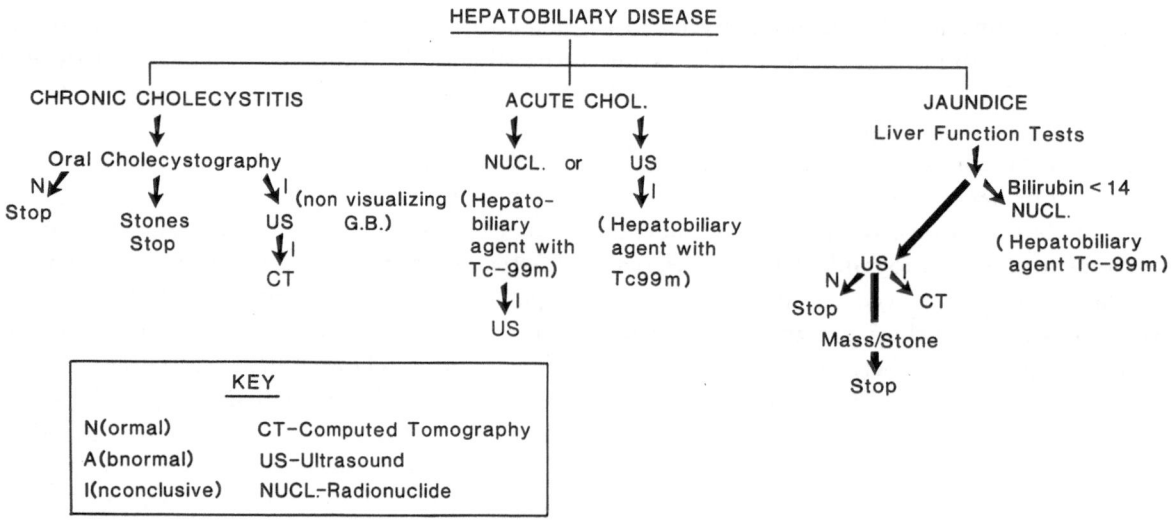

they are less dense than the surrounding hepatic parenchyma. However, on a few occasions when this is not very convincing, the contrast medium will accentuate the difference by increasing the opacification of the hepatic parenchyma. Very rarely, it is possible for the metastatic lesion to be isodense before the administration of contrast medium which when injected will produce a differential attenuation and, therefore, will demonstrate the presence of an unsuspected lesion.

The radionuclide study could be of value in vascular tumors such as hemangiomas, hepatomas, or melanomas when the rapid sequential perfusion image technique is used. While the static images show an area of filling defect, during the rapid perfusion the same area demonstrates an increased

density. Lymphomatous lesions by ultrasonography are many times sonolucent [53]. The echogenicity, however, of these lesions might change. More echogenic areas may develop after chemotherapy or radiation treatment. Computed tomography is accurate in the detection of nodular involvement, and the two examinations will yield a higher degree of accuracy.

Some of the benign hepatic lesions might be vascular, such as the adenomas, not infrequently seen among women using oral contraceptives for long periods of time. In the nonenhanced CT studies, the adenomas have a decreased attenuation in relation to the hepatic parenchyma. There is an increased density, however, following the intravenous administration of contrast medium. When such a lesion is suspected, hepatic arteriography might show a highly dense mass due to the increased vascularity of these benign lesions. Other benign vascular tumors include hemangiomas and hamartomas. Here we should also include the cases of nodular hyperplasia.

The use of ultrasound in detecting liver abscesses is very accurate. This is also the case with computed tomography where the abscess demonstrates an absorption coefficient lower than the one seen in metastatic desease surrounded by the denser wall, which is less sharply outlined than the metastatic lesions. Small abscesses could be missed by radionuclide study while the large ones might not demonstrate the exact size of the abscess, as the inflammation of the adjacent hepatic parenchyma frequently gives the impression of a larger abscess.

In diseases of the biliary tree, both computed tomography and ultrasonography represent highly accurate diagnostic methods. The two procedures can be considered complementary, particularly if the exact diagnosis is in doubt and the accuracy of the diagnosis is mandatory as part of a preoperative evaluation. We consider, in these cases, ultrasonography as the preliminary study.

When obstructive jaundice, due to a mass in the head of the pancreas, has to be evaluated, computed tomography will give the needed information accurately. The demonstration of the gallbladder by using ultrasonography is a reliable method and should be used routinely in cases of nonvisualizing gallbladder by oral cholecystography as already mentioned. CT should be used only in cases of an excessive amount of gas and when an intrahepatic gallbladder is obscured by the rib cage, making the sonographic examination difficult. Needless to say that barium sulfate used in the gastrointestinal study or the barium enema will handicap both modalities.

One of the newer radionuclide studies using agents that undergo biliary excretion such as the iminodiacetic acid analogues, which are labeled with technetium 99m, can adequately visualize the gallbladder and the biliary duct system when oral or even intravenous cholangiograms fail to do so [21, 22]. Even with a high bilirubin value of up to 14 mg/100 ml, the biliary system including the gallbladder might be visualized. This is a most reliable and valuable examination which should be used more widely, in cases of nonvisualizing gallbladder, by the oral method (Fig. 12a and b). The examination is more reliable and has less morbidity than the intravenous cholangiogram. One of the important applications is in the diagnosis of acute cholecystitis. The demonstration of the biliary duct system without the gallbladder indicates a positive diagnosis of cholecystitis while the simultaneous visualization of the gallbladder rules out this diagnosis.

In comparing the three basic imaging modalities for the examination of the liver, specifically the radionuclide, ultrasound, and computed tomography, we should state the following:

The radionuclide studies have the advantage of rendering some physiologic and functional information which the other two imaging modalities do not produce. On the other hand, a radionuclide examination can be considered only as a gross screening test for the detection of metastatic disease, which represents one of the main reasons for the radiologic exploration of the liver. The number of false-positive and false-negative radionuclide examinations makes it mandatory to complement this examination with one of the other more accurate imaging modalities, i.e., ultrasonography or computed tomography. In cases of suspected biliary disease, ultrasonography might represent the definitive diagnostic test without any need to resort to the more expensive and not always available CT study. While both the ultrasound and CT modalities, particularly the latter, can easily distinguish the extrinsic lesions of the liver, this is not frequently possible with the radionuclide studies. As mentioned above, there are occasional cases in which high accuracy is very important and all three modalities might have to be used [54]. For example, we may have a solitary lesion suspected as being metastatic in nature and demonstrated as a cold spot with the technetium 99m sulfur colloid study; the ultrasound might demonstrate a sonolucent lesion with a rather thin wall. If, however, on high-gain ultrasound there is some question of internal echoes and therefore the possibility of an abscess is raised with some clinical support, computed tomographic study will better demonstrate the thickness of the wall and its enhancement following contrast administration, thus diagnosing with high accuracy that the lesion under investigation indeed represents an abscess.

188

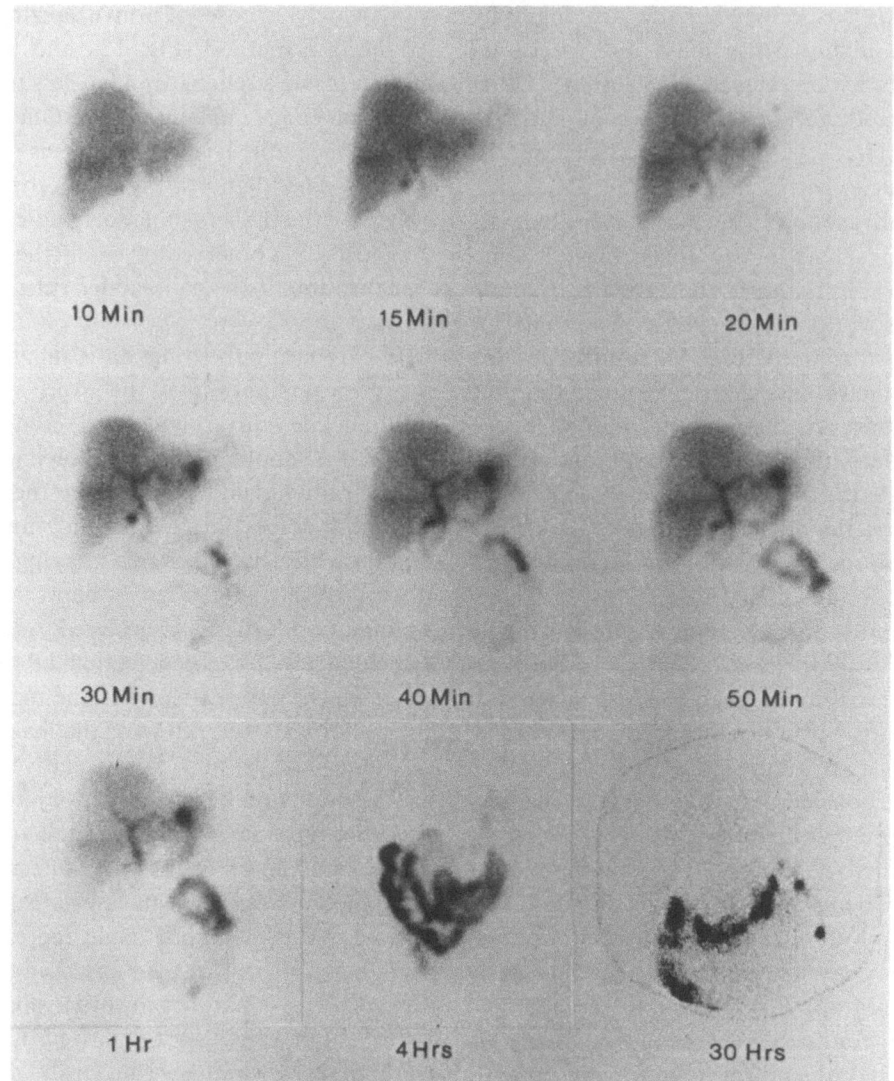

Figure 12a. Technetium 99m (PIPIDA) study. The isotope is excreted promptly and outlines a normal biliary tree. The duodenal bulb, (1) the C-loop, the small bowel, and the colon (30 h) are visualized. The gallbladder (2) is visualized promptly within 15 min.

As mentioned earlier, the cost of each examination should not be ignored, and whenever one expects approximately the same diagnostic accuracy, depending on the individual case, then the factor of time necessary for the examination, the radiation exposure involved, and the expense should be taken into consideration. When in doubt in establishing an accurate diagnosis important for the patient's treatment, all of the modalities in a logical sequence might have to be used when feasible, as the patient's well-being should be the most important consideration (Table 1).

Acknowledgment. The author wishes to thank Miss Faye Keen for her valuable assistance in preparing the illustrations in this chapter.

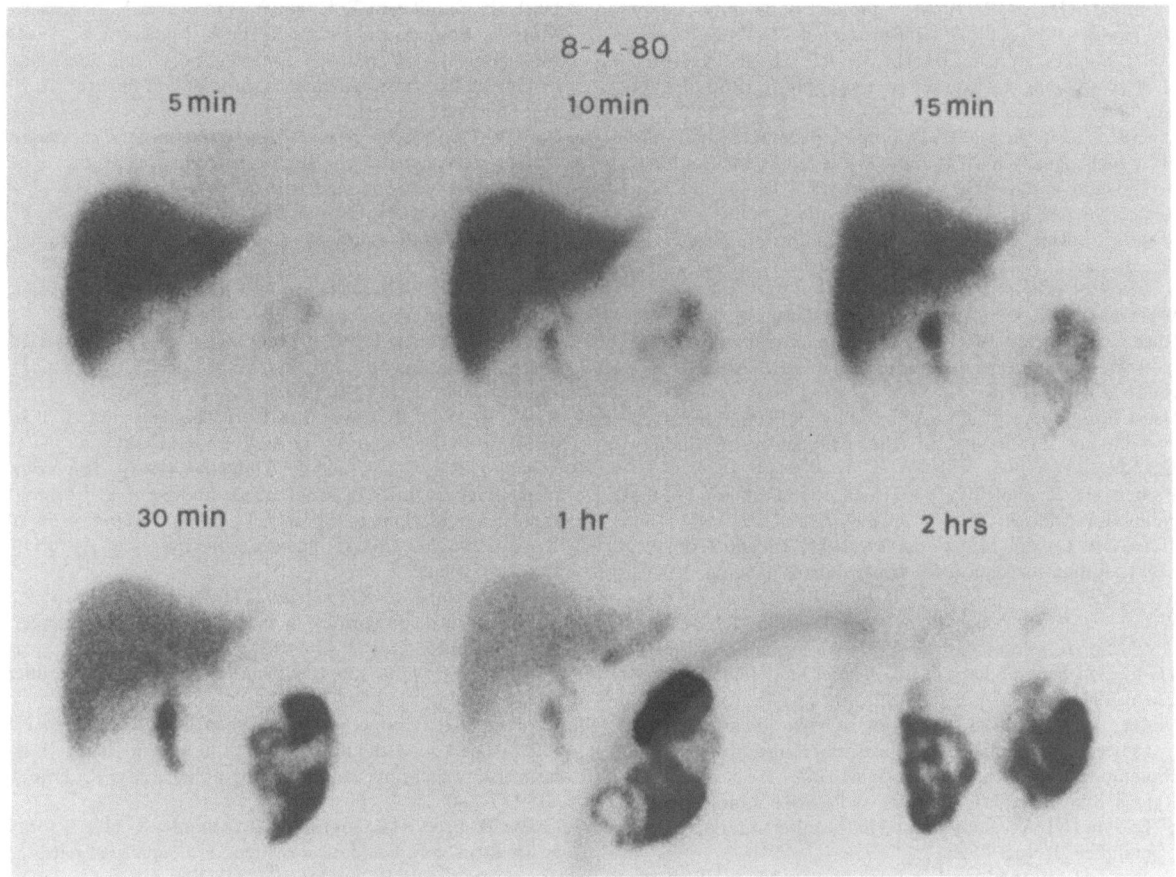

Figure 12b. Iminodiacetic acid analogue (PIPIDA) labeled with technetium 99m. The gallbladder is not visualized due to acute cholecystitis. Notice the uniform distribution of the isotope in the hepatic parenchyma, and the prompt excretion and opacification of the common biliary and common hepatic duct, the duodenum, and small bowel. The gallbladder is not visualized. Notice the almost complete elimination of the radionuclide from the liver in 2 h.

REFERENCES

1. Abrams HL, McNeil BJ (1978) Medical implications of computed tomographtyy. N Engl J Med 298:255–261, 310–318
2. Sheedy PF, Stephens DH, Hattery RR, Mouhm JR, Hartman GW (1976) Clinical trial with the EMI phototype. Am J Roentgenol 127:23–51
3. Sheedy PF, Stephens DH, Hattery RR, Brown LR, McCarty RL (1979) Computed tomography of the abdominal organs. Adv Intern Med 24:455–479
4. Stanley RJ, Sagel SS (1977) Computed tomography of the liver and biliary tract. In: Berk RN, Clement AR (eds) Radiology of the gallbladder and bile ducts. Philadelphia: WB Saunders, p 3652
5. Stanley RJ, Sagel SS, Levitt RG (1977) Computed body tomography of the liver. Radiol Clin North Am 15:331–348
6. Alfidi RJ, Haaga JR, Havrilla RTR, Pepe RG, Cook SA (1979) Computed tomography of the liver. Am J Roentgenol 127:69–74
7. Biello DR, Levitt RG, Siegel BA, Sagel SS, Stanley RJ (1978) Computed tomography and radionuclide imaging of the liver: a comparative evaluation. Radiology 127:159–163

8. McCarty RL Wahner HW, Stephens DH, Sheedy PF, Hattery RR (1977) Retrospective comparison of radionuclide scans and computed tomography of the liver and pancreas. Am J Roentgenol 129:23–28
9. Bryan PJ, Dinn WH, Grossman ZD, Wistow BW, McAfee JG, Kieffer SA (1977) Ultrasonography and radionuclide imaging of the liver in detecting space-occupying processes. Radiology 124:387–393
10. Grossman ZD, Wistow DW, Bryan PJ, Dinn WM, Mc Afee JG, Kieffer SA (1977) Radionuclide imaging, computed tomography and gray scale ultrasonography of the liver: a comparative study. J Nucl Med 18:327–332
11. Petasnick JP, Ram P, Turner DA, Fordham EW (1979) The relationship of computed tomography, gray scale ultrasonography, and radionuclide imaging in the evaluation of hepatic masses. Semin Nucl Med 9:8–22
12. Snow JH, Goldstein HM, Wallace S (1979) Comparison of scintigraphy, sonography, and computed tomography in the evaluation of hepatic neoplasms. Am J Roentgenol 132:915–918
13. Lomas F, Dibos PE, Wagner HN (1972) Increased specificity of liver scanning with the use of 67-gallium citrate. N Engl J Med 286:1323–1329

190

14. Alfidi RJ, Haaga JR (1976) Computed body tomography and cancer [Editorial]. Am J Roentgenol 127:1061

15. MacCarty RL, Sephens DH, Hattery RR, Sheedy PF (1979) Hepatic imaging by computed tomography. Radiol Clin North Am 17:137–155

16. Scherer U, Lissner J (1979) Computed tomography of the liver: high density mass lesions. Presented at International Symposium and Course on Computed Tomography, Las Vegas, Nevada

17. Scherer U, Rainer R, Eisenburg J, Schildberg GW, Meister P, Lissner J (1978) CT in circumscript liver disease. Am J Roentgenol 130:711–714

18. Wolgerson MK, Jagannadharao B, Sundaram M, Joyce PF, Riaz MA, Shields JB (1979) CT as a primary diagnostic method in evaluating intra-abdominal abscess. Am J Roentgenol 133:1089–1096

19. Hsu-Chong Y (1979) Ultrasonography and computed tomography of carcinoma of the gallbladder. Radiology 133:167–174

20. Finberg HJ, Birnholz JC (1979) Ultrasound evaluation of the gallbladder wall. Radiology 133: 699–702

21. Harvey E, Loberg M, Cooper M (1975) Tc-99m-HIDA: a new radiopharmaceutical for hepatobiliary imaging. J Nucl Med 16:533

22. Wistow BM, Subramanian G, Van Heertum RL, Gagne GM, Mall RC, McAffee JG (1977) An evaluation of 99m-TC-labeled hepatobiliary agent. J Nucl Med 18:455–461

23. Cheng TH, Davis MA, Seltzer SE, Jones B, Abbruzzese AA, Finberg HJ, Drum DG Evaluation of hepatobiliary imaging by radionuclide scintigraphy, ultrasonography, and contrast cholangiography. Radiology 133:761–768

24. Ryan J, Sikoff, Nagle C, Cooper M (1976) The combined use of Tc-99m HIDA and ultrasound in the differential diagnosis of jaundice. J Nucl Med 17:545

25. Ferrucci JT, Wittenberg J, Sarno RA, Dreyfuss FJ (1976) Fine needle transhepatic cholangiography: a new approach to obstructive jaundice. Am J Rontgenol 127:403–407

26. Ferrucci JT, Mueller PR, Harbin WP (1980) Percutaneous transhepatic biliary drainage: technique, results and applications. Radiology 135:1–13

27. Funaro AH, Ring AH, Freiman DB, Oleaga JA, Gordon RL (1979) Transhepatic obliteration of esophageal varices using the stainless steel coil. Am J Roentgenol 133:1123–1126

28. Gold RP, Casarella WT, Stern G, Seaman WB (1979) Transhepatic cholangiography: the radiological method of choice in suspected obstructive jaundice. Radiology 133:39–44

29. Gollin FF, Sims JL, Cameron JR (1964) Liver scanning and liver function tests, a comparative study. JAMA 187:111–116

30. Irish CR, Meaney TF (1980) Percutaneous transhepatic cholangiography: comparison of success and risk using 19- versus 22-gauge needles. Am J Roentgenol 134:137–140

31. Malini S, Sabel J (1977) Ultrasonography in obstructive jaundice. Radiology 123:429–433

32. Koenigsberg M, Wiener SN, Walzer A (1979) The accuracy of sonography in the differential diagnosis of obstructive jaundice: a comparison with cholangiography. Radiology 133:157–165

33. Levitt RG, Sagel SS, Stanley RJ Accuracy of computed tomography of the liver and biliary tract. Radiology 124:123–128

34. Okuda K, Tanikawa K, Emura T, Kuratami S, Jinnanchi S, Urabe K, Sumikoshi T, Kanda Y, Fukuyama Y, Musha H, Mori H, Shimakawa Y, Yakushiji F, Matsuura Y (1974) Non-surgical percutaneous transhepatic cholangiography: diagnostic significance in medical problems of the liver. Am J Dig Dis 19:21–36

35. Parbhoo K, Miller STK (1979) Experience with percutaneous transhepatic cholangiography in the diagnosis of biliary tract obstruction. J Irish Med Assoc 72:341–343

36. Purow E, Hadas N, Grosbery SJ, Waprick S, Suster B, Le Veen H (1979) Percutaneous transhepatic cholangiography: an experience with the Chiba needle. Am Surg 431–438

37. Haaga JR (1979) New techniques for CT guided biopsies. Am J Roentgenol 133:633–642

38. Haaga JR, Vanek J (1979) Computed tomographic guided liver biopsy using the Menghini needle. Radiology 133:405–408

39. Raval B, Wan R, Carey L (1979) The spectrum of liver disease on CT. J Can Assoc Radiol 30:211–215

40. Schapiro RL, Yiu-Chiu V, Chiu LC (1980) The complementary qualities of radionuclide and computed tomographic examinations of the liver. J Comput Tomogr 4:51–70

41. Rosenthal SN (1976) Are hepatic scans overused? Am J Dig Dis 21:659–663

42. Kawasaki H, Sakaguchi S, Irisa T, Hirayama C (1978) Value of B-scan ultrasonography in the diagnosis of liver cancer. Am J Gastroenterol 69:436–442

43. Parulekar SG: Ultrasound evaluation of common bile duct size. Radiology 133:703–708

44. Graham MR, Cooperberg PL Cohen MM, Burmenne HJ (1980) The size of the normal common hepatic duct following cholecystectomy: an ultrasonographic study. Radiology 135:137–140

45. Green B, Bree RL, Goldstein HM, Stanley C (1977) Gray scale ultrasound evaluation of hepatic neoplasms: patterns and correlations. Radiology 124:203–208

46. Callen PW, Filly R (1979) Ultrasonographic localization of the gallbladder. Radiology 133:677–686

47. Weissman HS, Frank M, Rosenblatt R, Goldman M, Freeman LM (1979) Cholescintigraphy, ultrasonography and computerized tomography in the evaluation of biliary tract disorders. Semin Nucl Med 9:22–36

48. McCarthy CF, Davies ER, Wells P, Ross FG, Follett DH, Muir KM, Read AR (1970) A comparison of ultrasonic and isotope scanning in the diagnosis of liver disease. J Radiol 43:100–109

49. Mulhern CB, Arger PH, Coleman BG, Stein GN (1979) Nonuniform attenuation in computed tomography study of the cirrhotic liver. Radiology 132:399–402

50. Whalen JP (1979) Caldwell lecture, Radiology of the abdomen: impact of new imaging methods. Am J Roentgenol 133:586–618

51. Lunia S, Parthasarathy KL, Bender MA (1975) An evaluation of 99mTc-sulphur colloid liver scintiscans and their usefulness in metastatic work-up: a review of 1,424 studies. J Nucl Med 16:62–65

52. Maztyck A, Holtsford RA (1980) Ultrasound and isotope correlation in perihepatic scanning. Med Ultrasound 4:28–30

53. Milder MS, Larson SM, Bagley CM, De Vita VT, Johson RE, Johnston GS (1973) Liver-spleen scan in Hodgkin's disease. Cancer 31:826–839

54. Margulis AR, Burhenne JH (1979) Alimentary tract radiology-abdominal imaging, vol 3. St. Louis: CV Mosby

11. CLINICAL ASPECTS OF MODERN HEPATOLOGY

L.I.M. Van Waes and L.H.F. Demeulenaere

1. INTRODUCTION

Recent advances in basic sciences and technology have had a considerable impact on clinical hepatology by increasing our understanding, improving diagnosis, and influencing the management of liver diseases. In the first part of this chapter, we will discuss several areas that most clearly illustrate the breakthrough of clinical hepatology from the empirism which for a long time has characterized it.

In the second part we will deal with the changing nature of liver diseases, especially the increasing prevalence of such 'modern' diseases as toxic injury and environmental diseases of the liver.

2. PROGRESS IN DIAGNOSIS AND MANAGEMENT OF LIVER DISEASES

2.1. Viral hepatitis

Traditionally, at least two distinct types of viral hepatitis [1] have been recognized: 'infectious hepatitis' with a short incubation period (3–6 weeks; mean 30 days), transmitted by the fecal–oral route and responsible for epidemic outbreaks of the disease; and 'serum hepatitis' with a longer incubation time (6 weeks–6 months; mean 60 days) and spread by parenteral exposure to infected blood or blood products. The existence of these separate entities was supported by the controlled experiments conducted at the Willowbrook school [2].

The incidental discovery of the Australia antigen by Blumberg in 1965 [3] and its linkage to viral hepatitis in 1968 by Prince [4] marked the start of a fascinating decade of research leading to the discovery of serological virus markers for hepatitis viruses A and B and their identification by immune electron microscopy.

2.1.1. Identification of hepatitis viruses A and B and serological markers for their detection. Hepatitis A virus (HAV) is a 27-nm cubic RNA virus, related to the picorna viruses [5]. After infection, HAV can be found in liver cells, where active replication takes place. At the end of the incubation, a transient viremia may occur, but its short duration and low concentration on infective particles explain why perenteral spread is hardly of any clinical significance in hepatitis A. By contrast, shedding of the virus in stool, probably derived from the bile, is most abundant several days before biochemical, clinical, and histological evidence of hepatitis and ends a few days after onset of jaundice. After contact with the virus (with or without clinically overt hepatitis), specific anti-HAV are formed, at first belonging to the IgM and later to the IgG class, which may persist for years after the acute disease [6]. Diagnosis of hepatitis A can be made by isolating the virus particles in stool during the late incubation period and early clinical stage, or more practically by demonstrating anti-HAV in the blood during the acute disease. Since, however, most of the adult population carries anti-HAV as a result of previous (sub-)clinical contact with the virus, diagnosis of a recent infection should depend on the demonstration of at least a fourfold increase in anti-HAV titers, or on the detection of specific IgM anti-HAV, by commercially available RIA or ELISA techniques.

Hepatitis B virus (HBV), a DNA virus, is by far more complex than HAV [7]. Its presence in liver cells can be directly demonstrated by immunofluorescence or electron microscopy. Indirect evidence can be obtained by light microscopy by the positive orcein staining [8] and spontaneous ground-glass appearance of infected cells [9]. The virion is also demonstrable in the blood by electron microscopy as the core of 42-nm spherical particles

(Dane particles). The envelope of these Dane particles and the associated smaller round particles and tubular forms do not contain infective material, but consist merely of proteins, lipids, and carbohydrates formed by the host in reaction to the virus. Viremia starts 2–8 weeks before the clinical and biochemical illness and persists for some weeks during convalescence. In some patients a chronic carrier state develops, sometimes lifelong. HBV has also been detected in urine, milk, saliva, semen, vaginal secretions, menstrual blood ... which may play a role in the spread of the disease.

HBV is antigenetically complex and at least three different antigen-antibody systems have been identified, which are presumably virus coded, i.e., hepatitis B surface antigen (HBsAg), hepatitis B core antigen (HBcAg), and hepatitis Be antigen, against which anti-HBs, anti-HBc, and anti-HBe, respectively, are formed. HBsAg is identical to the Australia antigen described by Blumberg and is associated with the envelope of the Dane particle and the other round and tubular particles in the blood [3]. It appears several weeks before clinical onset of the disease and is cleared during the clinical stage or early convalescence, at what time anti-HBs appear. However, production of these anti-HBs can be delayed for weeks and months after clearance of the antigen and, in one-third of patients, titers remain so low that they will escape detection by the conventional methods. Some patients develop a chronic carrier state with persistence of HBsAg and no detectable anti-HBs. Thus, the presence of HBsAg may indicate a recent infection or a chronic carrier state. HBcAg, which is associated with the core of the Dane particle, is not freely present in the blood, but viral DNA polymerase and HBeAg, associated with the virion, can be detected during the late incubation period and initial clinical stage as markers of active virus replication. Anti-HBc are formed during the clinical illness and may be the only hint to virus B infection after HBsAg has been cleared from the blood and before anti-HBs are formed. High titers of anti-HBc without HBsAg may indicate low HBsAg carriage and perhaps infectivity [10]. Anti-HBs without anti-HBc or HBsAg is indicative of active or passive immunization against virus B.

2.1.2. Redefinition of viral hepatitis. The routine application of serological virus markers in patients with clinical or biochemical evidence of liver disease made it necessary to redefine the natural course and epidemiology of acute hepatitis and the implication of hepatitis viruses in other liver diseases.

Thus it appeared that while 'infectious hepatitis' was mainly due to HAV and 'serum hepatitis' to HBV, some overlap made it impossible to make a clear-cut distinction between the two viruses based on the length of the incubation period and *modes of transmission*. In the case of hepatitis B, modes of transmission other than the inoculation with blood or blood products were recognized as equally important, i.e., spread by the genital–oral route [11] and vertical transmission from carrier mothers to their babies [12]. In fact, spread by intimate sexual contact seems to be the most frequent source of infection in household settings [13], and vertical transmission often resulting in subclinical liver disease in the recipient could play an important role in maintaining the human reservoir of the virus, particularly in developing countries.

In contrast to hepatitis A, which is a benign and self-limited disease, infection with HBV is complicated by *progression toward chronic hepatitis* and even cirrhosis in 5%–10% of cases, predictable by the persistence of HBsAg in the blood beyond the normal time [14], and perhaps the presence of piecemeal necrosis (not to be confused with mere spilling over of inflammatory cells, frequently seen in acute hepatitis), a large number of plasma cells in portal infiltrates, and portal–portal bridging necrosis in liver biopsy [15]. Conversely, serological markers of virus B infection are found in 0–81% of patients with chronic hepatitis and cirrhosis [16, 17], with a striking geographical variation. Most of these patients have no knowledge of a previous attack of acute hepatitis, again stressing the important role of subclinical forms of hepatitis as the onset of chronic liver disease (CLD). In other patients, treatment with steroids during the acute phase of the illness has played a predisposing role by suppressing the immunological defense mechanisms of the patients [17].

The finding of virus B markers in 16%–90% of patients with primary *liver cell carcinoma*, according to the geographic areas, has raised some questions about a possible oncogenic role of this virus. Indeed, evidence is now accumulating for a possible causal relationship between HBV infection (mostly subclinical) and hepatocellular carcinoma (HCC), i.e., the correlation of HCC incidence and the prevalence of HBsAg in different countries and even in different areas of the same country; the higher incidence of HBsAg among patients with HCC compared with controls; the increased risk of developing HCC in HBsAg carriers relative to HBsAg-negative controls; the higher incidence of HBsAg in HCC than in cirrhosis in some countries; the development of HCC in HBsAg-positive CLD at an earlier stage than in HBsAg-negative CLD... [18]. In some patients, transition from HBsAg-positive chronic hepatitis to cirrhosis and HCC has been documented [19].

2.1.3. Identification of 'non-A–non-B' hepatitis. The availability of reliable serological markers for HAV and HBV led to the identification of a third group of hepatitis, clearly unrelated to hepatitis A and B and not caused by other common hepatitis viruses, e.g., the Epstein-Barr virus or cytomegalovirus. There are several lines of evidence that even more than one agent may be responsible for 'non-A–non-B' hepatitis. Diagnosis is made by exclusion of other hepatitis viruses and nonviral hepatocellular injury. The clinical picture closely resembles that of HBV infection in that transmission is predominantly by parenteral routes, there is association with a chronic carrier state, and a high propensity to progression toward chronic hepatitis and cirrhosis [20]. The clinical illness is usually mild and anicteric forms are not unusual. Incubation periods are described to be intermediate between type A and type B hepatitis, perhaps representing the artificial means of a type with long and one with short incubation. 'Non-A–non-B' virus has been implicated as the causal agent of up to 90% of cases of posttransfusional hepatitis [20]. It is thought to be also responsible for 50% of all non-B hepatitis in adult patients.

2.1.4. Prevention of viral hepatitis. The *routine screening of blood donations* for HBsAg and avoidance of commercial blood preparations have reduced the incidence of posttransfusional hepatitis five- to tenfold, but have not resulted in its disappearance [20]. It is possible that screening also for anti-HBc would even further diminish the incidence

of this complication [10].

Passive immunization [21] by administration of immune serum globulins (ISG) is of proven effect in the prevention of hepatitis A. Their use is recommended for persons traveling to areas where hepatitis A is highly endemic (preexposure prophylaxis) and after intimate physical contact with patients in the early stage of hepatitis A (postexposure prophylaxis). By contrast, titers of antibodies against virus B are quite variable in different batches of standard gamma globulins, and although adequate prophylaxis against hepatitis B has occasionally been reported with ISG, their effect is unpredictable and hepatitis B immune serum globulins (HBIG) are required for safe prophylaxis. Use of HBIG is clearly indicated after a single acute exposure to HBV, e.g., accidental inoculation (needle stick), oral ingestion, or splashing on mucous membranes of infective material. In a large controlled study, HBIG was effective in preventing hepatitis B in at least 70% of patients with acute needle-stick exposure to HBV [22]. Sexual contact with a patient with acute hepatitis B within six weeks of onset may also be considered an indication, providing the partner is both HBsAg negative and anti-HBs negative and reexposure is unlikely. The use of HBIG in situations of chronic exposure, e.g., household contacts of HBsAg carriers, personnel of hemodialysis units, and staff of institutes for the mentally retarded, is not recommended. Indeed, the effect of a single dose is only temporary and the potential hazards and cost involved with repeated administration of HBIG do not justify its use. The passive immunization of HBsAg-negative babies born to HBsAg-positive mothers is still controversial and administration of HBIG shortly after birth may not always prevent antigenemia and hepatitis in the infant [23]. Immunoglobulins prophylactically given to patients who received large amounts of blood transfusions have reduced the incidence of chronic liver disease associated with non-A–non-B hepatitis [24], but definite conclusions about their use cannot be made until serological markers for 'non-A–non-B' virus become available.

Active immunization [25] through the development of vaccines clearly is the goal of prevention in cases of chronic exposure. Progress in this field has been hampered by the consistent failure to pass the virus in tissue cultures. However, purified and formalin-inactivated 20- to 25-nm spherical HBsAg particles obtained from infected persons have been used for preparation of a vaccine. Although this subunit vaccine is protective against hepatitis B by eliciting anti-HBs and is apparently safe, some doubts persist as to its oncogenic potential and purity, which preclude its distribution at the present time. Untoward immunological reactions due to contaminating host proteins are perhaps less likely with vaccines prepared from constituent polypeptides of the 22-nm spherical particles or with synthetic vaccines that are now under study. Once vaccination against hepatitis B will become available, it definitely will reduce the human HBV reservoir and help to control hepatitis B and perhaps HBV-associated liver cell carcinoma.

2.1.5. Treatment of chronic hepatitis B. Lack of clearance of HBV from the blood has been shown to predispose the patient to the development of chronic liver disease [14] and negativation of HBs-Ag has preceded cure in some patients with chronic hepatitis [17]. Based on this rationale, *antiviral agents* have been administered to patients with active virus B replication in an attempt to modify the course of the underlying liver disease [26]. Limited studies with interferon and synthetic antiviral drugs, e.g., adenine arabinoside, have documented suppression of virus replication by these agents. The effect in most cases, however, was transient and active virus replication resumed after withdrawal of the drug. No definite beneficial effect on the progression of the underlying liver disease has been noted, but perhaps further studies with prolonged virus suppression are needed to establish the value of these agents. Also, the cost of interferon and the possible side-effects of the synthetic agents may preclude their long-term use.

Other approaches to the treatment of patients with chronic HBV liver disease are aiming at stimulation of cell-mediated immunity by administration of levamisole or transfer factor [23]. In some patients, this has resulted in a transient increase of transaminases, possibly reflecting an increased destruction of infected cells. The clinical value of treatment with antiviral agents and immunostimulants is uncertain at this time, but the considerable theoretical interest in the hypotheses that are

the basis of these experiments fully justify further controlled studies.

2.2. *Jaundice*

Perhaps the most considerable progress in diagnostic methodology is concerned with the workup of the jaundiced patient. As differentiation between intrahepatic cholestasis and extrahepatic biliary obstruction is essential for the rational management i.e., medical versus surgical treatment, of these patients, an early and correct diagnosis is also of practical importance. The diversity of diagnostic tests that presently are at our disposition is in sharp contrast with the situation of only a few years ago, when 'exploratory laparotomy' not infrequently was the last resort after a lengthy, frustrating, and little contributive investigation.

2.2.1. Diagnosis. Visualization of the extrahepatic bile ducts plays a key role in the differential diagnosis of jaundice. In fact, although a meticulous history, physical examination, and biochemical tests may give a correct orientation in up to 90% of cases with obstructive jaundice [27], evaluation of the therapeutic possibilities – surgical and nonsurgical – requires the morphological definition of the exact site, extent, and perhaps nature of the obstruction. On the other hand, in some patients, especially those with known gallstones or previous cholecystectomy, definite diagnosis of intrahepatic cholestasis may be impossible without proof of patency of the bile ducts.

Since conventional oral and intravenous cholecystocholangiography are likely to fail when serum bilirubin exceeds 3 mg/100 ml, opacification will need direct filling of the bile ducts with contrast medium by endoscopic retrograde cholangiopancreatography (ERCP) or percutaneous transhepatic cholangiography (PTC). Older methods include cholecystocholangiography under laparoscopic control and operative cholangiography [28]. Alternate methods to study intra- and extrahepatic bile ducts, which are not influenced by the presence of jaundice, are now also available, i.e., ultrasound and computed axial tomography (CT scan) [29].

Technical aspects of PTC and ERCP are discussed in detail in chapter 10. Awareness of the specific information and limitations of each technique will greatly influence the diagnostic planning in a given patient [30]. Thus, the yield of percutaneous transhepatic cholangiography, which became very popular after introduction of the 'skinny needle,' depends a great deal on the caliber of the intrahepatic bile ducts, and failure to opacify nondilated ducts may be as high as 60% [31]. On the other hand, endoscopic retrograde cholangiography demands greater skill of the examiner and, even after successful cannulation, opacification of the bile duct system is obtained in only 75% of patients, which is attributed to the oblique angle with which the bile duct enters to papilla [32]. Both methods offer complementary information that is of invaluable importance to the surgeon in case of total obstruction of the main bile duct.

A practical guideline for the workup of the jaundiced patient, which we have been using with success in our unit, is shown in Figure 1. Based on history, clinical examination, and biochemical profile, cases can be classified as obviously extrahepatic obstruction, obviously intrahepatic cholestasis, or diagnosis undetermined. Second-step investigations include PTC and/or ERCP in the case of extrahepatic obstruction, and laparoscopy, with or without liver biopsy, when intrahepatic causes for jaundice are most likely [33]. In case the clinical data do not lead to a definite orientation in diagnosis, the choice of the second-step technique will depend on the results of ultrasound, a 'noninvasive' technique that in experienced hands may correctly differentiate between intra- and extrahepatic jaundice in 97% of the cases [34]. If the chosen technique fails or does not give the expected information, then the other techniques can be tried. Using this flow chart, we have been able to complete the workup of almost all patients with jaundice within one week after admission and begin adequate treatment without delay.

2.2.2. Nonsurgical treatment of obstructive jaundice. Refinements in the above-mentioned diagnostic endoscopic and catheterization techniques have led to the development of alternative nonsurgical treatments for some patients with extrahepatic biliary obstruction, i.e., endoscopic sphincterotomy and transhepatic external or internal bile drainage.

Retained common bile duct stones, among the most dreaded complications of biliary surgery, are responsible for up to 80% of biliary causes of the postcholecystectomy syndrome [35]. Reintervention carries an increased risk, especially in older patients and when bile ducts are not dilated. Nonsurgical methods have been tried in the past, e.g., retrieval of common bile duct stones with a Dormier catheter introduced in the bile duct via the T-tube tract, or instillation of solubilizing or fragmenting substances into the bile duct through a T-tube [36].

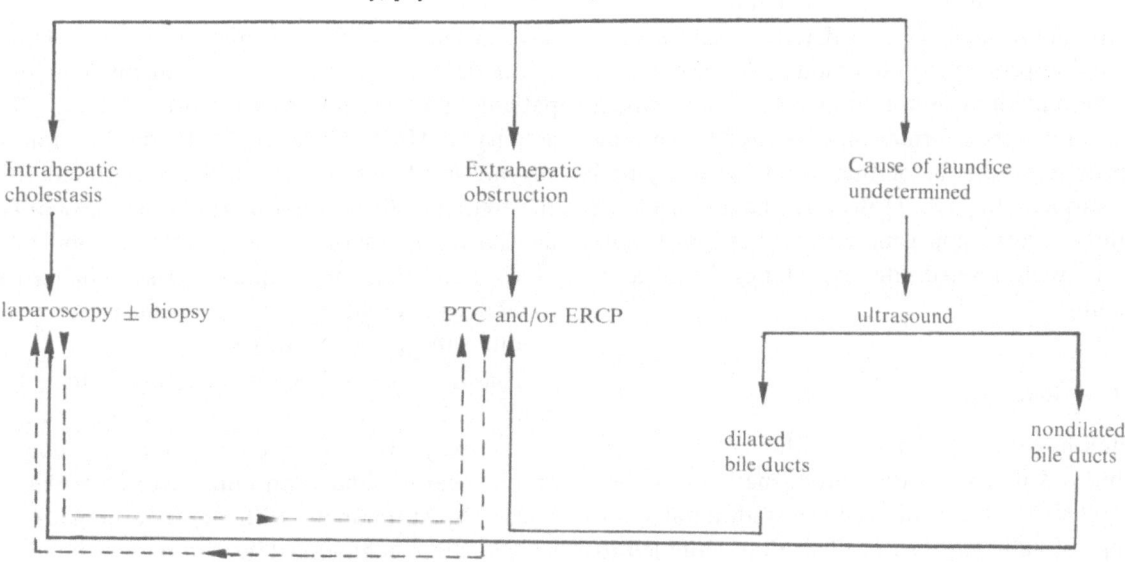

Figure 1. Flow chart for the workup of patients with jaundice (see text).

196

These methods, however, which now are mostly of historical interest, were not without risk for the patient and the success rate was low. By contrast *endoscopic sphincterotomy* (or rather papilloinfundibulotomy) now offers a safe alternative for surgical reintervention and even has become the method of choice for treating these patients. Technical aspects are discussed in chapter 10 of this book. Endoscopic papillotomy in experienced hands succeeds in 95% of patients, resulting in removal of the bile duct stones in about 90%, either spontaneously, after retrograde irrigation of the bile duct, or by introducing a Dormier catheter into the choledochus. The complication rate of this technique compares favorably with that of surgical reintervention: in a multicenter study compiling over 1100 procedures, mortality was 1% and morbidity 8.5%. The most common complication was bleeding in 3.5%, which in only rare instances required surgical intervention for hemostasis [37].

Based on the PTC technique, methods have been devised for prolonged *transhepatic biliary drainage* in patients with large bile duct obstruction and dilated intrahepatic bile ducts. Using prolonged preoperative bile drainage in patients with obstructive jaundice caused by resectable neoplasms, Nakayama et al. were able to reduce operative mortality form 28% to 8% [38]. In patients with inoperable bile duct obstruction, permanent external derivation or internal drainage of bile via an endoprosthesis maneuvered transhepatically beyond the obstruction can be considered to relieve pruritus and improve their life quality [39]. Experience with these methods is still limited to a few medical centers and more information is awaited concerning the benefits and risks of this technique compared with surgical bypass. However, the prospect of avoiding surgery and general anesthesia in fragile patients with limited life expectancy is at least appealing.

2.3. Gallstones

Insights into the dynamics of 'lithogenic bile' formation and its role in the pathogenesis of cholesterol gallstones have changed the traditional static concept of gallstone disease. This eventually led to the development of medical gallstone dissolution and revived the interest of internists in what was considered to be primarily a surgical problem.

2.3.1. Pathogenesis. The immense progress in this field was set in motion by the in vitro studies of Admirand and Small, who defined the maximal cholesterol-holding capacity of a bile-simulating system and introduced the concept of 'lithogenic bile,' i.e., bile supersaturated with cholesterol for the available amounts of lecithin and bile salts [40]. Under these conditions, cholesterol cannot be completely solubilized in the mixed micelles formed by the two other components, and free crystals may precipitate to form a cholesterol gallstone. This metabolic theory was validated by the finding that the bile of patients with cholesterol gallstones consistently showed supersaturation. As was pointed out, however, by Holzbach et al., supersaturated bile is not uncommon among patients without gallstones, especially after an overnight fast [41]. Thus, although lithogenic bile is a prerequisite, it is clear that presently ill-defined conditions favoring nucleation and stone growth must prevail before saturated bile leads to the formation of gallstones [42].

The mechanisms for the production of lithogenic bile have been extensively studied and have shed new light on the well-known risk factors for gallstone disease [43]. Thus, saturated bile may be the result of increased biliary excretion of cholesterol, decreased output of bile salts and phospholipids, or a combination of both. Increased output of cholesterol in bile is most often due to increased hepatic synthesis such as has been documented in obese patients and during hypercaloric feeding. Also, activity of HMG-CoA reductase, the rate-limiting enzyme in cholesterol synthesis, was found to be elevated in gallstone patients. Other mechanisms have also been invoked, e.g., increased mobilization of cholesterol from peripheral tissues in patients treated with clofibrate, or diminished cerebrotendinous xantomathosis (CTX).

Abnormalities in bile salt metabolism have been implicated in the pathogenesis of gallstones in various ways. Biliary secretion of bile salts depends on bile acid pool size and number of enterohepatic cycles. Most patients with cholesterol gallstones have an abnormally low bile acid pool, which could be the result of a primary defect in synthesis (e.g., in CTX: effect of estrogens), an enhanced negative feedback on hepatic synthesis, or an uncompensated loss of bile salts. Increased intestinal loss of bile salts, e.g., during treatment with cholestyramine or in Crohn disease of the terminal ileum, is normally compensated for by an increased hepatic synthesis. Only when the loss exceeds 20% of hepatic excretion is synthesis insufficient to maintain an adequate pool size. The role of the gallbladder function in regulating pool size has recently been emphasized [44]. Sequestration of bile salts in a noncontracting gallbladder causes interruption of the enterohepatic circulation and is held responsible for the production of lithogenic bile through a decreased output of bile salts after an overnight fast. On the other hand, enhanced emptying (increased gallbladder response to cholecystokinin has been documented in gallstone patients) could have a similar effect by an augmented negative feedback on bile acid synthesis exerted by the increased recycling frequency [45].

From the foregoing, it is obvious that cholesterol gallstone disease has to be regarded as the result of chronic and complex alterations in cholesterol and bile salt metabolism in which both hepatic and gallbladder factors are interwoven. Whereas the conditions leading to the formation of lithogenic bile are now relatively well understood, factors that determine cholesterol precipitation and gallstone formation in patients with lithogenic bile remain to be clarified.

2.3.2. Medical dissolution of gallstones. Once the metabolic basis for cholesterol gallstone formation was understood, it was tempting to try to dissolve gallstones by medically interfering with bile composition. Although several substances were shown to improve bile lithogenicity, dissolution of stones has succeeded so far only with cheno- and ursodeoxycholic acid, both naturally occurring bile salts in man.

Based on the rationale that expansion of the bile acid pool would result in a better solubilization of cholesterol, different bile acids were fed to patients with gallstones. As was expected, chenodeoxycholic acid (but not cholic acid) resulted in a rapid decrease in bile saturation and more slowly in dissolving gallstones in some of these patients [46]. The therapeutic effect of chenodeoxycholic acid (CDC) was afterward confirmed on more ample series of patients [47, 48].

Although the clinical effect of CDC treatment seems now well established, the mechanism of action of the drug remains incompletely understood [49]. Contrary to the working hypothesis, no constant expansion of pool size was seen as the increase in CDC pool was counteracted by a negative feedback on cholic acid synthesis. A decrease in cholesterol output, presumably by depression of HMG-CoA reductase activity, seems to be the main mechanism whereby CDC decreases saturation of bile. Also, intestinal absorption of cholesterol is decreased under CDC treatment, but the clinical relevance of this finding is equivocal.

From a clinical point of view, it became important to identify factors that could impede the efficacy of CDC [48]. Failure of stones to dissolve under CDC therapy has been attributed to poor patient compliance, use of a dosage insufficient to bring bile back to an unsaturated state, or presence of counteracting factors, e.g., obesity and contraceptives. The most important drawback, however, is related to poor patient selection. Indeed, current radiological selection criteria for cholesterol stones, based on radiolucency of stones, may falsely include up to 15% pigment stones, which will not benefit from CDC treatment [50]. As the dissolution of gallstones is the result of long-term interaction with the newly formed unsaturated bile, a functioning gallbladder is a *conditio sine qua non* for CDC treatment. Small stones may be easier to dissolve than large ones, as their surface–volume ratio is more favorable for the exchange process.

Based on these data, CDC treatment should be most effective in patients with multiple small stones (microlithiasis) in a functioning gallbladder. A dosage of 10–15 mg/kg body weight is sufficient in most patients to produce nonsaturated bile [51]. During treatment, patients may still suffer from complications of the gallstones and this long-term treatment is therefore not indicated for patients with frequent attacks of biliary pain. By contrast, atypical so-called biliary dyspepsia and even migraine may be alleviated by this treatment, possibly due to the choleretic action of the drug.

The question of whether all asymptomatic patients with radiolucent stones and functional gallbladder should be treated with CDC remains largely unsettled. Possible benefits, i.e., prevention

198

of potential complications, should be weighed against possible side-effects and risks. Patients may complain of diarrhea and abdominal cramps, in which case the treatment may need to be occasionally interrupted. Liver damage from the increased production of its toxic metabolite lithocholic acid is apparently prevented by increased sulphation of the latter [52], and the slight elevation of transaminases in some patients at the start of treatment has not been associated with histological proof of liver damage. Ursodeoxycholic acid (UDC), which has similar effects on bile saturation and gallstone dissolution as CDC at two-thirds of the dose and does not have adverse effects on colonic function nor cause transaminitis, may be of benefit in replacing CDC in some of these patients [53, 54].

After discontinuation of treatment, the bile returns to its supersaturated state, and recurrence of gallstone formation has been documented in some patients. It is our policy to continue with a maintenance dose after dissolution, although others interrupt treatment and reserve maintenance therapy for those patients with proven recurrence of stones after dissolution. Obviously, long-term follow-up studies are required to answer this question.

3. INCREASED PREVALENCE OF LIVER INJURY FROM DRUGS AND ENVIRONMENTAL AGENTS

There has been an increased awareness in recent years of the role of hepatotoxins as a cause of liver injury in man and animals. Since drug-induced lesions may closely mimic the entire spectrum of liver diseases from other etiologies, a thorough search for exposure to drugs and environmental toxins should be part of the routine workup on all patients with liver problems. Questions should be explicit because certain drugs, e.g., ethanol, oral contraceptives, laxatives, and vitamins, are no longer considered as such by the patients. Whereas the list of agents incriminated as the cause of liver injury is expanding every day, little progress has been made in the understanding of the mechanism whereby liver injury is induced by these drugs.

3.1. Ethanol

Although association between liver disease and chronic drinking has been recognized for many years, definite proof incriminating ethanol (and not associated malnutrition) as the responsible hepatotoxin was only given in 1975, based on studies in the baboon model of alcohol liver disease [55]. The wide spectrum of alcohol-induced liver injury has been amply documented and the principal mechanisms of ethanol hepatotoxicity established, i.e., metabolic disturbances due to alterations in the redox potential of the liver cell by ADH-mediated ethanol oxidation: adaptive changes due to induction of the microsomal ethanol-oxidizing system (MEOS) [55]. However, evidence is now accumulating about additional mechanisms of liver toxicity:
- The in vivo role of acetaldehyde, which is an established toxin for liver cells in vitro.
- Increased susceptibility of chronic drinkers to the toxic effect of other drugs (by an enhanced formation of their toxic metabolites) such as has been demonstrated for carbon tetrachloride.
- Increased susceptibility of chronic drinkers to the effect of carcinogens.
- Autoimmune reactions that could perpetuate alcohol-induced liver damage after abstinence [56].

3.2. Other drugs

Virtually all drugs may be liver toxic, either directly (in which case the effect is constant, predictable, dose-related, and reproducible in animals), or indirectly by causing an allergic reaction in the host (in which case toxic effects are rare, unpredictable, dose independent, and not reproducible in animals). Agents with an intrinsic hepatotoxic action have mostly been banned from clinical use. Some clinically stable drugs, however, are metabolized in the liver into potent alkylating or arylating agents, which by covalent binding to vital cellular proteins may produce liver cell necrosis. Liver injury through the intermediate of toxic reactive metabolites may be a common denominator of a number of direct toxic drug reactions, as has been demonstrated for acetaminophen, phenacetin, acetanilid, and furosemide [57]. The explanation for the fact that most of these drugs are safe in the normal therapeutic dose range is not univocal and illustrates the complexity of the drug problem. Among the protective mechanisms, effective at low doses but insufficient in overdoses of the drug, are plasma protein binding (furosemide) and captation of the reactive metabolites by glutathione (acetaminophen).

Production of reactive metabolites and hence toxicity of a drug in a given patient may also be influenced by induction of the microsomal biotransformation system by such commonly used agents as ethanol and tranquilizers, and by genetic predisposition. The latter has been demonstrated for isoniazid, which in 'slow acetylators' is less converted to the toxic acetylhydrazine than in genetically 'fast acetylators.' The finding that drugs are converted into chemically reactive metabolites that form covalent bonds with tissue macromolecules raises the interesting hypothesis that this biotransformation could be also the initial step in allergic drug reactions. Thus, both the direct-toxic and the hypersensitivity type of drug reactions may not be as strongly opposed as traditionally thought. This is perhaps illustrated in halothane- and isoniazid-induced liver injury in which both mecnanisms seem to be involved.

The spectrum of drug-induced liver injury is wide and, although some drugs may produce different kinds of liver lesions, the clinical pattern associated with a given drug is quite stereotypic (Table 1). Drug-induced liver disease may be clinically, biochemically, and histologically indistinguishable from acute and chronic liver diseases of another etiology. Diagnosis largely depends on careful history and epidemiologic data, although final proof that a certain drug is the cause of the observed liver lesions in a given patient is often difficult, if not impossible, to obtain. Rechallenge might be useful, but is not recommended in allergic drug reactions because of the risk of fatal liver necrosis. Recognizing hepatic drug reactions is important because

Table 1. Liver injury induced by drugs and environmental agents

Type of lesion	Agents responsible (not limitative)
Steatosis	L-Asparaginase, ethanol, glucocorticosteroids, methotrexate, tetracycline
Toxic hepatitis	
Acute	Carbon tetrachloride, DDT, dinitrophenol, phosphorus, tannic acid, phalloidin, TNT, toluene Actinomycin D, 6-mercaptopurine, mithramycin Alpha-methyldopa, furosemide, halothane, indomethacin, isoniazid, paracetamol, salicylates
Chronic	Alpha-methyldopa, ethanol (?), iproniazid, isoniazid, nitrofurantoin, oxyphenisatin, paracetamol, perhexiline maleate, propylthiouracil, sulfonamides
Cholestatic	Azathioprine, chlorpromazine, erythromycin estolate, PAS, penicillin
'Alcoholic'	Ethanol, perhexiline maleate
Fibrosis/cirrhosis	Inorganic arsenicals, ethanol, methotrexate, thorotrast, urethane, vinyl chloride, perhexiline maleate, vitamin A
Biliary cirrhosis	Organic arsenicals, phenothiazines, tolbutamide
Granulomas	Beryllium, diphenylhydantoin, ethanol, phenylbutazone, halothane, hydralazine, quinidine, sulfonamides, methotrexate, nitrofurantoin, probenicid, procainamide
Cholestasis	Anabolic and contraceptive steroids
Thesaurismosis	Thorotrast, polivinyl pyrrolidone
Tumors	
Focal nodular hyperplasia, adenoma, hamartoma	Androgens (?), estrogens, oral contraceptives
Hepatocellular carcinoma	Aflatoxin, anabolics/androgens, ethanol, estrogens, oral contraceptives
Angiosarcoma	Inorganic arsenicals, thorotrast, vinyl chloride
Vascular lesions	
Peliosis	Anabolic steroids, androgens, azathioprine, chenodeoxycholic acid, corticosteroids, oral contraceptives
Budd-Chiari syndrome	Oral contraceptives, pyrrolizidine alkaloids
Venoocculisive disease	Azathioprine, irradiation, oral contraceptives, pyrrolizidine alkaloids, urethane
Hepatoportal sclerosis	Inorganic arsenicals, azathioprine, methotrexate, vinyl chloride
Idiopathic portal hypertension	Azathioprine

200

toxic liver injury has a far better prognosis than liver injury from another etiology, with usually a rapid clinical and even histological improvement after withdrawal of the drug [58].

3.3. Environmental toxins

There has been an increased exposure to environmental toxins in recent years [59]. Among the most toxic *occupational agents* are the synthetic halocarbons [60], universally used in industry as solvents, propellants, or refrigerants (e.g., carbon tetrachloride, dichloromethane, and perchloroethylene). Other members of this family of chemicals are used as insecticides (DDT, o-dichlorobenzene), local anesthetics (chloroethane, chloromethane), or for the production of plastic polymers (vinyl chloride). Exposure to the toxic effects of these agents goes far beyond an occupational hazard (factory workers) or ingestion (suicide). In fact, we all have probably been inadvertently contaminated since these agents have become ubiquitous constituents of our environment (food, drinking water, air) as the result of pollution.

Other examples of environmental liver injury have been traced back to *toxins in food* [61]. Among the most notorious are venoocclusive disease and Budd-Chiari syndrome due to pyrrolizidine alkaloids in herbal infusions ingested as tea (*Senecio*) or for their medicinal properties (*Crotalaria*); massive hepatitis following poisoning with phalloidin, a mushroom toxin from *Amanita phalloides*; hepatoma due to (?) aflatoxin from the mold *Aspergillus flavus* contaminating cereals [62]. Concern has

been expressed that the currently revived interest in obscure 'health foods' and herbal medicines also in Western countries might become a source of environmental liver injury.

The increasing trend toward uncontrolled self-medication probably represents another hazard, as is illustrated by liver fibrosis associated with chronic overdose of vitamin A; CALD (chronic active liver disease) due to abuse of laxatives containing oxyfenisatin (now banned from use in most countries); the spectrum of liver injury (including benign liver tumors) from oral contraceptives.

Environmental liver injury often develops insidiously, in patients with long-term continuous or intermittent exposure to low doses of toxins [59]. Symptoms (if any) and morphologic liver lesions are often atypical and resemble liver disease of other, e.g., viral etiology. Epidemiologic observations therefore are frequently the keystone to diagnosis, i.e., clustering of a rare type of liver disease in a relatively closed group with known exposure to a toxic agent should raise suspicions of a causal relationship. Well-known examples are the high prevalence of angiosarcoma in a group of vinyl-chloride workers, and increased incidence of benign liver tumors in women who use oral contraceptives. Similar observations in animals exposed to the same agent may give additional support to its hepatotoxicity. On the other hand, it may be impossible in an individual case to link with certainty the observed liver lesions to a known environmental toxin, and diagnosis is often partially by exclusion.

REFERENCES

1. WHO Expert Committee on Viral Hepatitis (1977) Advances in viral hepatitis. WHO Tech Rep Ser 602
2. Krugman S, Giles JP, Hammond J (1967) Infections hepatitis: evidence for two distinctive clinical, epidemiological and immunological types of infection. JAMA 200:365–373
3. Blumberg BS, Alter HJ, Visnich S (1965) A 'new' antigen in leukemia sera. JAMA 191:541–546
4. Prince AM (1968) An antigen detected in the blood during the incubation period of serum hepatitis. Proc Natl Acad Sci USA 60:814–821
5. Dienstag JL (1980) Viral hepatitis type A: virology and course. Clin Gastroenterol 9:135–154
6. Frösner GG (1977) Nachweis von Hepatitis-A-Antigen und -Antikörpern zur Diagnose der Hepatitis-A-Infektion,
Muench Med Wochenschr 119:825–828
7. Burrell CJ (1980) Serological markers of hepatitis B infection. Clin Gastroenterol 9:47–63
8. Shikata T, Uzawa T, Yoshiwara N, Akatsuka T, Yamazaki S (1974) Staining methods of australia antigen in paraffin section. Detection of cytoplasmic inclusion bodies. Jpn J Exp Med 44:25–36
9. Hadziyannis S, Gerber MA, Vissoulis C, Popper H (1973) Cytoplasmic hepatitis B antigen in 'ground-glass' hepatocytes of carriers. Arch Pathol 96:327–330
10. Hoofnagle JH, Seeff LB, Bales ZB, Zimmerman HJ (1978) VA Hepatitis Cooperative Study Group: type B hepatitis after transfusion with blood containing antibody to hepatitis B core antigen. N Engl J Med 298:1379–1393
11. Zuckerman AJ (1977) Sexual transmission of hepatitis B. Nature 266:14–15

12. Buffet C, Larouze B (1977) Transmission maternelle du virus de l'hépatite B. Gastroenterol Clin Biol 1:1053–1062
13. Perillo RP, Gelb L, Campbell C, Wellinghoff W, Ellis FR, Overby L, Aach RD (1979) Hepatitis Be Antigen, DNA polymerase activity and infection of household contacts with hepatitis B virus. Gastroenterology 76:1319–1325
14. Yamada G, Nakane PK (1979) Hepatitis B core and surface antigens in liver tissue. Lab Invest 36:649–659
15. Dietrichson O, Juhl E, Christoffersen P, Elling P, Faber V, Inversen K, Nielsen JO, Petersen P, Poulsen H (1975) Acute viral hepatitis: factors possibly predicting chronic liver disease. Acta Pathol Microbiol Scand [A] 83:183–188
16. Wright R (1980) Type B hepatitis: progression to chronic hepatitis. Clin Gastroenterol 9:97–115
17. Van Waes L, Segers J, Van Egmond J, Van Nimmen L, Barbier F, Wieme R, Demeulenaere L (1974) Chronic liver disease and hepatitis-B antigen: a prospective study. Br Med J 3:444–446
18. Hadziyannis SJ (1980) Hepatocellular carcinoma and type B hepatitis. Clin Gastroenterol 9:117–134
19. Dudley FJ, Scheuer PJ, Sherlock S (1973) Natural history of hepatitis-associated antigen-positive chronic liver disease. Lancet 2:1388–1393
20. Alter HJ (1980) The dominant role of non-A, non-B in the pathogenesis of post-transfusion hepatitis: a clinical assessment. Clin Gastroenterol 9:155–170
21. Seeff LB, Hoofnagle JH (1979) Immunoprofylaxis of viral hepatitis. Gastroenterology 77:161–182
22. Veterans administration cooperative study (1978) Type B hepatitis after needle-stick exposure: prevention with hepatitis B immune globulin. Ann Intern Med 88:285–293
23. Beasley RP, Stevens CE (1978) Vertical transmission of HBV and interruption with globulin. In: Vyas GN, Cohen SN, Schmid R (eds) Viral hepatitis. Philadelphia: Franklin Institute, pp 333–345
24. Knodell RG, Conrad ME, Ishak KG (1977) Development of chronic liver disease after acute non-A,non-B post-transfusion hepatitis: role of gamma globulin prophylaxis in its prevention. Gastroenterology 72:902–909
25. Zuckerman AJ (1980) Prophylaxis of hepatitis type B: immunoglobulins and vaccines. Clin Gastroenterol 9:65–83
26. Thomas HC, Bassendine MF (1980) Immunological and anti-viral therapy of chronic hepatitis B virus infection. Clin Gastroenterol 9:85–95
27. Schenker S, Balint J, Schiff L (1962) Differential diagnosis of jaundice. Am J Dig Dis 7:449–463
28. Elias E (1976) Cholangiography of the jaundiced patient. Gut 17:801–811
29. Wheeler PG, Theodossi A, Pickford R, Laws J, Knill-Jones RP, Williams R (1979) Non-invasive techniques in the diagnosis of jaundice – Ultrasound and computer. Gut 20:196–199
30. Elias E, Hamlyn AN, Jain S, Long RG, Summerfield JA, Dick R, Sherlock S (1976) A randomized trial of percutaneous transhepatic cholangiography with the Chiba needle versus endoscopic retrograde cholangiography for bile visualization in jaundice. Gastroenterology 71:439–443
31. Okuda K, Tanikawa E, Kuratomi S, Jinnouchi S, Urabe K, Sumikoshi T, Kanda Y, Fukuyama Y, Hirotaka M, Mori M, Shimokawa Y, Yakushiji F, Matsuura Y (1974) Nonsurgical, percutaneous transhepatic cholangiography, diagnostic significance in medical problems of the liver. Am J Dig Dis 19:21–36
32. Cotton PB (1977) Progress report: ERCP. Gut 18:316–341.
33. Van Waes L, Versieck J, Barbier F, Demeulenaere L (1973) Laparoscopy in the differential diagnosis of jaundice. Acta Gastroenterol Belg 36:624–631
34. Taylor KJW, Carpenter DA, McCready VR (1974) Ultrasound and scintigraphy in the differential diagnosis of obstructive jaundice. J Clin Ultrasound 2:105–115
35. Bodvall B (1973) The postcholecystectomy syndromes. Clin Gastroenterol 2:103–126
36. Classen M, Ossenberg FW (1977) Non-surgical removal of common bile duct stones. Gut 18:760–769
37. Liguory C, Coffin JC, Familiari L, Di Matteo G (1979) La sphinctérotomie par voie endoscopique dans le traitement de la lithiase biliaire. Rev Med 22:1191–1195
38. Nakayama T, Ikeda A, Okuda K (1978) Percutaneous transhepatic drainage of the biliary tract. Gastroenterology 74:1286–1294
39. Hoevels J, Ihse I (1979) Percutaneous transhepatic insertion of a permanent endoprosthesis in obstructive lesions of the extrahepatic bile ducts. Gastrointest Radiol 4:367–377
40. Carey MC, Small DM (1978) The physical chemistry of cholesterol solubility in bile. J Clin Invest 61:998–1026
41. Holzbach RT, Marsh M, Olszewski M, Holan K (1973) Cholesterol solubility in bile. Evidence that supersaturated bile is frequent in healthy man. J Clin Invest 52:1467–1479
42. Holan KR, Holzbach RT, Hermann RE, Cooperman AM, Claffey WJ (1979) Nucleation time: a key factor in the pathogenesis of cholesterol gallstone disease. Gastroenterology 77:611–617
43. Bennion LJ, Grundy SM (1978) Risk factors for the development of cholelithiasis in man. N Engl J Med 299:1221–1227
44. Lamorte WW, Schoetz DJ Jr, Birkett DH, Williams LF Jr (1979) The role of the gallbladder in the pathogenesis of cholesterol gallstones. Gastroenterology 77:580–592
45. Northfield TC, Kupfer RM, Maudgal DP, Zentler-Munro PL, Meller ST, Garvie NW, McCready R (1980) Gallbladder sensitivity to cholecystokinin in patients with gall stones. Br Med J 1:143–144
46. Danzinger RG, Hofmann AF, Schoenfield LJ, Thistle JL (1972) Dissolution of cholesterol gallstones by chenodeoxycholic acid. N Engl J Med 286:1–8
47. Hofmann AF, Paumgartner G (eds) (1975) Chenodeoxycholic acid therapy of gallstones. Progress report 1975. Stuttgart: FK Schattauer
48. Van Waes L, Nachtegaele P, Demeulenaere L (1979) Traitement de la lithiase biliaire par l'acide chénodésoxycholique. Indications, facteurs de succès, résultats. Rev Med 22:1171–1179
49. Andersen JM (1979) Chenodeoxycholic acid desaturates bile – but how? Gastroenterology 77:1146–1150
50. Trotman BW, Petrella EJ, Soloway RD, Sanchez HM, Morris TA, Miller WT (1975) Evaluation of radiographic lucency or opaqueness in identifying cholesterol or pigment stones. Correlation of lucency or opaqueness with calcium and mineral content. Gastroenterology 69:1563–1566
51. Mok HYI, Bell GD, Dowling RJ (1974) Effect of different doses of chenodeoxycholic acid on bile lipid composition and on frequency of side effects in patients with gallstones. Lancet 2:253–257
52. Allan RN, Thistle JL, Hofmann AF, Carter JA, Yu PYS (1976) Lithocholate metabolism during chemotherapy for gallstone dissolution. Serum levels of sulphated and unsulphated lithocholates. Gut 17:405–412
53. Maton PN, Murphy GM, Dowling RH (1977) Ursodeoxycholic acid treatment of gallstones. Dose-response study and possible mechanism of action. Lancet 2:1297–1301

54. Stiehl A, Czygan P, Kommerell B, Weis HJ, Holtermüller KH (1978) Ursodeoxycholic acid versus chenodeoxycholic acid. Comparison of their effects on bile acid and bile lipid composition in patients with cholesterol gallstones. Gastroenterology 75:1016–1020

55. Van Waes L, Lieber CS (1979) Toxic effects of alcohol on the liver. In: Farber E, Fisher MM (eds) Toxic injury of the liver. New York: Marcel Dekker, pp 629–653

56. Lieber CS (1978) Pathogenesis and early diagnosis of alcoholic liver injury. N Engl J Med 298:888–893

57. Mitchell JR, Nelson SD, Thorgeirsson SS, McMurtry RJ, Dybing E (1976) Metabolic activation: biochemical basis for many drug-induced liver injuries. In: Popper H, Schaffner F (eds) Progress in liver diseases, vol 5. New York: Grune and Stratton pp 259–279

58. Maddrey WC, Boitnott JK (1979) Drug-induced chronic hepatitis and cirrhosis. In: Popper H, Schaffner F (eds) Progress in liver diseases, vol 6. New York: Grune and Stratton, pp 595–603

59. Popper H, Gerber MA, Schaffner F, Selikoff IJ (1979) Environmental hepatic injury in man. In: Popper H, Schaffner F (eds) Progress in liver diseases, vol 6. New York: Grune and Stratton, pp 605–638

60. Reynolds ES, Moslen MT (1980) Environmental liver injury: halogenated hydrocarbons. In: Farber E, Fisher MM (eds) Toxic injury of the liver. New York: Marcel Dekker, pp 541–596

61. McLean EK, Mattocks AR (1980) Environmental liver injury: plant toxins. In: Farber E, Fisher MM (eds) Toxic injury of the liver. New York: Marcel Dekker, pp 517–539.

62. Editorial (1975) More on the aflatoxin-hepatoma story. Br Med J 2:647–648

12. TRENDS AND DEVELOPMENTS IN HEPATIC SURGERY

D.C. MARTIN, JR., and W.S. BLAKEMORE

> In injuries of the liver, as well as in resections of this organ, hemostasis presents the greatest difficulties.
>
> Prof. Carl Garrè, 1907*

1. INTRODUCTION

This chapter is written to bring into focus some of the recent trends and developments in important areas of hepatic surgery. The choice of topics is limited, and no attempt is made to provide comprehensive coverage in a single chapter of the vast field of hepatic surgery. For this, the interested reader is referred to the recent survey of hepatic surgery edited by Madding and Kennedy [1] and to the short, basic monograph of McDermott [2]. It should be added that although surgical conditions involving the extrahepatic biliary system and portal circulation might properly be included in such a discussion, they too will be omitted inasmuch as consideration of these areas, however important clinically, is beyond the scope of this book. Throughout the discussion an attempt will be made to point out recent findings and new approaches and to call attention to those areas where results are discouraging and renewed effort needed; additionally, recent review articles of particular relevance and merit will be cited.

2. TRAUMA TO THE LIVER

Modern man's penchant for fast driving and for wielding weapons of one sort or another has generated, among other things, an increasing number of blunt and penetrating injuries of the liver. The current popularity of the motorcycle, encouraged by rising gasoline costs, further aggravates the problem.

Situated directly under the right dome of the diaphragm and protected externally only by fragile ribs and thin intercostal muscles, the liver is vulnerable to injuries from above, as well as from below, where the fleshy and often flabby abdominal wall offers the only resistance. Moreover, the impressive mass of the organ, translated into kinetic energy by the equation $\frac{1}{2}$(mass) (velocity)^2, assures that substantial deformation of liver substance will take place in acceleration/deceleration injuries, and that tearing, fracturing, shattering, and crushing of this friable, highly vascular organ, with two inflow systems and a fluid-filled ductal system, are all possible in the context of blunt injuries to this area. Additionally, the supporting structures are easily torn, and when tears involve the posteriorly situated hepatic veins, which attach the liver to the inferior vena cava, exsanguination can rapidly occur. With regard to penetrating injuries, whether stab wounds, gunshot wounds, shotgun wounds, shrapnel wounds, or the like, the generous dimensions of the organ make it a choice target located right at the midsection. Further, the proximity to other vital, unpaired structures – notably the aorta, inferior vena cava, pancreas, duodenum, portal vein, and common bile duct, as well as the expendable but treacherous ascending and transverse colon – provides a setting for multiple, severe injuries in a contaminated field. When, as so often occurs in patients with liver trauma, combined injuries of the chest and abdomen are present, with or without major injuries elsewhere, the chance of a favorable outcome is further diminished.

With these brief facts as a background, one can appreciate to some extent the challenge faced by the trauma surgeon in dealing with injuries of the liver. Although recent retrospective reviews of liver injuries [3–5] reveal a preponderance of relatively *simple* injuries, ranging from isolated capsular tears

---

* Garrè, Prof. Dr. C. (1907) On resection of the liver. *Surg. Gynecol. Obstet.* 5:331–341.

to moderate-sized lacerations with active but readily controllable bleeding, a sizable proportion of liver injuries are the *complex* variety, with profuse bleeding, deep and often irregular tears, significant areas of devitalization, and a high incidence of associated intra- or extraabdominal injuries. In this latter group of patients, who very often are in a state of shock, postoperative complications develop in the vast majority of patients, with respiratory problems, sepsis, and bleeding heading the list. The mortality rate of 20%–25% for these complex injuries of the liver [3, 5] is equally alarming; when the liver and five other intraabdominal organs are injured or when major hepatic resection is required to control the bleeding, the mortality exceeds 50%.

The immediate assessment and resuscitation of the trauma victim follows the time-honored ABCs of trauma: establishment of an adequate AIRWAY, control of brisk external BLEEDING, and support of the general CIRCULATION. Depending upon circumstances, one or two large (14 g) intravenous catheters are appropriately placed for the administration of Ringer lactate solution or, in urgent situations, O-negative whole blood, while a sample of the patient's blood is sent to the laboratory for immediate typing and cross-matching, complete blood count, baseline electrolyte determinations, and, in the case of suspected abdominal trauma, serum amylase determination. Arterial blood gas analysis can be done quickly, and, if time allows, appropriate x-rays are taken, together with an electrocardiogram when chest trauma is suspected. (In abdominal trauma, and especially in suspected liver injuries, intravenous infusions should not be given in the lower extremities to avoid pooling of fluids in the retroperitoneum in the event of traumatic tears of the inferior vena cava.)

The astute examiner will meanwhile have noted in a matter of seconds the character of the pulse and the integrity of movements of the chest wall, while placing an ear close to the patient's nose and mouth to judge the force and frequency of the ventilatory effort [7]

Expeditious but thoughtful assessment of the abdomen is prompted by obvious wounds of the torso and, deductively, by circumstances enumerated by Lord Smith [8]: (1) head injury with fracture or fractures of the lower extremities, which raises the question as to what has happened between these two regions, (2) an unconscious patient with hypovolemic shock, which directs attention to the torso, rather than the head, as the cause of the shock, and (3) multiple rib fractures, which focus attention on the liver on the right, the spleen on the left, and the diaphragm bilaterally.

The concept of 'torso trauma' [9] deserves further comment. Although, anatomically, the diaphragm rather neatly divides the torso into thorax and abdomen, the division in situations involving major trauma is largely artificial inasmuch as the wounding agent or agents, and the forces generated by them, infrequently respect the thin barrier presented by the diaphragm. In considering liver injuries, the importance of this concept cannot be overemphasized.

In the presence of liver trauma the examination of the abdomen, which may be unreliable in the unconscious or obtunded patient, yields nonspecific findings. Abdominal tenderness, involuntary guarding, and loss of bowel sounds are often elicited. According to Thal et al. [10], 'abdominal rigidity, or involuntary guarding, is the most helpful sign, and even when present alone, warrants exploratory celiotomy.' A false-positive or false-negative examination occurs in 10%–20% of cases.

In assessing abdominal trauma, the homely adage 'two tubes and a finger' is also helpful: a nasogastric tube empties the stomach and detects blood, a Foley catheter monitors urine output and reveals hematuria, and a finger in the rectum identifies recent bleeding from the colon or rectum.

In the comatose patient [11], or when findings in the alert patient are equivocal, peritoneal tap, supplemented when necessary by peritoneal lavage, is appropriate when time allows. The tap is preferably done in the midline two fingerbreadths below the umbilicus, and lavage, which takes approximately 20 min, is accomplished with 1 liter of saline or Ringer lactate solution. False-positive results are rare and usually reflect poor technique; false-negative results are more common and justify caution in interpreting the negative result.

Angiography, although sometimes applicable to the patient with multiple injuries [12], is usually omitted in cases of suspected liver trauma, owing to the urgency of the situation.

Operation is carried out with appropriate monitoring after an attempt at hemodynamic stabilization, which may prove futile in the patient with major hepatic injury. Operative draping of the patient allows for possible extension of the abdominal incision into the chest, and entry into the peritoneal cavity is gained by a generous midline incision. Should thoracic extension of the incision become necessary, median sternotomy [13] is currently the preferred approach in trauma cases; access to both pleural spaces and the pericardium is provided, exposure of the supradiaphragmatic and retrohepatic inferior vena cava is facilitated, and postoperative respiratory problems are fewer than with the traditional thoracoabdominal incision that extends into the seventh or eighth intercostal space and traverses a larger segment of diaphragm.

The basic principles in the operative treatment of liver injuries are hemostasis, debridement, and drainage, the manner of application depending upon circumstances. Certainly the most urgent problem on opening the abdomen of a patient with liver trauma is the control of bleeding. With superficial wounds it can be minimal and of little concern, but with larger wounds it is often relentless and massive. Apart from the immediate threat to life that major, uncontrolled hemorrhage represents, rapid deterioration of the clotting mechanism occurs in liver injuries after the transfusion of 4000–5000 cc of whole blood [14, 15]. Indeed, fresh whole blood is highly desirable beyond this point, underlining the importance of access to an unlimited blood supply in institutions definitively treating hepatic trauma. In this connection, Calne et al. [16] have recently proposed that in situations where such facilities do not exist, or where expertise in anesthesia and critical care are lacking, primary packing of the massively injured liver (after failing to control bleeding with sutures or hepatic artery ligation), with transfer of the patient to a large medical center for definitive treatment, is a worthy option.

Two patterns of bleeding have been identified [8]. In the first, sudden deterioration does not occur when the abdomen is opened, blood replacement can keep up with loss, and there are no tears or splits extending across the dome of the liver into the region of the hepatic veins. In the second, sudden deterioration does occur on entering the abdomen, unmanageable blood loss is encountered, and severe disruption of the liver is noted, with tears extending back toward the hepatic veins and in-

ferior vena cava. An entirely abdominal approach is usually adequate in the first situation. In the second, if the Pringle maneuver (temporary inflow occlusion at the porta hepatis by means of manual compression or atraumatic vascular clamp) fails to control the bleeding, prompt extension of the incision into the chest is indicated to provide exposure of the retrohepatic space and to permit, if necessary, vascular isolation of the liver [17], a technically difficult procedure prone to failure [6].

The application of specific methods of controlling hemorrhage depends upon the operative findings. Capsular tears very often can be left alone. Similarly, superficial lacerations that have stopped bleeding by the time the abdomen is opened require nothing more than an appropriately placed Penrose drain. With deeper lacerations, which usually bleed actively, the favored approach is to resist the temptation of bridging the gap with large mattress sutures and to ligate individual bleeders and major ducts with nonabsorbable suture ligatures or metallic clips. Occasionally this requires enlarging the defect to obtain proper exposure, or, in stab wounds or gunshot wounds, unroofing the tract of the penetrating object. The interposition of synthetic hemostatic agents such as gelatin foam or oxidized cellulose is thought to retard healing and to favor abscess formation, but Morgenstern [18] has advocated the topical application of microfibrillar collagen for diffuse small vessel bleeding in superficial liver lacerations, after major bleeders have been ligated.

Complex liver injuries require more demanding techniques. Gross areas of devitalization, which characteristically occur in irregular and stellate lacerations, missile injuries, and crush injuries, require some form of debridement to avoid subsequent abscess formation, fistulation, and recurrent bleeding. The favored technique, known as 'resectional debridement,' consists of elevation and manual compression of the liver while piecemeal removal of devitalized tissue is carried out by the 'finger-fracture' technique, with ducts and bleeding vessels individually suture-ligated as they are encountered. The resulting irregular, raw surface, which does not conform to defined anatomic planes, is left open or covered with omentum, with multiple drains brought out through the skin.

Occasionally, in bursting injuries of the liver,

206

which have a tendency to follow the path of least resistance through the liver – namely, along the intersegmental and interlobar planes, which transmit the fragile branches of the hepatic veins, rather than branches of the portal vein or hepatic artery, which are wrapped in the more sturdy fibrous matrix of the portal triads – the resulting low-pressure backflow venous bleeding responds, after appropriate debridement, to the placement of one or two pedicle flaps of omentum, tucked into the depths of the wound and secured with overlying sutures placed across the crevice. With sump suction added, Stone and Lamb [19] claim success in stopping bleeding in 37 of 37 cases, with only two late deaths in the series, both from renal failure.

When brisk bleeding from the injured liver is largely arterial, selective hepatic artery ligation has been advocated [20]. The portal vein, which supplies 70%–80% of the blood and 50%–70% of the oxygen to the liver, is left undisturbed, and additional blood flow to the liver takes place through the numerous collateral pathways, 26 in all, demonstrated by the meticulous anatomic studies of Michels [21]. Indeed, collateral flow to a devascularized lobe of the liver can be shown radiographically to occur as early as 10 h after interruption of the corresponding hepatic artery or the common hepatic artery [22]. Certainly, former fears about hepatic artery ligation – generated in the 1930s by the fulminant septic hepatic necrosis seen in the dog when the hepatic artery is ligated experimentally – have abated with the appreciation that the dog liver differs from the normally sterile human liver in harboring a resident population of anaerobic organisms, notably clostridia, which account for the lethal course of events in the dog.

While most surgical centers, by Walt's estimate [23], presently employ hepatic artery ligation in no more than 4%–5% of cases of liver trauma, which is considerably less than the 31% rate of use in 178 consecutive liver injuries at the University of Louisville hospitals [24], there can be no doubt that the procedure has demonstrable value in the non-cirrhotic patient with difficult arterial bleeding from the severely injured liver. In other words, in a deteriorating situation in which judicious application of local methods of hemostasis has failed, hepatic artery ligation should be tried. The important technical features of the procedure are: (1)

avoidance of extensive dissection of supporting structures of the liver to minimize disruption of collateral vessels, (2) placement of ligatures on the right or left hepatic arteries as close to the liver as possible to avoid disturbing the hilar collateral flow, and (3) removal of the gallbladder when the right or common hepatic artery is ligated and, debatably, when the left hepatic artery is ligated. The common hepatic artery is preferably ligated *proximal* to a major collateral, such as the right gastric artery or the gastroduodenal artery, to provide some flow through the distal hepatic artery; if such flow proves too much, a second ligature is placed more distally [25].

Rebleeding after hepatic artery ligation occasionally occurs in the postoperative period [6, 24], and there are isolated reports of hepatic necrosis [26] and intrahepatic abscess [27] following the procedure. The most consistent sequelae are transient, pronounced elevations of hepatic enzymes (4–6 times above normal) and decreased levels of serum albumin, prothrombin, and cholesterol [28]. Hypoglycemia is prevented by the infusion of 5% dextrose, and hyperbilirubinemia when present suggests perihepatic sepsis, rather than acute liver damage. In general, the prime requisites for success with hepatic artery ligation are the avoidance postoperatively of hypovolemia, fever, sepsis, and hypoxia, and to reduce metabolic demands on the liver by putting the bowel at rest for 7–10 days. In this connection, the use of total parenteral nutrition in limited amounts may be helpful.

Formal hepatic lobectomy in the management of acute liver trauma is done infrequently [3, 4, 6, 15, 29, 30, 171], the two indications for its use being: (a) major shattering wounds of the liver, with massive bleeding and extensive areas of devitalization, and (b) juxtahepatic venous injuries that cannot be managed by other methods. Mainly, such injuries result from severe blunt torso trauma and from shotgun wounds. The right lobe of the liver, by virtue of its bulk, is more often affected than the left, although occasionally wounds involve both lobes in a manner that makes trisegmentectomy feasible.

Probably the most important thing that can be said about hepatic resection for trauma is that the operative decision for or against it should be made *early* in the course of the operation, before excessive blood loss has occurred. This is because, as mentioned earlier, the clotting mechanism rapidly deteriorates after 4000–5000 cc of blood has been replaced, with a corresponding sharp rise in the mortality rate. It is not a procedure which, like hepatic artery ligation, can be adopted as an afterthought after local methods of hemostasis have failed. The overall situation should be assessed rapidly, and if the liver is massively damaged or retrohepatic bleeding is not amenable to other methods of control, lobectomy or trisegmentectomy is carried out without further delay.

Technical aspects of hepatic resection are discussed in the section of this chapter entitled 'Hepatic resection.' What should be emphasized here is the need postoperatively for expert multidimensional care and monitoring. The patient is placed in an intensive care unit where skilled nursing care, continuous hemodynamic monitoring, respiratory physiotherapy, sequential blood gas determinations, and full nutritional support are all available. Hypoglycemia and hypoalbuminemia are aggressively combated, as well as hypovolemia, fever, infections, and other conditions that place metabolic demands on the liver. Even with the provision of quality care in the setting of a large medical center, the mortality rate for this procedure averaged greater than 50% in three recent series of civilian patients with major liver trauma [4, 29, 30]. Experience with hepatic resection for liver injuries in the Viet Nam War was also discouraging [31], although the mortality data were not presented.

Returning to juxtahepatic venous injuries, it needs to be acknowledged that, even with the availability of techniques for internally shunting the inferior vena cava through an incision in the right atrium [32], the results with this procedure, scattered among various centers over the past 12 years, have been dismal. Walt [6] frankly admitted failure in nine out of nine patients on whom the technique was tried at the Wayne State University Hospitals, and success elsewhere has been largely anecdotal. Not infrequently, the patient with major retrohepatic bleeding dies on the operating table from exsanguination, cardiac arrhythmias, or air embolism caused by the unwary surgeon who rotates the liver anteromedially to investigate the bleeding. Should the patient survive the operation, death from sepsis or sepsis-related organ failure, respiratory pro-blems, cardiovascular problems, renal failure, rebleeding, and a variety of other problems too often occurs. Technically, cross-clamping the aorta above the celiac trunk, and the inferior vena cava above and below the liver, is probably the simplest way to achieve vascular isolation of the liver [17], but the procedure induces cardiac arrhythmias in a majority of patients and usually has to be abandoned in favor of placement of an internal shunt, which is technically more difficult to do and has a higher associated blood loss, whether the shunt is inserted through the right atrium or via the intrahepatic inferior vena cava.

Confronted with a nonexpanding hematoma behind the liver, the surgeon is generally well advised to leave it alone. If the hematoma is expanding, it should not be explored until the incision is extended into the chest and fuller access to the retrohepatic space obtained.

Finally, mention should be made of subcapsular and intrahepatic hematomas, which have often gone unrecognized in the past but which have become increasingly detectable in recent years with the aid of hepatic scintiscans, arteriography, ultrasonography, and computed tomography. In the world literature, 45 such cases have been reported, and four new cases – all diagnosed with computed tomography – have been seen at the Medical College of Ohio Hospital (White and Howard, personal communication, 1980). Typically, the lesions contain blood, bile, and necrotic debris in varying proportions, and there is a demonstrated potential for evolution into chronic traumatic cysts or into abscesses. Except in cases where hemobilia is present, hematomas of the liver are generally not clinically apparent unless they reach generous proportions, with diameters greater than 10 cm and volumes well in excess of 1 liter. Jaundice is the most frequent finding in intrahepatic hematomas but is absent in subcapsular hematomas. Hemobilia, which has been seen with intrahepatic hematomas as small as 3 cm in diameter, is much less frequent. Treatment of hematomas of the liver depends on symptoms, location of the lesion, size, and accompanying conditions. Observation (with or without antecedent laparotomy), selective embolization with gelatin foam [33], evacuation and drainage, and lobectomy have been used with success in acute cases, and evacuation and drainage, with occasional resort to lobectomy, has been employed in chronic cases. In the rare case of hemobilia [6], selective hepatic artery ligation has emerged as the favored procedure [34, 35], although observation, selective gelatin foam embolization [36], hepatotomy with ligation of the bleeding vessel, and lobectomy have proved effective in some cases.

3. PRIMARY TUMORS OF THE LIVER

In the Western world, primary tumors of the liver, whether benign or malignant, occur infrequently, in contrast to Africa and Asia where in some areas, for reasons poorly understood, carcinoma of the liver is the most commonly encountered visceral malignancy. Even with the inclusion of secondary malignancies of the liver, increasingly detectable in recent years with the aid of improved scanning techniques, the incidence of surgically resectable hepatic tumors remains small, so that few individuals or institutions in this part of the world have accumulated sizable experience with these lesions. Indeed, Foster, in collaborating with Berman on *Solid liver tumors* [37], a comprehensive and much cited monograph, was obliged personally to visit 98 hospitals across the United States in order to acquire a 'critical mass' of information about surgically resectable liver tumors.

Nevertheless, despite the paucity of resectable tumors and the technical demands of extirpative procedures, there has been heightened interest in recent years in methods of diagnosis and treatment of liver tumors. There are several reasons for this. First, aids in diagnosis, the chief of which are radioisotope scanning of the liver, ultrasonography, computed tomography, and, in some cases, determination of serum alpha-fetoprotein levels, have increased in accuracy while becoming available on a massive and possibly extravagant scale. Second, the apparent increased incidence in women of tumors of the liver – specifically, hepatic cell adenoma, focal nodular hyperplasia, and, more rarely, hepatic malignancies of various types – in association in many cases with the use of oral contraceptives, has generated much discussion and raised interesting questions about tumor biology and about the practical management of these curious tumors. Thirdly, with respect to primary and secondary

malignancies of the liver, continuing disappointment with the results of chemotherapy and radiotherapy as primary or ancillary treatment for these tumors has focused attention on surgical resection as the therapeutic mainstay [178]. Finally, refinements and innovations in operative and anesthetic techiques, and in methods of postoperative care, to the point where over the past two years operative mortality rates of less than 10% for elective major hepatic resections have been reported from several centers [38–41], have helped dispel the pessimism these tumors once generated. Much of the advance, it should be noted, derives from a fuller understanding, ripening in the post World War II era, of the intricacies of hepatic architecture and metabolism.

Of the benign tumors of the liver, *cavernous hemangiomas* are the most common, occurring in approximately 2% of necropsies [42]. For the most part they are found incidentally at laparotomy or necropsy, usually as small, asymptomatic, solitary lesions, although occasionally lesions on the surface of the liver bleed intraperitoneally, necessitating laparotomy and local resection. Larger lesions, known as 'giant hemangiomas,' measure as much as several centimeters in diameter and are typically solitary. They too can be incidental findings or can present in a variety of ways: as an asymptomatic abdominal mass, as acute hemoperitoneum with shock, as intestinal or gastric obstruction, or in infants (rarely in adults) as thrombocytopenia secondary to platelet trapping. Hepatic angiography is helpful diagnostically, characteristic features being pooling of contrast material and a persistent 'tumor stain' throughout the capillary and venous phases of the angiogram, and Barnett et al. [43] have recently reported that computed tomography, which shows delayed contrast enhancement of the lesion, may be helpful in warning against biopsy. The preferred treatment is resection when feasible [44, 45], although extensive or inaccessible lesions have sometimes responded to radiotherapy. In infants and children in whom cardiac failure may develop secondary to multiple arteriovenous fistulas, corticosteroids have proved effective on occasion.

A rarer benign lesion, of some interest surgically, is *bile duct adenoma*. Usually less than 0.5 cm in diameter and grayish-white in color, these asymptomatic tumors typically are solitary, firm, and sub-

209

capsular in location. Their importance stems chiefly from the ease with which they may be confused at operation with metastatic carcinoma, with possible adverse influence on the choice of operation for the primary malignancy [46]. Frozen section usually clarifies the issue, but in confusing cases, where active bile duct proliferation is seen microscopically, an appreciation of the gross characteristics of bile duct adenoma – principally the small size and subcapsular location – aids in the correct diagnosis.

The association between tumors of the liver in women and the use of oral contraceptives was first reported by Baum et al. in 1973 [47] in a series of seven cases, all with benign tumors. Since then, several hundred additional cases have been reported from various centers, with documentation of both brief and prolonged use of oral contraceptives; over half the patients reported using birth control pills for more than five years, while 10% used them for only 6–12 months [43]. An early report suggested that oral contraceptives containing mestranol had greater oncogenic potential than those containing ethinyl estradiol [49] but valid statistical evaluation is made difficult by the shorter span of use of the later compounds. Of the tumors encountered, over 90% have been benign, with the rest malignant. Despite confusion in the literature about the nomenclature of these tumors, benign tumors of the liver, with few exceptions, appear to be of two types, *hepatic cell adenoma* and *focal nodular hyperplasia*; malignant tumors include *hepatocellular carcinoma*, *hepatoblastoma*, and *mixed hepatocellular carcinoma*.

Despite intensive, ongoing research, the etiologic role of oral contraceptives in the formation of these tumors remains to be elucidated. Certainly, the incidence of liver tumors in women taking oral contraceptives is very small indeed, Vessey et al. [50] having concluded, after scrutinizing several large data bases in the United Kingdom, that 'benign tumors of the liver are extremely rare in both users and non-users of oral contraceptives.' On the other hand, two recent studies – one tabulating published case reports of contraceptive-related hepatic tumors over a three-year period and numerically comparing them with the total number of published reports of similar tumors in non-pill-users between 1937 and 1976 [48], and the other surveying by questionnaire 477 hospitals in the United States to determine the

incidence of oral contraceptive use in patients undergoing resection of benign hepatic tumors [51] – strongly support the impression that tumors of the liver have increased in frequency in recent years in women taking birth control pills. Additionally, Klatskin, in his detailed review [48], notes that: (1) benign hepatic tumors are known to regress completely following cessation of contraceptive therapy, although, oppositely, they can also persist or become manifest years after stopping therapy, cases having been discovered as late as ten years after stopping the pill; (2) benign tumors of the liver have recurred following resection in women who have continued to use birth control pills; (3) in women who do not develop liver tumors, oral contraceptives can promote hepatomegaly and periportal and midzonal congestion; (4) benign hepatic tumors in women on oral contraceptives tend to bleed intraperitoneally and intramurally more often than similar tumors in non-pill-users. These clinical findings, which represent rather tenuous circumstantial evidence, by no means establish a causal relationship between the use of oral contraceptives and the development of hepatic tumors, but they do tentatively hint at a promoting, if not initiating, role for oral contraceptives in the production of liver tumors, with, possibly, hormone-induced vascular changes in the liver participating in some important way. Also, it should be remembered that focal nodular hyperplasia and hepatic cell adenoma have been found in children and in elderly female patients, as well as in male patients in approximately 10% of cases, although hepatic cell adenoma, it should be added, is extremely rare in the adult male [37]. On the ultrastructural level, long-term use of oral contraceptives induces only nonspecific changes in the hepatocyte, specifically, the appearance of paracrystalline inclusions in the hepatocyte mitochondria [50].

The evidence for possible malignant transformation of benign hepatic tumors is even more meager. Davis et al. [53] describe a benign hepatic tumor in a woman taking oral contraceptives in which there was unmistakable evidence of carcinoma within the tumor, and Klatskin ([48], personal communication from Bagenstoss) calls attention to two cases seen at the Mayo Clinic with unequivocal areas of hepatocellular carcinoma within a hepatic cell adenoma in women on birth control pills, further mentioning that no examples suggesting malignant transformation have been found in nonusers of oral contraceptives.

Pathologically, focal nodular hyperplasia and hepatic cell adenoma display contrasting features, with rare instances of overlap [37, 54, 55]. Focal nodular hyperplasia typically occurs as a firm, grossly nodular mass, usually less than 5 cm in diameter, which may vary in color from dark red-brown to tan. The tumor is often evident on the surface of the liver, sometimes as a pedunculated mass, and approximately 20% are double or multiple. Prominent surface vessels are commonly seen. Microscopically, the distinguishing characteristic of focal nodular hyperplasia is fibrous septation, often emanating from a prominent central scar, with criss-crossing fibrous bands creating a pattern resembling macronodular cirrhosis; foci of proliferating bile ducts, blood vessels (often thick-walled), and lymphocytes are seen within the fibrous septae.

Hepatic cell adenomas, on the other hand, are often soft and bulky, frequently in excess of 10 cm in diameter, with variations in color from white to orange-yellow to light brown. Surface vessels are often prominent, and approximately 30% are double or multiple. As with focal nodular hyperplasia, pedunculation is sometimes seen, occurring in approximately 10% of cases. The histologic picture in hepatic cell adenoma (Fig. 1) is one of monotonous sheets of mature hepatocytes arranged in abnormally thick cords, with areas of hemorrhagic necrosis a common feature; the stellate fibrosis and bile duct proliferation seen in focal nodular hyperplasia are conspicuously absent in hepatic cell adenoma, and, in most cases, the only nonhepatocyte elements seen traversing the substance of the tumor are scattered, thin-walled vessels. In a few reported cases, features of both focal nodular hyperplasia and hepatic cell adenoma have been present in the same tumor, making classifi-

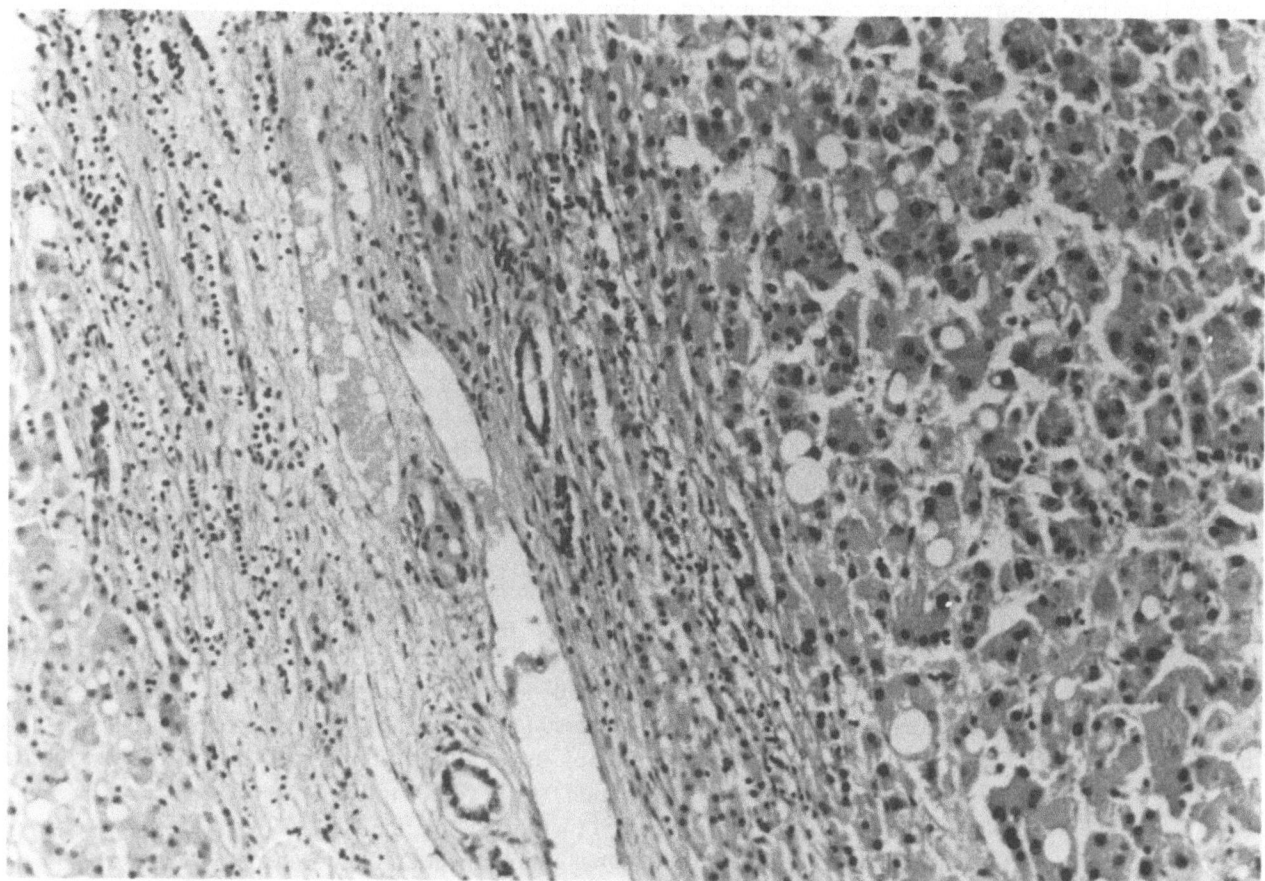

Figure 1. Hepatic cell adenoma. At the right, section shows a monotonous pattern of mature hepatocytes arranged in abnormally thick cords, bordered, in the center, by a fibrous capsule. At the left, vacuolated normal hepatocytes can be seen; × 354. Courtesy of Dr. J. Patrick, Medical College of Ohio.

cation difficult and raising suspicions about the relatedness of these tumors. Indeed, Klatskin [48] has suggested that the stimulus to tumor growth may affect entodermal and mesenchymal elements in the liver to a variable degree in different tumors, although Foster and Berman [37] favor the view that focal nodular hyperplasia, for whatever reason, is largely a regenerative process, in contrast to hepatic cell adenoma, which they regard as a true neoplasm.

With respect to hepatocellular carcinoma, the pathologic features of this lesion are reviewed later in this chapter and are similar in pill users and non-pill-users, with the exception that hypervascularity is more prominent in the former group of patients [56].

Clinically, prior to operation, there is no good way to differentiate focal nodular hyperplasia from hepatic cell adenoma. Statistically, hepatic cell adenoma is far more likely to present as acute abdominal pain with shock, and focal nodular hyperplasia much more often presents as an asymptomatic finding picked up unexpectedly on liver scan or at laparotomy for another condition. But in the individual patient, either lesion can present in either of these two ways, or, alternatively, it can present as a palpable mass in the upper abdomen or as a vague, gnawing pain in the epigastrium or right upper quadrant. Liver function tests and alpha-fetoprotein determinations are usually unremarkable, and radioisotope scans of the liver are unreliable in these cases, false-negative scans being particularly common in focal nodular hyperplasia [37, 54, 55]. Indeed, tumors less than four centimeters in diameter uniformly escape detection by radioisotope scans of the liver [48]. However, a high sensitivity and specificity has been reported for computed tomography in the diagnosis of hepatic neoplasms [57], and the combination of scintography and computed tomography appears to be an accurate, albeit expensive, screening plan. The most important diagnostic study, when time allows, is arteriography, which fairly reliably identifies single or multiple lesions and helps evaluate resectability; focal nodular hyperplasia frequently displays more prominent vascular changes than hepatic cell adenoma, characteristically showing prominent enlargement of the hepatic artery, hypervascularity of the tumor, displacement of vessels, and a distinct

tumor 'blush' on the venous phase, but the arteriographic differences between the two tumors are not consistent enough to be of differential value. Finally, it should be pointed out that percutaneous needle biopsy of the liver is considered hazardous in view of the vascularity of these tumors.

The treatment of hepatic cell adenoma and focal nodular hyperplasia varies according to the mode of presentation. In an emergency situation in which blood loss is severe, confirmatory studies such as arteriography are usually omitted, and the surgeon proceeds with laparotomy simply on the basis of abdominal findings and peritoneal tap. Indeed, if the bleeding is intrahepatic rather than intraperitoneal, the diagnosis is often obscure; in either case, unless there is a high index of suspicion, it is not uncommon for a hepatic origin of the bleeding to be completely overlooked in the preoperative diagnosis [58]. At operation, after the situation has been quickly assessed and the site of bleeding identified, it is well in most instances to do as little as possible to stop the bleeding, in view of the documented high risk of extensive hepatic resection in an emergency setting. Initially, manual compression of adjacent normal liver tissue and packing of the bleeding site are tried, while the anesthesiologist attempts to catch up with blood loss; if this fails to control the bleeding, the Pringle maneuver, as described in section 2 on 'Trauma to the liver,' is carried out. After the situation has stabilized, local resection of the tumor by using methods described later may be carried out, depending upon the condition of the patient, blood bank resources, and the experience of the operator. Alternatively, if local resection is not feasible for whatever reason, careful biopsy of the tumor is done together with ligation of the appropriate hepatic artery. Definitive treatment is then carried out at a later date.

If, on the other hand, the bleeding episode at the time of presentation is not severe, preliminary angiography is often helpful. Indeed, there is currently some interest in radiologic embolization of the right or left hepatic artery as a technique for controlling modest hemorrhage [59], but data relating to this approach are scant.

In the situation where an asymptomatic liver tumor is encountered at laparotomy for another condition, excisional biopsy should be done in the case of a small, accessible mass and generous wedge

212

biopsy in the case of a large, firm, accessible mass. If the mass is inaccessible or soft, needle biopsies may be tried, with definitive treatment planned for a later time.

In the situation where there has been time for a deliberate preoperative workup in a woman taking birth control pills, there is lingering controversy as to the correct therapeutic approach. Edmondson et al. [60], on the basis of three cases in which regression of hepatic cell adenoma was observed after cessation of oral contraceptive therapy, recommend percutaneous needle biopsy of the mass and interdiction of birth control pills as the preferred way to manage these patients, and there is some agreement that this approach is justified in the high-risk patient [61]. However, the potential problems associated with percutaneous needle biopsy in these patients – i.e., the risk of major bleeding from the tumor, the frequent inadequacy of the biopsy specimen, and the possibility of malignant seeding – as well as the substantial risks of *not* doing a biopsy – i.e., the demonstrated tendency of hepatic cell adenoma to bleed spontaneously with an associated 6% mortality [48], and the possibility of a fatal delay in treating a malignant primary tumor [56] – make the expectant approach in the good-risk patient unattractive to many clinicians. Instead, there is more appeal in doing a carefully planned laparotomy with open liver biopsy and possible hepatic resection: the risk is modest, the information more certain, and the treatment in most cases more definitive. If at laparotomy a small, peripheral tumor is identified, excisional biopsy is done; if the tumor is large or less accessible, a generous wedge biopsy with frozen section is carried out. If the frozen section report comes back focal nodular hyperplasia, the decision whether or not to proceed with resection is based upon the case of resectability. If microscopic examination is inconclusive or reveals hepatic cell adenoma or primary carcinoma, local resection with a margin of normal tissue is recommended [37], although others [38, 39, 62] are inclined, when the tumor is resectable, to carry out formal lobectomy or trisegmentectomy. If multiple benign tumors are encountered, the largest or most threatening is resected, possibly by formal hepatic resection or trisegmentectomy if other benign lesions are present in the same lobe, and tumors of the opposite lobe, if

present, are followed postoperatively by sequential scans of the liver.

Primary cancer of the liver in the adult consists of three main epithelial types – *hepatocellular carcinoma, cholangiocellular carcinoma,* and *mixed hepatocellular cholangiocellular carcinoma* – and very rare *cystadenocarcinomas, angiosarcomas,* and *embryonal sarcomas.* Hepatic malignancies of infancy and childhood include *hepatoblastomas,* which are embryonal tumors of epithelial or 'mixed' character occurring in children under the age of five, adult-type *hepatocellular carcinomas,* and *embryonal or rhabdomyoblastic sarcomas.* Much has been written about the epidemiology and peculiar geographic distribution of adult hepatic malignancies, and there is now impressive evidence that (1) liver cell carcinoma has an intimate association with hepatitis B virus infection and exposure to aflatoxin (commonly found as a contaminant of foodstuffs in sub-Saharan Africa and Southeast Asia); (2) bile duct carcinoma is associated in the Orient with liver fluke infestation of the bile ducts (*Clonorchis sinesis, Opisthorchis felineus, Opisthorchis viverrini*), and in Western countries with gallstones, congenital biliary cysts, chronic biliary diseases such as primary sclerosing cholangitis, and the carrying of typhoid; and (3) angiosarcoma of the liver is associated in developed areas of the world with distant exposure to Thorotrast, vinyl chloride, and arsenicals (see review by Lefkowitch [172]). Strikingly, the most consistent finding, common to almost all areas where primary liver cancer is found, is the frequent association with nutritional and posthepatitic cirrhosis. One notable exception is Norway, where only 7% of cases of primary liver cancer (including pediatric cases) had preexisting cirrhosis [63], but in most areas of the West, including Hawaii [64], which demographically represents an interface between the East and West, the incidence of associated cirrhosis varies from approximately 50% to 85% (see literature survey by Foster and Berman [37]). The same high incidence of cirrhosis in patients with primary liver cancer is seen in other parts of the world, especially in populations with a high incidence of liver cancer, such as native tribesmen in Uganda, the Japanese in Indonesia, and the Chinese and Malaysians in the Malaysian Peninsula. Overall in the Western world approximately 4% of patients with cirrhosis

213

eventually develop primary carcinoma of the liver. The etiologic role of cirrhosis is poorly understood, but it is tempting to speculate that the sustained regenerative response of liver cells in the cirrhotic patient, involving possibly some degree of de-differentiation of normally nondividing hepatic cells, engenders a state of vulnerability in these cells that, with continuing cycles of injury and exposure to oncogenic stimuli, eventually leads to unrestrained growth.

Hepatocellular carcinomas are typically soft and bulky, with a dull gray to tan-yellow coloration and marked vascularity. Patterns of liver involvement are described as massive, nodular, or diffuse. Areas of necrosis, sometimes with disruption of the Glisson capsule and attendant intraperitoneal hemorrhage, are commonly seen, and there may be conspicuous invasion of adjacent structures such as the diaphragm, hepatic veins, or portal vein. Regional lymph node metastases are unusual at the time of presentation, but blood-borne pulmonary

metastases are common and can occur relatively early. Microscopically, hepatocellular carcinoma exhibits a variety of structural patterns and cellular features (Fig. 2), ranging from a common trabecular pattern with thick cords of well-differentiated cells resembling normal hepatocytes, to less common types described as adenoid, giant cell, anaplastic, and pseudoepitheliomatous.

Cholangiocellular carcinomas tend to be firmer, less vascular, and more nodular in configuration than hepatocellular carcinomas, but gross patterns of liver involvement are similar. Gray-white coloration is typical, and an umbilicated external contour, resulting from invasion of the Glisson capsule, may be evident. Features such as necrosis, venous invasion, and early distant metastasis are uncommon, but spread to regional lymph nodes is a frequent finding at operation. Microscopically, the characteristic appearance of these tumors (Fig. 3) is one of disorganized acinar or ductular structures within a dense, fibrous stroma. In chol-

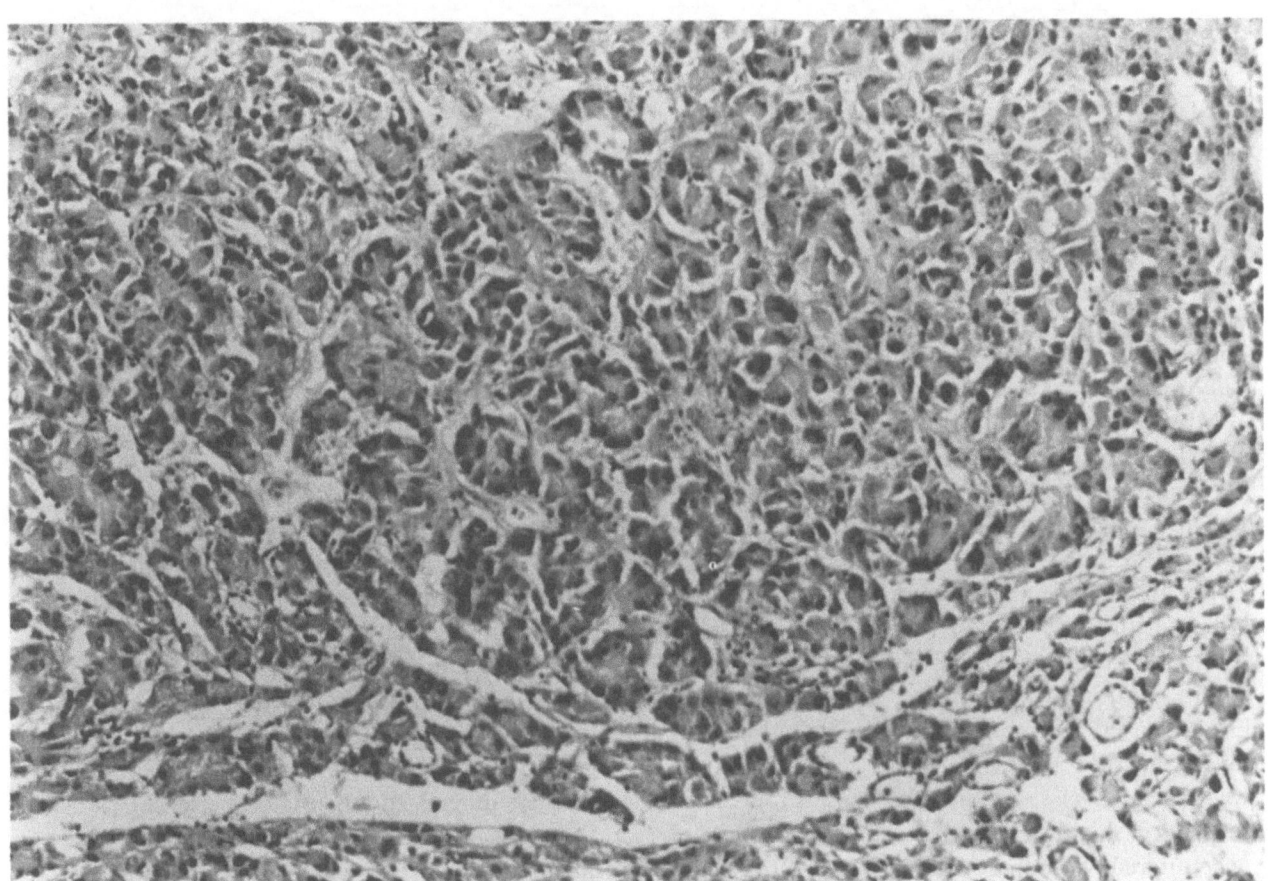

Figure 2. Hepatocellular carcinoma. Section shows thick cords of well-differentiated cells resembling normal hepatocytes; × 354. Courtesy of Dr. J. Patrick, Medical College of Ohio.

214

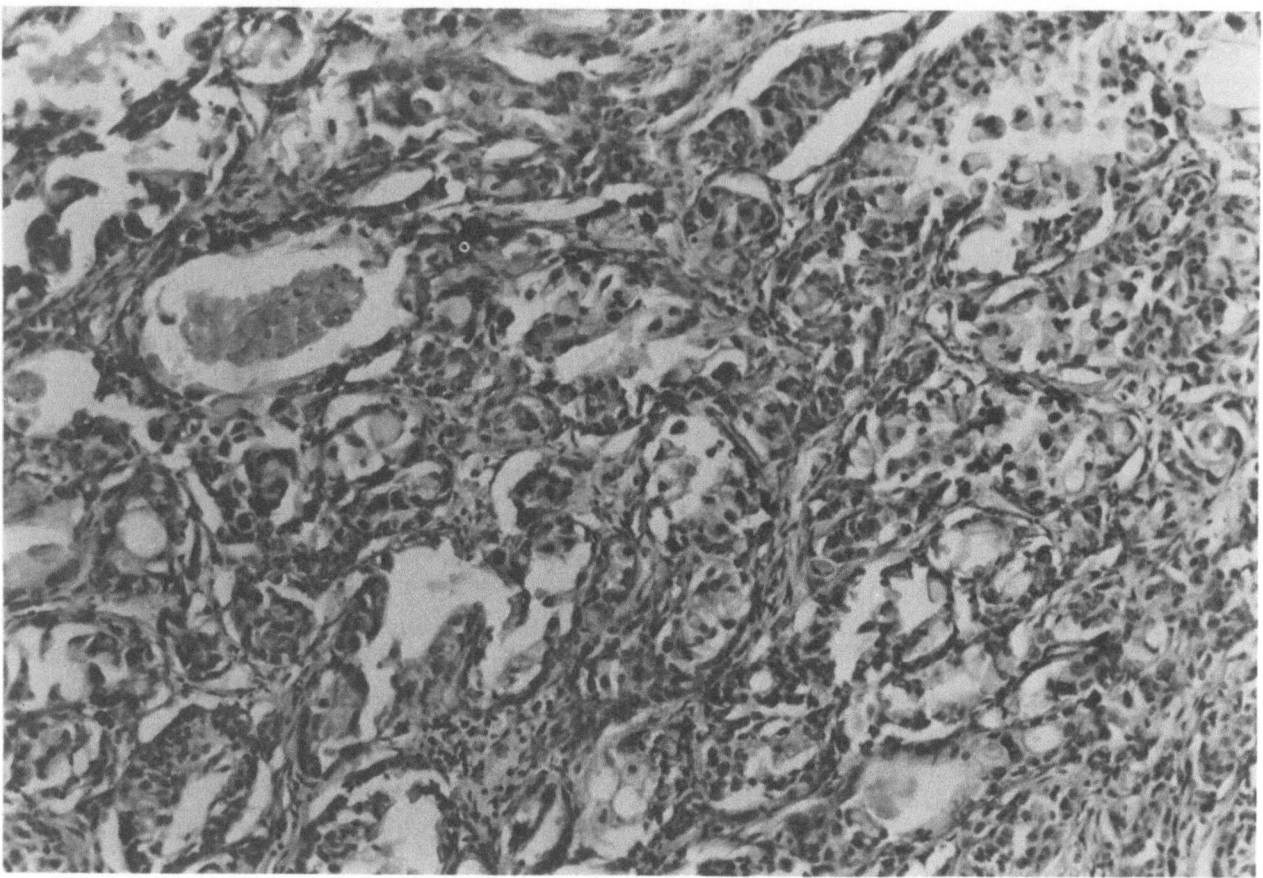

Figure 3. Cholangiocellular carcinoma. Section shows disorganized acinar and ductular structures within a fibrous stroma; × 354. Courtesy of Dr. J. Patrick, Medical College of Ohio.

angiocellular carcinomas associated with the ingestion of Thorotrast, atypical proliferation of bile ducts and diffuse portal scarring are characteristically seen.

Mixed hepatocellular cholangiocellular carcinomas grossly and microscopically combine in varying proportions features of both types of epithelial tumors, without creating a distinct appearance.

The main signs and symptoms of primary liver cancer at the time of presentation are the presence of a mass, pain, weight loss, epigastric distress, signs of intraperitoneal hemorrhage, and hepatomegaly [37]. A variety of other nonspecific findings such as fever, diarrhea, anorexia, nausea and vomiting, weakness, malaise, itching, and jaundice are also seen. Occasionally, paraneoplastic syndromes are encountered with these tumors – erythrocytosis, hypercalcemia, hypoglycemia, hyperlipidemia, dysfibrinogenemia, and virilizing and feminizing ef-

fects being mentioned in the review by Margolis and Homcy [65]. Indeed, they consider erythrocytosis in a patient with cirrhosis to be a reliable indicator of neoplastic transformation. Weight loss, wasting, ascites, jaundice, splenomegaly, and palpable lymphadenopathy signify a preterminal state [37], and gastrointestinal bleeding as a presenting complaint also bodes poorly for the patient [64]. In contrast, the isolated finding on physical examination of a palpable abdominal mass or hepatomegaly offers some hope of cure. Although early detection understandably is regarded as the 'conditio sine qua non' of curability, it is discouraging that Malt et al. [66] reported no improvement in survival in patients diagnosed early in their clinical course compared with others diagnosed much later, perhaps because of the multifocal origin of the disease or early intrahepatic or distant spread. Tumor multicentricity is indeed the rule in the presence of underlying cirrhosis, and Tompkins et al. [67] have called attention to the frequent bilobar involvement in cholangiocellular carcinoma, urging that chole-dochoscopy be done prior to embarking upon a major curative resection in these patients.

The most important diagnostic tests for evaluating patients with suspected primary liver cancer are radioisotope scanning, angiography, ultrasonography, and computed tomography. Radioisotope scanning remains the preferred method of screening for liver tumors [68], but computed tomography, although recognized to have limitations in detecting isodense tumors, has a high sensitivity and has detected tumors as small as 1.5–2.0 cm in diameter when contrast enhancement techniques are used [69, 70]. However, the computed-tomographic appearance of hepatocellular carcinoma is nonspecific and cannot be distinguished from that of hepatic abscesses, hepatic metastases, or involvement by malignant lymphoma [71]. In assessing resectability, Kim et al. [72], using arteriography in combination with technetium-99 m colloid scans of the liver, noted an error rate of 20%–30% and concluded that laparotomy was the only reliable way to make this determination. However, portal venography and inferior vena cavography in association with hepatic arteriography have recently been advocated as a means of detecting involvement of hilar vessels and the inferior vena cava [73], there being no false-positive and no false-negative results in a series of 25 patients; accordingly, when either or both of these findings is present, resection is deemed unfeasible. Liver function tests, such as serum alkaline phosphatase, glutamic oxalacetic transaminase, glutamic pyruvic transaminase, lactic dehydrogenase, and Bromsulphalein retention, are not as a rule meaningfully abnormal in patients with potentially curable liver tumors, but serum albumin and serum bilirubin determinations, together with other clinical factors, are known to be valuable in assessing the severity of cirrhosis. Evaluation of coagulation factors should be done, and, as emphasized in a later section, preoperative nutritional assessment is important in the patient in whom major hepatic resection is planned. Serum alpha-fetoprotein determinations, although positive in approximately 30% of patients with hepatocellular carcinoma, are negative in patients with cholangiocellular carcinoma. Determination of hepatitis-associated antigen is of questionable diagnostic value [37], but epidemiologically it may be a useful thing to do inasmuch as Blumberg et al. [74] have proposed a causal relation between hepatitis B virus, cirrhosis, and liver cancer. Needle biopsy of the liver is generally ill-advised, Linder et al. [75] having reported three cases of fatal hemorrhage among 27 patients with liver cancer subjected to percutaneous needle biopsy. Fortner [76] emphatically states that needle biopsy in these cases is 'unnecessary, unreliable, and unsafe.'

The treatment of primary liver cancer in appropriate cases is resection. Mention has been made of various physical and angiographic findings that weigh against an aggressive surgical approach, and there is general agreement that the presence of cirrhosis warrants operative restraint for at least three reasons: (1) the poor regeneration of the remaining liver and the poor tolerance for major hepatic resection, leading to a high incidence of postoperative liver failure, (2) the multicentricity of hepatocellular carcinoma in cirrhosis, and (3) the very early invasion of the vascular system in cirrhosis. Overall, the rate of resectability of primary liver cancer in the Western world, on the basis of reported series, is approximately 20% [37].

The long-term results of hepatic resection in adult patients operated upon for cure of primary malignancies is moderately favorable for noncirrhotic patients but dismal for cirrhotic patients, the 1974 Liver Tumor Survey revealing a 35% five-year survival rate for the former group of patients and no surviors beyond *three* years for the latter group. Surprisingly, the size of the tumor in resected cases appeared to have no relation to the outcome, and patients with multiple tumor nodules encompassed by dissection fared as well over a five-year period as did those with clinically solitary nodules.

In pediatric patients, in whom the operative mortality rate for major hepatic resection is approximately 20% [37], the long-term survival, in the absence of multicentricity and lymph node involvement, is substantially better than in adults undergoing hepatic resection for primary hepatic malignancies. Calculated five-year survivals in pediatric patients, derived from documented three-year 'cures', are 65% for hepatoblastoma and 51% overall, excluding operative deaths [37]. Adjuvant chemotherapy in these patients appears promising, and in unresectable cases the use of combined radiotherapy and chemotherapy may allow subsequent 'curative' resection.

4. METASTATIC TUMORS OF THE LIVER

What to do about hepatic metastasis is a complex matter involving the physical and mental state of the patient, the philosophical and biological perspective of the responsible physician or surgeon, and the oncologic capabilities of the institution where care is rendered.

In contrast to the 1950s when there was some confidence about the correctness of an aggressive surgical approach in most malignancies, with radical operations generally being 'de rigueur' in potentially curative situations, in recent years the results of long-term follow-up studies on a variety of surgically treated cancer patients, and a growing clinical impression that many malignancies represent systemic, or at least multifocal disease, have tended to deprecate the notion that cancer can be encompassed, and therefore cured, by timely and thoughtful dissection. In its place, although poorly understood by many clinicians, the concept of 'tumor immunology' has increasingly been looked upon as the Rosetta Stone for understanding and ultimately controlling tumor behavior in humans [77, 78], despite clear warnings [79] that conspicuous differences exist between the animal models on which this concept is based and the human patient afflicted by an aggressive tumor; Bray [79] further points out that the *in vitro* tests for detecting tumor immunogenicity in cancer patients, on which so much of the evidence rests in support of the notion of 'immune surveillance' [80] of human tumors, are often technically difficult to do, unstandardized, imprecise, and hard to interpret. Additionally, various clinical trials of immunotherapy for presumed 'immunogenic' tumors such as melanoma, with or without hepatic metastasis, have so far been largely disappointing [81].

With respect to metastatic tumors to the liver from whatever source, there is the further realization that these implants represent the growth of blood-borne tumor emboli and that, very likely, widespread dissemination of tumor has occurred by the time hepatic metastasis is detected. Indeed, metastatic tumors to the liver from the pancreas, breast, lung, stomach, kidney, reproductive organs, and skin (melanoma) are so consistently associated with metastatic seeding elsewhere that even when seemingly adequate resection of solitary or unilobar liver implants is carried out either synchronously or metachronously (i.e., after a period of observation) in relation to curative resection of the primary lesion, patient survival of five years or longer is exceedingly rare [37].

Nevertheless, despite constraints on the aggressive use of hepatic resection in the treatment of metastatic tumors of the liver, selective employment of this approach appears warranted in two situations: (a) in patients with clinically solitary or unilobar hepatic tumors secondary to carcinoma of the colon and rectum [37, 41, 82, 83], and (b) in patients with resectable hepatic metastases from Wilms tumor. The latter group of patients are usually given vigorous combinations of chemotherapy and radiotherapy in addition to operative treatment (which sometimes includes pulmonary resection for metastatic nodules), and the five-year survival rate in these young patients approaches 50% [83]. The former group of patients – those with primary carcinoma of the colon and rectum – are found to have clinically solitary or unilobar hepatic metastases in approximately 5% of cases, and when these and the primary tumor are resected, five-year survival rates of 30% are seen in cases with solitary hepatic nodules and 13% in cases with unilobar lesions [37]. If the liver implants are less than 5 cm in diameter, survival rates are further improved. Contrary to Pack's vanguard views [84], synchronous resection, it now appears, yields five-year survival rates comparable to those seen following metachronous resection, and hepatic lobectomy offers no better chance of cure than does wedge resection, provided an adequate margin of normal tissue is obtained. Case selection requires that: (1) the patient be noncirrhotic and in reasonably good condition; (2) there be no demonstrable metastatic tumors elsewhere; (3) the hepatic tumor be amenable, in terms of size and location, to resection; and (4) the surgeon possess the requisite level of technical skill.

The difference in survival rates between patients undergoing hepatic resection for liver tumors secondary to carcinoma of the colon and rectum and those undergoing the same operation for liver tumors secondary to other types of cancer is attributable, it would appear, to well-appreciated pathologic and anatomic features of colorectal carcinoma. It has been known for some time that long-term survival following curative resection for carcinoma of the colon and rectum correlates strongly with microscopic demonstration of intravascular invasion within the primary tumor [85, 86], and Dukes and Bussey [87, 88], in refining the concept of venous embolization in colorectal carcinoma, were led after detailed pathologic study to regard the primary growth as the main source of tumor emboli, rather than lymphatic metastases, from which venous emboli can also occur. There is thus ample data supporting the notion that liver implants in carcinoma of the colon and rectum arrive there via the portal circulation, with the primary tumor being the main source of migratory tumor cells. Accordingly, a tumor-trapping phenomenon within the liver is readily envisioned since the portal blood flow feeds directly and exclusively into this organ, except when portal hypertension is present; other tumors do not have this unique arrangement. That this trapping mechanism is efficient to a degree that makes hepatic resection for liver metastasis reasonable in selected patients is affirmed by the painstaking necropsy studies of Willis [89], which show that in patients with fatal cancer of the colon in whom liver metastasis is found, the liver is the sole site of demonstrable metastasis in 30% of cases.

Certainly, if no treatment is provided, the outlook is bleak. Jaffe et al. [90] in a classic study of 177 patients with metastasis to the liver from colon carcinoma found an overall median survival time of five months from the time of diagnosis of metastasis; when metastasis in the liver appeared subsequent to curative resection, the median survival time was nine and a half months from the time of diagnosis of metastasis; when resection was palliative, the median survival time was six months; when palliative diversion was done, the median survival time was three and a half months; when only laparotomy was done, the median survival time was five weeks.

Attempts to prolong survival in patients with hepatic metastasis, using systemic chemotherapy and/or radiotherapy, have done little to improve the outlook. The liver, after modest doses of external beam radiation, is subject to radiation hepatitis, the hepatic venules being particularly susceptible to injury, and the kidneys may also be damaged in the course of liver irradiation. With respect to systemic chemotherapy, a great variety of agents and protocols have been tried over the past two decades, with response rates of only 10%–14% and survival times of 7–9 months [91]. At present it appears that a program of single-agent 5-fluorouracil is as effective as combination therapy using some of the newer agents.

Because of the liver's unique ability to detoxify excess quantities of cancerostatic drugs, and since delivery of these agents via the hepatic artery or portal vein tends to reduce the systemic effects of large doses, there has been considerable interest in recent years in infusion chemotherapy as a means of treating hepatic metastases. In most reports, including the important study by Watkins et al. [92], the hepatic artery, cannulated via the gastroduodenal artery at the time of laparotomy [93] or percutaneously via the femoral or brachial artery by using the Seldinger technique, is used for delivery of the desired cytotoxic agent, most commonly 5-fluorouracil or floxuridine. Remission criteria [94], four of which must be present, include: (1) reduction of tumor size by at least 50% at repeat laparotomy, (2) reduction of tumor size by at least 50% at hepatic angiography, (3) reduction of liver size by 50% at palpation, (4) reduction of liver enlargement by 50% at scintiscanning of the liver, (5) reduction of liver enzyme, CEA, and alpha-fetoprotein levels, and (6) symptomatic improvement. Using these strict criteria, Sundqvist et al. [94] in a recent retrospective study of 46 patients who received infusion chemotherapy with 5-fluorouracil (500 mg per day for an average of six weeks) achieved remission rates of 43% with overall median survival from onset of treatment of six months; the quality of life, they felt, was improved in 63% of the patients studied. Cady and Oberfield's study [95], which adopted less strict criteria, showed a clinical response rate of 71% in 55 consecutive patients who received regional infusion chemotherapy with 5-fluoro-2′ deoxyuridine (5-FUDR) (20 mg per day for interrupted periods over 6–9 months), with a median survival time of 16 months in responders and five months in nonresponders. Somewhat counter to this experience, a recent report from the

218

Central Oncology Group in the United States of a prospective randomized study of hepatic artery infusion with 5-fluorouracil versus intravenous 5-fluorouracil in 61 acceptable patients with hepatic metastasis from colorectal carcinoma failed to show a significant difference in the response rate, time to progression, duration of the response, and survival rate [96]. Other methods of treatment, recently reported, include: (a) combined hepatic artery infusion chemotherapy, radiotherapy, and systemic chemotherapy [97]; (b) combined hepatic artery ligation, hepatic artery infusion chemotherapy, and portal vein infusion chemotherapy [98]; (c) hepatic artery infusion of *Corynebacterium parvum* and chemotherapy [99]; and (d) adjuvant cytotoxic liver perfusion for colorectal carcinoma [100, 101].

Unfortunately, regional infusion chemotherapy for liver metastasis, by whatever means, involves significant morbidity and some mortality. Ansfield et al. [102] reported a total of 109 complications in 419 patients receiving hepatic artery infusion chemotherapy and listed as complications, in descending order of occurrence: catheter displacement, catheter cracking or leaking, infection at the site of percutaneous catheter entry, upper gastrointestinal bleeding, infected mycotic aneurysms or peripheral septic embolization, catheter clotting, hepatic artery occlusion, and nonfatal stroke. Death from sepsis has occurred [94], and at the University of Iowa Hospitals two of six patients who developed pyogenic liver abscesses following hepatic artery infusion chemotherapy died prematurely [103].

In summary, except for the 5% of patients with hepatic metastasis from colorectal carcinoma who are candidates for hepatic resection (13%–30% of whom will live five years or longer following curative resection of the primary and hepatic tumors), the overall results of treatment for metastatic liver disease remain discouraging. Hopefully, with increased use of serial carcinoembryonic antigen (CEA) determinations following curative resection of colorectal carcinoma [104, 105] – a simple and inexpensive method of detecting local or distant (particularly hepatic) metastasis [106] – hepatic spread will be identified sooner so that chemotherapy, commenced earlier with better agents or more effective combinations of agents, can offer improved results. Too, the early detection of solitary or unilobar hepatic metastases from carcinoma of the colon and rectum should marginally improve the long-term results of hepatic resection for metastatic disease.

5. HEPATIC RESECTION

The various techniques of major hepatic resection are described in detail in several recent accounts [37, 41, 108–110, 173]. The account by Foster is particularly rich in detail and contains pithy advice for the operating surgeon on a number of problematic technical points. It hardly needs mentioning that the institution where elective major hepatic resection is performed should have adequate support facilities, including a well-supplied blood bank, refined respiratory support facilities, a well-staffed Intensive Care Unit with advanced monitoring capabilities, and, in terms of attending and house staff support, depth in anesthesia, surgery, and internal medicine. It bears emphasis that although the surgeon who undertakes to perform major hepatic resection assumes the main responsibility for the outcome, *teamwork* involving the coordinated efforts of a variety of medical and paramedical personnel is clearly crucial to the success of these operations, and, in general, where the overall experience of the team is greatest, the results are best [37]. The surgeon who performs the operation should be well trained in thoracic as well as abdominal surgery, not only because of the usefulness of thoracoabdominal incisions in many cases, but because an inadvertent tear of the retrohepatic inferior vena cava requires a transpericardial approach to the retrohepatic inferior vena cava to gain superior (distal) control of the bleeding in this very difficult situation.

Because there are no avascular planes in the liver along which one can easily dissect, an inviolable requirement for the performance of these operations is a detailed knowledge of the anatomy of the liver, particularly of the complexities of the hepatic vasculature and of the frequent anomalies of these vessels [25, 107]. The hepatic veins, it should be noted, run independently of the portal triads and intersect them at right angles, and the minimizing of blood loss, which technically is the main strategy of hepatic resection, requires the avoidance of these veins, whether or not lobar inflow occlusion has been obtained [170]. In this connection, it is important to remember that: (a) drainage of the middle hepatic vein is bilobar, with major tributaries coming from the medial segment of the left lobe and from the anterior segment of the right lobe; (b) the right and left hepatic veins at their junction with the inferior vena cava are partially encased by liver substance, making extrahepatic ligation of these veins extremely hazardous; (c) the umbilical fissure of the left lobe, seemingly the natural place to carry out left lateral segmentectomy, directly overlies major triadal structures in the anterior portion of the intersegmental plane and a lengthy segment of the left hepatic vein in the posterior portion of the plane. Further difficulties with anatomy are generated by the vascular distortions caused by bulky tumors, so that interlobar 'planes' are often angulated and contoured, rather than flat, as depicted in anatomy textbooks. Accordingly, preoperative hepatic angiography, which to some extent reveals these distortions and anomalies, should be done, with care taken to avoid intimal disruption of the common hepatic artery.

Positioning of the patient and the choice of incision depend upon the type of resection to be performed. Right lobectomy, extended right lobectomy, and right trisegmentectomy (maximally extended right lobectomy) require thoracoabdominal incisions in adults and right subcostal or bilateral subcostal incisions in infants and children. Wedge resection, left lobectomy, left lateral segmentectomy, and central or 'middle' hepatectomy are usually done through an abdominal incision – either a right subcostal incision extended from the right iliac crest to the left subcostal margin or a bilateral subcostal or 'dome' incision. Preliminarily, assessment of resectability is usually carried out through a right subcostal incision large enough to freely admit two hands; after systematic exploration of the entire peritoneal cavity, thorough exploration of the retroperitoneum and posterior regions of the liver at the hilum and diaphragm is done, followed by bimanual palpation of the right and left lobes. Resection in cases of primary hepatic malignancy is precluded by: (1) evidence of disease outside the liver, (2) involvement of the inferior vena cava, (3) intraluminal or adventitial involvement of the portal vein at the level of its

bifurcation, (4) certain patterns of bilobar involvement, and (5) the presence of diffuse cirrhosis. In the event that the tumor is resectable, the incision is extended appropriately, thoracic entry being gained through the seventh or eighth intercostal space, and the avascular attachments of the right or left lobe, but *not* both (to avoid displacement and angulation of the remaining lobe or segment), are cut. Hilar ligation of the right or left hepatic duct, artery, and portal vein are then carried out, except in wedge resections when this step is omitted. (Some operators prefer median sternotomy for thoracic entry, as we do in some trauma cases involving the liver, or, alternatively, an entirely abdominal approach [38]. However, in the more deliberate setting of, say, elective right hepatic lobectomy, a right thoracoabdominal incision seems to provide better exposure of the posterior aspect of the liver, the inferior vena cava, and the hepatic vein/inferior vena cava junction; the right lung can also be thoroughly evaluated for evidence of metastasis.) Again, anomalies must be kept in mind, and if there is any question about bile duct anatomy, an 8-10 F soft rubber catheter or filiform catheter should be inserted into the common hepatic duct and directed superiorly into the right or left hepatic ducts, after very limited dissection of the common hepatic duct. If the lesion calls for right lobectomy or trisegmentectomy, with ligation of the right branch of the portal vein, it is well to approach this branch from its lateral aspect at the hilus, where troublesome side branches are absent, and to be especially alert for a large posterior segmental branch of the portal vein that begins at or just after the bifurcation of the portal vein, creating what is regarded as a dangerous 'trifurcation.' When hilar ligation is completed, transection of liver substance is commenced, omitting in most instances preliminary extrahepatic isolation and ligation of the major hepatic veins, for reasons mentioned earlier. The Glisson capsule is sharply incised along the desired line of resection, and the underlying liver substance is separated by careful blunt dissection, using a scalpel handle or the tip of an unsheathed Pool abdominal sucker to gently tease the parenchyma away from an assortment of vessels and ducts.

Throughout this phase of the operation, which is carried out in a controlled but expeditious manner,

220

there is reliance first on *feel* – i.e., on the soft, yeilding character of normal hepatic parenchyma and on the firmer consistency of vessels and ducts – to detect points of resistance, and then on direct *visualization* to identify precisely where metal clips or fine silk ligatures should be placed *prior* to cutting the variously oriented vessels and ducts. If cut prior to ligation, the smaller vessels within the liver will rapidly retract and prove difficult to retrieve, and the larger vessels, especially if cut tangentially, may require large, devitalizing mattress sutures for control of hemorrhage – a technique which, together with electrocautery and the use of crushing clamps, is now widely decried in most spheres of hepatic resection. (The distinguished unit at Kuala Lumpur advocates the use of a specially designed large hemostatic liver clamp [171, 173].) Intrahepatic ligation of major hepatic veins requires special care and is accomplished with fine silk ligatures carefully placed under direct vision after ascertaining the direction and caliber of the vessel. Importantly, the placement of ligatures for the control of potential bleeding must also avoid compromising the vascular inflow and the venous and ductular drainage of the remaining segments. Diffuse oozing usually stops by itself or with gentle pressure from a moist gauze pack held patiently against the raw surface, although persistent arterial bleeding may require an occasional, small figure-of-eight suture ligature. Attempts at capsular reapproximation are generally ill-advised because of their tendency to promote necrosis, hematoma, and dead-space formation. As a means of filling the space occupied by the resected lobe or segment, it is sufficient to place omentum, stomach, or colon against the raw surface of the liver. The gallbladder is removed in major resections involving the right lobe, and T-tube drainage of the common bile duct is employed when there is concern about angulation, patency, or injury of the remaining ductal system. In other situations, T-tube drainage of the common bile duct is presently considered meddlesome. A closed system of drainage, employing several large, soft suction drains brought out through separate stab incisions, provides exit for the blood, bile, and detritus that emanate from the raw surface of the liver in the immediate postoperative period, although the decision when and how to use drains

must necessarily be individualized.

Postoperatively, the patient is cared for in the Intensive Care Unit until hemodynamic stability has been achieved and, if a thoracoabdominal incision has been employed, until the chest tube is out and the respiratory status is satisfactory. In patients with borderline cirrhosis and in those who have undergone right trisegementectomy, it is especially important to avoid hypovolemia and hypoxia during the first postoperative week and to reduce metabolic demands on the liver by cautious resumption of oral feedings and by aggressively treating proven infection. However, low-grade fever is very common in the first few days following major hepatic resection, and if the patient is otherwise doing well and there is no demonstrable cause for the fever, there should be no cause for alarm or precipitous action. The use of prophylactic antibiotics is controversial. With the development of improved methods of hemostasis in liver surgery, which minimize the amount of bacteriophilic necrotic slough coming from the raw surface of the liver, and with the effective employment of closed systems of drainage that appear to reduce the ingress of bacteria via drain tracts, there has been a more confident avoidance of prophylactic antibiotics in recent years, although individual factors such as nutritional status, coexisting illness, and the length and difficulty of the procedure have to be taken into account. The hemoglobin level for a variety of reasons tends to drift downward in the first postoperative week, and in this connection it is well to keep a nasogastric tube in place for 3–4 days for the detection of stress ulceration, which is common in patients who have undergone hepatic resection [111]. To prevent or treat stress ulceration, antacids administered via the nasogatric tube, rather than intravenous Cimetidine, are currently recommended [112, 113, 180]. The prothrombin time usually remains prolonged for a week or so postoperatively, and if massive intraoperative replacement of blood loss has been required, complex clotting problems can develop. Specifically, deficiencies of factors V and VII, fibrinogen, and platelets have been identified after major hepatic resection [114], and recourse to fresh whole blood is helpful in both preventing and treating this difficult problem. Jaundice is common postoperatively, serum bilirubin levels often reaching 10 mg % or more, but unless the serum bilirubin persists at this level for longer than ten days, there is no need for concern. Serum albumin levels start to fall within 24 h after operation, reaching their lowest level on about the seventh day, and this is combated with infusions of salt-poor albumin, usually 50–75 mg a day for the first few days, to keep the serum albumin level somewhere near 3.5 mg%, although the need for this extra albumin has been questioned by Vajrab-ukka et al. [115]. Failure of the patient to increase endogenous albumin synthesis by the third week is considered a bad prognostic sign, especially if compounded by ascites formation. Hypoglycemia, which can also occur soon after operation, is countered by intravenous infusions of 10% dextrose in water. Recently, the serial measurement after major hepatic resection of the blood ketone body ratio (ratio of acetoacetate to 3-hydroxybutyrate), which correlates with the energy status of the remnant liver, has been recommended as a method of detecting incipient hepatic insufficiency and failure [181].

As mentioned earlier, the mortality rate for elective major hepatic resection has fallen below 10% in several centers, although the 1974 Liver Tumor Survey by Foster and Berman [37] revealed an overall operative mortality rate of 13% for a variety of procedures ranging from wedge resection to extended right lobectomy. Remarkably, in a recent series [116], there was only one operative death from among 30 patients subjected to right trisegmentectomy, and Adson and Beart [117], reporting on a personal experience with more than 70 partial hepatic resections, noted an operative mortality rate of only 4%. In the 1974 Liver Tumor Survey [37], the most frequent primary cause of death was intraoperative and postoperative hemorrhage, followed by liver failure, 'judgment errors' (operations on patients with cirrhosis, preexisting liver failure, and/or perihepatic sepsis), sepsis, gastrointestinal hemorrhage, cardiopulmonary problems, and probable air embolism. In patients with cirrhosis undergoing major hepatic resection, the operative mortality rate was approximately 55%.

6. HEPATIC REGENERATION

Following major hepatic resection, with removal of

40% or more of noncirrhotic liver, there is a prompt, vigorous, seemingly orchestrated proliferation of cells throughout the hepatic remnant until at 3–6 months, depending upon the age and fitness of the patient and the type of liver disease for which the resection was performed, the normal hepatic mass is regained or exceeded; at this point, again in a seemingly orchestrated way, the proliferative process comes to a halt and the characteristically low preoperative rates of cell division resume. This remarkable process of 'hepatic regeneration,' which grossly begins in the human within two or three days of major resection [115], is not, strictly speaking, a true regrowth of the resected lobe or segment in the sense that normal preoperative hepatic architecture is faithfully restored. Rather, in its finished form it represents a diffuse compensatory hyperplasia of parenchymal and nonparenchymal elements within the remnant, with the vascular and ductal pattern of the restored mass conforming to that of the remnant itself rather than to that of the original intact liver. A full regenerative response is seen with hepatic resections of as much as 80%–90% [118, 119], and, even following massive resections, liver function tests have usually returned to normal by the end of the third postoperative week. In the cirrhotic patient, on the other hand, regeneration in those patients who survive major resection is either abortive or absent, regardless of the duration of the postoperative interval, and liver function tests and protein manufacture by the liver remain seriously deranged [120].

Experimentally, because of its relevance to fundamental problems of stimulated nucleic acid metabolism and cell division in higher organisms as well as to practical aspects of liver function in sick patients, hepatic regeneration has been studied in great detail, notably in the rat, mouse, and dog, in which the segmental anatomy of the liver favors quantifiable and technically easy major hepatic resection, and there is much of value pertaining to this vast and biologically complex field in the reviews of Bucher and Malt [121, Hays [122], and Karran and Eagles [123]. Additionally, tissue culture studies of hepatic regeneration, recently reviewed by Leffert et al. [124], provide, under more precisely defined conditions, insights into the basic mechanisms controlling hepatic regeneration.

The overall sequence of events following experimental hepatic resection has been summarized succinctly by Hays [122]:

Following removal of 30 to 70 percent of the liver, after a short interval, extremely rapid liver cell hypertrophy occurs. This is promptly followed by cell division which probably involves all of the hepatocytes once and some several times. Ductal and littoral cells follow the same course at a somewhat slower rate. The process gradually decelerates, and all cellular elements return to the normal state of almost complete inactivity in respect to cell division. Whether the factor or factors which control this unique phenomenon are single or multiple, pulselike or continuing throughout the response, even stimulatory or repressive relative to normal growth regulators, is unknown. The sequence of events in which new hepatocytes are formed initially, followed by ductal cells and stromal cells in sequence, as well as the somewhat independent regeneration of littoral cells, suggest that there may be organizing or other secondary regulators within the regeneration system. [By permission, *Surgery, Gynecology and Obstetrics*.]

Inasmuch as liver cells are normally in the G_0 or resting pase of the cell cycle for prolonged periods, possibly in the unprovoked liver for the adult life of the animal, it is of considerable interest that immediately following partial (68%) hepatectomy in the rat they somewhat asynchronously pass into the active phases of the cell cycle, culminating, with respect to hepatocytes, in peak levels of mitosis after 28–30 h; with respect to nonparenchymal cells, which comprise 35%–40% of the cell population, the same stimulation of cell growth and division takes place but with a lag of about 24 h.

In an effort to decipher this profound, sudden change in the direction of liver cell metabolism, and to at least partially identify the subcellular and transcriptional/translational events accompanying mitogenic stimulation, much attention has been focused on the morphological and biochemical changes in liver cells during the first 72 h after partial hepatectomy [121]. Such scrutiny has resulted in the identification of an initial phase of cell *hypertrophy* and a second phase of cell *hyperplasia*, which appear to be under somewhat separate influences.

During the phase of hypertrophy, which in the rat lasts 20–24 h, the liver enlarges and becomes paler, the latter change being occasioned by glycogen depletion and by extensive fatty vacuolization of hepatocytes, and the former change by a diffuse doubling (or more) in size of individual cells prior to mitosis. Histologically, these changes are first seen in cells adjacent to the portal triads where,

presumably, the constituents of portal and systemic inflow are most concentrated and where oxygen levels are probably highest, and then later in the central zone of the hepatic lobules. At the subcellular level, there is an important increase during this phase in ribosome production and in the amount of smooth endoplasmic reticulum, and very early after partial hepatectomy there is a change in patterns of protein synthesis by hepatocytes, certain proteins being critical – in ways that are poorly understood – to eventual DNA replication, which begins in periportal hepatocytes at about 16 h after partial hepatectomy and peaks for the entire population of hepatocytes at 20–24 h. Varieties of newly synthesized RNA also appear soon after operation and participate in ribosome formation, translation, and, in some obscure way, DNA synthesis.

The phase of hyperplasia is characterized by a burst of mitotic activity which lags behind DNA replication by about 6–8 h and reaches peak activity in hepatocytes at 28–30 h after partial hepatectomy and in ductal and littoral cells at 42–54 h after operation. As with DNA replication, mitosis begins in cells closest to the portal triads and then sweeps toward the central veins. During this first cycle of cell division, the G_1 interval is lengthened from 9 h to 21–24 h, but subsequently in the small percentage of cells that are stimulated to divide at least twice the G_1 interval is shortened to 5 h. Curiously, the proportion of binucleate hepatocytes (normally 20%–30% of rat hepatocytes) decreases to 10% after partial hepatectomy, with a corresponding increase in the polyploidy of these cells. The meaning of these changes is unclear.

Although it has been shown that hepatic regeneration will take place in the partially hepatectomized rat when portal blood flow is diverted from the liver by side-to-side or end-to-side portacaval shunt, it has been known for a long time that deprivation of portal flow to the regenerating lobe leads to measurable loss of mass of that lobe [125]. It was assumed initially that the stunted growth of these lobes was the result of a deficient proliferative response by the remnant, but recent work has shown that the regenerative impulse of the remaining liver cells is not thwarted by portal deprivation, just made more sluggish – there being slightly delayed but ample DNA synthesis and mitotic activity following partial hepatectomy in portally deprived animals [126–128]. Rather, the loss of liver mass in these preparations appears to be due to diffuse atrophy of individual hepatocytes, which nonetheless retain the ability to divide. (The histologic appearance of these atrophic cells is quite normal; electron microscopy reveals only depletion of rough endoplasmic reticulum and glycogen granules.) In other words, the proliferative potential of liver cells persists, whether cell atrophy or cell hypertrophy has occurred, the implication being that hepatocyte mass and hepatocyte dividing capability are independent variables and that portal blood flow seems to have a separate effect on each.

Precisely how the portal circulation exerts an influence on hepatic regeneration has been the subject of prolonged and exhaustive study. Following the demonstration that experimental procedures that increase portal flow to the liver do not significantly stimulate cell division [129], just as procedures that reduce total blood flow or portal flow to the liver do not thwart hepatic regeneration, the proposition that hemodynamic factors have a prime influence on hepatic regeneration [125] has been largely depreciated in favor of a search for hepatotrophic factors, even though there is in fact an impressive increase in the 'specific' blood flow (ml blood/g tissue) to the remnant immediately after partial hepatectomy [130]. This shift in emphasis from quantitative to qualitative aspects of portal blood flow was reinforced by the experiments of Marchiora et al. [131], which showed that partial portacaval transposition in the dog – i.e., anastomosing the supraadrenal inferior vena cava to either the right or left branch of the portal vein while leaving portal flow through the opposite branch of the portal vein undisturbed – resulted in gross and microscopic atrophy and deglycogenation in the portion of the liver receiving systemic venous blood, compared with no change in the portally perfused liver – the measured flow rates after reconstruction being comparable for the two sides.

This led to further experiments in dogs in which portal venous flow to the liver was anatomically partitioned so that one lobe received pancreatic-gastroduodenal-splenic flow and the other intestinal flow – so-called splanchnic flow division procedures [132]. In these studies, liver specimens were obtained at autopsy one to five and a half months after operation in three groups of dogs –

one with partial portacaval transposition, one with splanchnic flow division, and one with total portacaval transposition – with multifactorial morphologic and biochemical determinations done on the specimens. The conclusion of this study was that the dominant hepatotrophic influence was derived from blood returning from the pancreas, duodenum, stomach, and spleen and that pancreatic hormones, specifically insulin and glucagon, were the main hepatotrophic factors.

Extensions of these experiments on dogs rendered diabetic by alloxan administration or by total pancreatectomy revealed a significant alteration in the differential effects of splanchnic flow division on the right or left lobe, with or without accompanying 30% or 60% hepatectomy; the key observation was that the lobes previously protected either by pancreatic-gastroduodenal-splenic flow or by total splanchnic flow now partly, or completely, lost this advantage in both short-term (3–5 days) and long-term (two months) experiments on hepatectomized and nonhepatectomized dogs [133, 134]. In other words, some component or components of pancreatic-gastroduodenal-splenic flow that fostered hypertrophy and hyperplasia of hepatocytes in nondiabetic dogs, with or without hepatectomy, was removed, inactivated, or counteracted in the diabetic animal. A further set of experiments in which the left lobe of the liver was perfused with systemic venous blood from the hindquarters, kidneys, and adrenal glands, and the right lobe with the entire splanchnic flow, revealed an advantaged status of the right lobe compared with the left, which was diminished but not eliminated by total pancreatectomy or alloxan-induced diabetes. The conclusion of these crude but well-conceived experiments was that the most favorable situation was portal perfusion with splanchnic venous blood containing normal amounts of endogenous insulin; the least favorable was perfusion with systemic venous blood; intermediately favorable was perfusion with splanchnic venous blood deficient in endogenous insulin but rich in other elements. Such findings lent support to the view that of the interreacting hormones arriving at the liver via portal blood flow insulin has the most influential hepatotrophic role. Later experiments in eviscerated dogs portally infused with insulin, glucagon, or epidermal growth factor reinforced this view [135].

However, in other studies glucagon, despite its reputation as a catabolic hormone, was identified with insulin as an important hepatotrophic factor. Bucher and Swaffield [127] subjected rats to resection of the gastrointestinal tract, pancreas, and spleen, and maintained them with intravenous infusions of glucose and electrolytes. Although the animals were portally deprived by this procedure, they responded to partial hepatectomy with a delayed and diminished, but nevertheless significant, rise in hepatic DNA synthesis, which was restored to normal by the infusion of insulin and glucagon, but not by either hormone alone; further, the ability of insulin and glucagon to restore DNA synthesis to normal was not decreased by delaying the start of hormone treatment for 6–7 h after partial hepatectomy. These findings – namely, that significant regenerative activity is inducible in the absence of pancreatic hormones, and that delayed administration of insulin and glucagon after partial hepatectomy is as effective as prompt administration in restoring regeneration to normal in eviscerated rats – suggested that in spite of the pronounced influence of these two hormones, one or more additional factors are required to initiate cell proliferation. This interpretation was reinforced, in their view, by the finding that portal vein insulin levels in normal rats fall abruptly after partial hepatectomy [136], and that insulin and glucagon fail to appreciably activate DNA synthesis in eviscerated, nonhepatectomized rats.

Similarly, studies by Dugay et al. [137] in the pancreatectomized dog showed that insulin supplementation without glucagon resulted in significantly delayed hepatic regeneration, compared with supplementation with insulin plus glucagon. They further demonstrated, using a rat bioassay model consisting of 30% nonregenerating liver isografts, that perfusion of the graft with pancreas extract or with an insulin and glucagon mixture stimulated hepatic regeneration compared with no perfusion or perfusion with saline or with spleen extract.

A number of studies have suggested a nonportal origin of the factor(s) initiating hepatic regeneration. Experiments by Fisher et al. [138] in rats subjected to segmental small intestinal resection at various levels prior to partial hepatectomy, with or without end-to-side portacaval shunt, either singly or in cross-circulated pairs of rats, implicated the intestinal tract as a source of hepatotrophic factor. Similarly, Chandler [139] demonstrated that the insulin-containing pancreaticoduodenal component of portal blood is not adequate by itself to prevent liver atrophy or to stimulate DNA replication selectively, and that the hepatotrophic activity of rabbit portal blood is either markedly volume dependent or derived from splanchnic viscera other than the pancreas and duodenum. More recently, important studies by Griesler et al. [140], in which normal rats were cross-circulated with totally hepatectomized rats – half of which had also undergone excision of all of the portal organs – showed that after 48 h of cross-circulation, active DNA synthesis and evidences of hepatic regeneration were found in normal rats cross-circulated with the hepatectomized/portally eviscerated rats, demonstrating a blood-borne factor not arising from the portal organs that is capable of stimulating hepatic regeneration. Interestingly, when a normal rat was cross-circulated with a hepatectomized rat having intact portal organs, hepatic regeneration took place but with less exuberance than when portal organs had been removed – a finding for which no compelling explanation could be found. It should be added that in these experiments it was not determined whether DNA synthesis in the normal member of the pair was stimulated in organs other than the liver – information that might have shed light on the specificity of the unidentified stimulatory factor.

Within the context of growth control mechanisms of mammalian cells in cell culture [141], tissue culture studies of hepatocytes provide a still different perspective on liver regeneration. Leffert et al. [142] showed that stationary phase adult rat hepatocytes, obtained from normal liver and permitted to undergo one growth cycle in primary monolayer culture, can be made to synthesize DNA and to divide by the addition to fresh growth medium of only insulin, glucagon, and epidermal growth factor [143], although there is a curious, unexplained stimulatory effect in these experiments of the serum component of growth medium; indeed, increasing the amount of serum in the medium 24–28 h post-plating enhances the effect. More recent experiments [144] show that the stimulatory effect of insulin, glucagon, and epidermal growth factor on primary liver cell cultures grown in serum free media is reversibly blocked by Amiloride, a Na^+ influx inhibitor.

A further fragment of the puzzle, recently reported by Terblanche et al. [145], is that a cytosol extract prepared from 48-h, and especially 72-h, regenerating dog liver [146] when infused intraportally into another dog over a 6-h period beginning 4–6 h after partial hepatectomy, has the ability to significantly augment the regenerative response normally seen. The effect becomes manifest 48 h after the infusion begins and peaks at 72 h. No effect is seen in normal controls infused intraportally with the cytosol extract, and there is no significant response in normal or hepatectomized dogs to a 6-h intraportal infusion of insulin or to a cytosol extract prepared from normal dog liver.

Much of this data needs to be looked at very carefully, not only because the experiments for the most part are complex and unavoidably crude, often with conflicting conclusions, but because there is much in them that still needs to be digested. What can be said at this point is that there is improved definition of the portal blood factors which appear importantly to modify the regenerative response to hepatic resection, but that there is very little information about the initiating or trigger factor(s). It is at least reasonable to assume, on the basis of elegant nuclear transplantation studies in cultured cells [147], that the conditioning or stimulation of the nucleus to divide comes from a signal provided by the cytoplasm, and this to some extent narrows the range of possibilities. Whatever the mode of action of the elusive hepatotrophic factor, it would seem that it has to react in some way with the cytoplasm before its influence can be felt in the nucleus.

7. LIVER TRANSPLANTATION

Although at present clinical transplantation of the liver remains experimental, mention should be made of four recent reports of long-term experience with this formidable undertaking – two from the University of Colorado Medical Center [116, 148] going back 16 years, one from Addenbrooke's Hospital (Cambridge)–King's College Hospital [149] going back 11 years, and one from Memorial Sloan-Kettering Cancer Center in New York [108] going back eight years. The first three reports present the experience of two centers where massive effort has gone into the development and clinical application of orthotopic liver transplantation (removal of the diseased liver and replacement in the same anatomic location of a liver allograft) in a total for the two centers of 238 patients; the fourth report analyzes in the context of 43 cases from the ACS/NIH Organ Transplant Registry experience with seven patients on whom heterotopic liver grafting (placement of an auxiliary liver within the confines of the body, leaving the diseased liver in place) was carried out by a technically accomplished surgeon.

In circles where there is clinical acceptance of the procedure, the indications for orthotopic liver grafting include biliary atresia, primary hepatic malignancy (mainly hepatocellular carcinoma), advanced cirrhosis of various forms [150], chronic aggressive hepatitis, and certain inborn errors of metabolism. Starzl et al. [116] prefer not to perform the operation on patients more than 50 years old and, indeed, have performed 53 of their 164 liver transplants on infants and children with biliary atresia; Calne [151], on the other hand, has carried out liver transplantation on patients as old as 65 and has been reluctant to perform the operation on infants and children because of concern about the quality of life of these young patients after the operation. Donor livers, which are obtained from cases of brain death where there has been an intact circulation and no evidence of infection or systemic malignancy, are provided without reference to tissue typing (in contrast to renal transplantation) and have been found to tolerate cold preservation by various methods for periods of up to 12 h. The recipient operation, which is technically difficult, consists of removal of the diseased liver – which may entail massive bleeding, coagulation problems, electrolyte disturbances (notably potassium flux in and out of the liver), acidosis, and hemodynamic instability when various vascular-clamping maneuvers are carried out – followed by insertion of the donor liver by using a variety of anastomotic techniques. Immunosuppression, most recently with cyclosporin A and prednisone [183], is begun on the day of transplantation and continued indefinitely.

Early experience with 93 patients [152] included a 34% incidence of biliary obstruction and bile fistula formation, but more recently, with choledochocholedochostomy having replaced cholecystoduodenostomy as the preferred method of accomplishing biliary reconstruction at the University of Colorado, results have significantly improved [116]; a similar decrease in these complications has been effected at Addenbrooke's Hospital using the donor gallbladder as a pedicle graft conduit in reconstructing the common bile duct. Immediate postoperative complications include hepatic dysfunction, sepsis, hemorrhage, cardiopulmonary problems, fistulation, ascending cholangitis, and acute rejection; long-term problems leading to death include liver failure (secondary grafts, with removal of the first graft, are sometimes placed), overwhelming systemic infections [153], recurrent tumor, biliary obstruction (sometimes from extensive biliary cast formation), and chronic rejection of the graft. Survivals following the procedure have been as long as seven and a half years [116] and five years [149], with an average one-year survival rate of 32% for the University of Colorado series and 16% for the Cambridge–King's College Hospital series. Somewhat disturbingly, although 30 consecutive patients undergoing orthotopic liver transplantation at the University of Colorado Medical Center between July 1976 and January 1978 experienced a one-year survival rate of 50% [116], a subsequent set of 23 similar patients at the same institution had only a 26% one-year survival rate following the procedure [40]. Faulty case selection, technical complications, the use of damaged organs, and complications of immunosuppression were given as the reasons for the decline in survival.

Heterotopic transplantation of the liver appears to have a very limited role in the treatment of severe liver disease. Fortner's view [108], based on personal experience with seven such operations, one of which resulted in a continuing survival of five and a half years, is that it is useful in the management of the cirrhotic patient with a shrunken liver; in this setting, he feels, heterotopic liver grafting can materially augment hepatic function, without causing excessive crowding within the abdomen (where the second liver is placed) and with avoidance of the substantial trauma of recipient hepatectomy. Starzl et al. [116], having done five such procedures,

believe it should be reserved for patients with acute hepatic disease in whom the objective is temporary life support while recovery of the native liver is in progress.

8. NUTRITION IN SURGICAL CONDITIONS OF THE LIVER

Increasing awareness that malnutrition adversely affects surgical results, particularly in high-risk patients undergoing major procedures, has led in recent years to heightened interest in the nutritional assessment and support of the surgical patient [175]. Such concern applies particularly to surgical conditions of the liver. The posttrauma or posthepatectomy patient or the patient with hepatic malignancy, biliary atresia, or cirrhosis very often is, or becomes, nutritionally depleted and immunoincompetent to a significant degree [154], and it behoves the surgeon to assess the deficit and, if possible, to promote positive nitrogen balance.

Beginning with the report of Blackburn et al. [155], work at a number of centers has identified clinically useful nutritional 'markers' (objective indicators of malnutrition), which reliably predict states of increased risk or morbidity and mortality in the surgical patient. Of these, serum albumin levels, serum transferrin levels, delayed hypersensitivity reactivity to skin testing [174], and triceps skinfold measurements have, in descending order of importance, gained the widest acceptance although rapid-turnover transport proteins such as thyroxine-binding prealbumin and retinol-binding protein appear to be truer indicators of subclinical protein-energy malnutrition and to respond earlier to nutritional manipulation [176]. Indeed, Buzby et al. [156] recently formulated a linear predictive model which relates the risk of operative morbidity, mortality or both to nutritional status. The attractiveness of the model, despite the length and complexity of the equation, relates to its applicability to the *individual* patient. [The equation: prognostic nutritional index (PNI) (percent) = 158 − 16.6 (ALB) − 0.78 (TSF) − 0.20 (TFN) − 5.8(DH), where ALB is serum albumin level (g/100 ml), TSF is triceps skinfold (mm), TFN is serum transferrin level (mg/100 ml), and DH is cutaneous delayed hypersensitivity reactivity to any of three recall antigens (mumps, streptokinase-streptodornase, Candida), graded as 0 (nonreactive), 1 (less than 5 mm induration) or 2 (5 mm or greater induration).] Thus, it is now possible to approximately classify patients, using this model, as low, intermediate, or high risk prior to operation, and to design and implement with some precision an individual program of nutritional support in the pre- or postoperative period.

It should be noted that of the aforementioned nutritional 'markers,' those known as 'visceral proteins' – serum albumin, serum transferrin, serum prealbumin, and serum retinol-binding protein – are manufactured in the liver and correspondingly reflect acute and chronic derangements of protein metabolism in the liver. For example, cirrhosis, septic states, and hepatocellular carcinoma all lead sooner or later to decreased levels of 'visceral' protein, the implication being that patients with these conditions are particularly vulnerable to complications and death in the postoperative period, however technically adequate a particular procedure may have been. It follows that pre-operative nutritional repletion by whatever means has special impetus in such patients.

The components of the nutritional program and the route or routes used to deliver the nutrients, whether pre- or postoperatively, depend largely on the availability of the gastrointestinal tract, the dictum being that when the gastrointestinal tract is available and functionally intact, it should be used. The advantages of this route are safety, simplicity, and cost effectiveness. Moreover, it is clear that portal blood flow delivers nutrients to the liver by the most anatomically direct route and in the most physiologically correct admixture; the liver then takes what it needs for its myriad metabolic processes and allows the rest to filter through. When parenteral routes are used to administer nutrients, the nutrients arrive at the liver after a circuitous passage through the rest of the body, and in large part they represent the 'leftovers' that other organs have not utilized.

A variety of methods are available for 'gut feeding.' In an outpatient setting, commercially available dietary supplements are often well tolerated and effective. In an inpatient setting, if the patient cannot accept oral feedings, balanced nutritionally complete diets and elemental diets can be given via a small bore feeding tube, easily inserted through the nose [157]. In such cases, it is important that the rate of instillation be carefully regulated to avoid the diarrhea known to be associated with the sudden deposition in the small intestine of large, hyperosmolar loads.

When vigorous nutritional therapy is required following a major abdominal operation, fine needle catheter jejunostomy at the end of the procedure [158, 159, 182], with graduated, around-the-clock instillation of an elemental diet, has been shown to be an effective method of promoting positive nitrogen balance over periods of ten days or more. Recent reports [160, 161] emphasize the safety and simplicity of the technique, and it is remarkable that such feedings can be begun in most instances on the first or second postoperative day except in cases of generalized peritonitis, small bowel obstruction, extensive small bowel adhesions, intrinsic small bowel disease, or extensive retroperitoneal dissection. It is particularly useful in nutritionally problematic patients undergoing operations on the liver, biliary system, or pancreas. The general rule is that feedings should be started slowly in dilute form and advanced gradually, the most common complication, diarrhea, being controllable by reducing the rate and concentration of the elemental diet. Distention and vomiting, which may also occur, are managed by stopping the feedings, either temporarily or permanently, and catheter problems, such as slippage or intraperitoneal leakage, are rare when the loop of jejunum is affixed to the parietal peritoneum. In the typical adult patient, 1700–1800 calories a day can be provided by this route.

In situations where the gut, for whatever reason, is inactivated for prolonged periods, effective methods of *parenteral feeding* are available. The clinical use of intravenous fat emulsions, which had to await the development of preparations free of the disturbing side effects of earlier emulsions, is now widely practiced, a variety of safe emulsions presently being available in Europe and the United States. Ease of administration, usually via peripheral vein, is one of the advantages of this approach, and a number of studies attest to the attainability of positive nitrogen balance when fat emulsions are used as the primary source of calories. Although the optimal fat to carbohydrate ratio has not been determined, the administration of fat emulsions is customarily accompanied by the infusion of a mixture of 10% dextrose and 5% crystalline L-amino acids given via a Y-connector through the same intravenous catheter as the fat emulsion. In patients with liver disease, it is probably wise to do a triglyceride clearance test prior to the administration of fat emulsions, although even in patients with advanced alcoholic cirrhosis, fat emulsions have been shown to be cleared from the plasma at a normal rate [179].

The most high-powered method of nutritional support when the gastrointestinal tract is not available for feeding is intravenous hyperalimentation, or 'total parenteral nutrition.' This technique, developed by Dudrick and co-workers at the University of Pennsylvania [162], employs concentrated hyperosmolar mixtures of glucose and crystalline L-amino acids, with calorie to nitrogen ratios of 100–150 to 1; it safely provides as much as 3000–4000 calories a day through a catheter inserted via the subclavian or internal jugular vein into the superior vena cava. Metabolic and technical considerations, as well as a variety of complications, are succinctly discussed in the recent review by Ota et al. [163]. What is germaine to this brief discussion is the intensified interest over the past few years in *qualitative* aspects of intravenously administered amino acid mixtures. In particular, the anticatabolic properties of branch chain amino acids – valine, leucine, and isoleucine – are receiving increased attention, and, following preliminary animal studies [164–166], clinical trials have been conducted that reveal the ability of these amino

acids, with or without other essential amino acids, to promote positive nitrogen balance even in the first postoperative week when accentuated urinary nitrogen loss ordinarily occurs [167]. The effect is noted whether the branch chain amino acids are administered intravenously or via the gut. Present evidence suggests that skeletal muscle selectively utilizes branch chain amino acids as an energy source and as substrate for gluconeogenesis via the glucose-alanine cycle; additionally, it appears that leucine acts as a regulator of protein turnover in skeletal muscle by inhibiting protein synthesis. Whatever the mechanism of action, it is apparent that the demand for branch chain amino acids is pronounced during sepsis, when they become the major determinant of gluconeogenesis and protein catabolism, and in advanced cirrhosis, when aromatic amino acids can no longer be metabolized by the liver and the peripheral utilization of branch chain amino acids becomes the dominant metabolic event [168]. Accordingly, in the septic or cirrhotic patient, with or without a superimposed surgical insult, the provision of branch chain amino acids by either enteral or parenteral means appears to offer significantly improved nutritional support even in the presence of liver failure, particularly since these patients tend to be hyperglucagonemic and glucose intolerant [169, 177].

Acknowledgment. The authors gratefully acknowledge the help of Dr. Leonard Heintz on aspects of computed tomography of the liver.

REFERENCES

1. Madding GF, Kennedy PA (eds) (1977) Hepatic surgery. Surg Clin North Am 57:229–474
2. McDermott WV Jr (1974) Surgery of the liver and portal circulation. Philadelphia: Lea and Febiger
3. Aldrete JS, Halpern NB, Ward S, Wright JO (1979) Factors determining the mortality and morbidity in hepatic injuries. Ann Surg 189:446–474
4. McInnis WD, Richardson JD, Aust JB (1977) Hepatic trauma. Arch Surg 112:157–161
5. Pachter HL, Spencer FC (1979) Recent concepts in the treatment of hepatic trauma. Ann Surg 190:423–429
6. Walt AJ (1978) The mythology of hepatic trauma – or Babel revisited. Am J Surg 135:12–18
7. Rutherford RB (1973) Thoracic injuries. In: Ballinger WF, Rutherford RB, Zuidema GD (eds) The management of trauma. Philadelphia: WB Saunders, pp 336–337
8. Smith R (1978) Injuries of the liver, biliary tree and pancreas. Br J Surg 65:673–677
9. Freeark RJ (1977) Blunt torso trauma. Surg Clin North Am 57:1317–1333
10. Thal ER, McClelland RN, Shires GT (1979) Abdominal trauma. In: Shires GT (ed) Care of the trauma patient. New York: McGraw-Hill, p 291
11. Butterworth JF, Miller JD, Kimball IM, Becker DP (1980) Detection of occult abdominal trauma in patients with severe head injuries. Lancet 2:759–762
12. Freeark RJ (1969) Role of angiography in the management of multiple injuries. Surg Gynecol Obstet 128:761–771.
13. Miller DR (1972) Median sternotomy extension of abdominal incision for hepatic lobectomy. Ann Surg 175:193–196
14. Donovan AJ, Michaelian MJ, Yellin AE (1973) Anatomical hepatic lobectomy in trauma to the liver. Surgery 73:833–847
15. Lim RC, Lau G, Steele M (1976) Prevention of complications after liver trauma. Am J Surg 132:156–162
16. Calne RY, McMaster P, Pentlow BD (1979) The treatment of major liver trauma by primary packing with transfer of

the patient for definitive treatment. Br J Surg 66:338–339

17. Yellin AE, Chaffee CB, Donovan AJ (1971) Vascular isolation in treatment of juxtahepatic venous injuries. Arch Surg 102:566–573

18. Morgenstern L, Michel SL, Austin E (1977) Control of hepatic bleeding with microfibrillar collagen. Arch Surg 112:941–943

19. Stone HH, Lamb JM (1975) Use of pedicled omentum as an autogenous pack for control of hemorrhage in major injuries of the liver. Surg Gynecol Obstet 141:92–94

20. Mays ET (1972) Lobar dearterialization for exsanguinating wounds of the liver. J Trauma 12:397–407

21. Michels NA (1960) Newer anatomy of the liver – variant blood supply and collateral circulation. JAMA 172: 125–132

22. Mays ET, Wheeler CS (1974) Demonstration of collateral arterial flow after interruption of hepatic arteries in man. N Engl J Med 290:993–996

23. Walt AJ (1979) Discussion of 'Hepatic artery ligation' by ET Mays et al. Surgery 86:536–543

24. Flint LM, Mays ET, Aaron WS, Fulton RL, Polk HC (1977) Selectivity in the management of hepatic trauma. Ann Surg 185:613–618

25. Madding GF, Kennedy PA (1971) Trauma to the liver. Philadelphia: WB Saunders

26. Lucas CE, Ledgerwood AM (1978) Liver necrosis following hepatic artery transection due to trauma. Arch Surg 113:1107

27. Aust JB (1977) Discussion of 'Selectivity in the management of hepatic trauma' by LM Flint et al. Ann Surg 185:618

28. Aaron S, Fulton RL, Mays ET (1975) Selective ligation of the hepatic artery for trauma of the liver. Surg Gynecol Obstet 141:187–189

29. Defore WW, Mattox KL, Jordan GL, Beall AC Jr (1976) Management of 1,590 consecutive cases of liver trauma. Arch Surg 111:493–497

30. Levin A, Gover P, Nance FC (1978) Surgical management of hepatic injury: a review of Charity Hospital experience. J Trauma 18:399–404

31. Carroll CP, Cass KA, Whelan TJ (1973) Wounds of the liver in Vietnam. Ann Surg 177:385–392

32. Schrock T, Blaisdell FW, Mathewson S Jr (1968) Management of blunt trauma to the liver and hepatic veins. Arch Surg 96:698–704

33. Lambeth W, Rubin BE (1979) Nonoperative management of intrahepatic hemorrhage and hematoma following blunt trauma. Surg Gyncol Obstet 148:507–511

34. Taylor SA, Dawson JL (1978) The treatment of haemobilia. Br J Surg 65:252–253

35. Mays ET, Conti S, Fallahzadeh H, Rosenblatt M (1979) Hepatic artery ligation. Surgery 86:536–543

36. Bass EM, Med M, Crosier JH (1977) Percutaneous control of post-traumatic hepatic hemorrhage by gelfoam embolization. J Trauma 17:61–63

37. Foster JH, Berman MM (1977) Solid liver tumors. Philadelphia: WB Saunders

38. Fortner JG, Kim DK, Maclean BJ, Barrett MK, Iwatsuki S, Turnbull AD, Howland WS, Beattie EJ Jr (1976) Major hepatic resection in neoplasia. Ann Surg 188:363–371

39. Cady B, Bonneval M, Fender HR Jr (1979) Elective hepatic resection. Am J Surg 137:514–521

40. Starzl TE, Koep LJ, Porter KA, Schroter GPJ, Weil R III, Hartley RB, Halgrimson CG (1980) Decline in survival after liver transplantation. Arch Surg 115:815–819

41. Adson MA, Van Heerden JA (1980) Major hepatic resections for metastatic colorectal carcinoma. Ann Surg 191:576–583

42. Ochsner JL, Halpert B (1958) Cavernous hemangioma of the liver. Surgery 43:577–582

43. Barnett PH, Zerhouni EA, White RI Jr, Siegelman SS (1980) Computed tomography in the diagnosis of cavernous hemangiomas of the liver. Am J Radiol 134:439–447

44. Grieco MB, Miscall BG (1978) Giant hemangiomas of the liver. Surg Gynecol Obstet 147:783–787

45. Starzl TE, Koep LJ, Weil R III, Fennell RH, Iwatsuki S, Kano T, Johnson ML (1980) Excisional treatment of cavernous hemangioma of the liver. Ann Surg 192:25–27

46. Cho C, Rullis I, Rogers LS (1978) Bile duct adenomas as liver nodules. Arch Surg 113:272–274

47. Baum JK, Holtz F, Bookstein JJ, Klein EW (1973) Possible association between benign hepatomas and oral contraceptives. Lancet 2:926–929

48. Klatskin G (1977) Hepatic tumors: possible relationship to use of oral contraceptives. Gastroenterology 73:386–394

49. Edmondson HA, Henderson B, Benton B (1976) Liver-cell adenomas associated with the use of oral contraceptives. N Engl J Med 294:470–472

50. Vessey MP, Kay CR, Baldwin JA, McLeod IB (1977) Oral contraceptives and benign liver tumors. Br Med J 1:1064

51. Vana J, Murphy GP, Aronoff BL, Baker HW (1977) Primary liver tumors and oral contraceptives. JAMA 238:2154–2158

52. Perez V, Gorosdisch (1969) Oral contraceptives: long-term use produces fine structural changes in liver mitochondria. Science 165:805–807

53. Davis M, Portmann B, Searle M, Wright R, Williams R (1975) Histological evidence of carcinoma in a hepatic tumor associated with oral contraceptives. Br Med J 4:496–498

54. Ishak KG, Rabin L (1975) Benign tumors of the liver. Med Clin North Am 59:995–1013

55. Guzman IJ, Gold JH, Rosai J, Schneider PD, Varco RL, Buchwald H (1977) Benign hepatocellular tumors. Surgery 82:495–503

56. Neuberger J, Nummerley HB, Davis M, Portmann B, Laws JW, Williams R (1980) Oral-contraceptive-associated liver tumors: occurrence of malignancy and difficulties in diagnosis. Lancet 1:273–276

57. Snow JH Jr, Goldstein HM, Wallace S (1979) Comparison of scintigraphy, sonography, and computed tomography in the evaluation of hepatic neoplasms. Am J Roentgenol 132:915–918

58. Catalano PW, Martin EW, Ellison C, Carey LC (1979) Reasonable surgical treatment for tumors of the liver associated with the use of oral contraceptives. Surg Gynecol Obstet 148:759–763

59. Terblanche J (1978) Liver tumors associated with the use of contraceptive pills. S Afr Med J 53:439–442

60. Edmondson HA, Reynolds TB, Henderson B, Benton B (1977) Regression of liver cell adenomas associated with oral contraceptives. Ann Intern Med 86:180–182

61. Anderson PH, Parker JT (1976) Observations after estrogen withdrawl. Arch Surg 111:898–900

62. Weil R III, Koep LJ, Starzl TE (1979) Liver resection for hepatic adenoma. Arch Surg 114:178–180

63. Flatmark A, Fretheim B, Knutrud O, Lande G (1977) Surgical treatment of primary liver carcinoma. Scand J Gastroenterol 12:571–575

64. Inouye AA, Whelan TJ (1979) Primary liver cancer: a

230

review of 205 cases in Hawaii. Am J Surg 138:53–61

65. Margolis S, Homcy C (1972) Systemic manifestations of hepatoma. Medicine 51:381–391

66. Malt RA, Van Vroonhoven TJ, Kakumoto Y (1972) Manifestations and prognosis of carcinoma of the liver. Surg Gynecol Obstet 135:361–364

67. Tompkins RK, Johnson J, Storm FK, Longmire WP (1976) Operative endoscopy in the management of biliary tract neoplasms. Am J Surg 132:174–182

68. Bryan PJ, Dinn WM, Grossman ZD, Wistow BW, McAfee JG, Kieffer SA (1977) Correlation of computed tomography, gray scale ultrasonography, and radionuclide imaging of the liver in detecting space-occupying processes. Radiology 124:387–393

69. Itai Y, Nishikawa J, Tasaka A (1979) Computed tomography in the evaluation of hepatocellular carcinoma. Radiology 131:165–170

70. Kunstlinger F, Federle MP, Moss AA, Marks W (1980) Computed tomography of hepatocellular carcinoma. Am J Roentgenol 134:431–437

71. Dunnick NR, Ihde DC, Doppman JL, Bater HR (1980) Computed tomography in primary hepatocellular carcinoma. J Comput Assist Tomogr 4:59–62

72. Kim DK, McSweeney J, Yeh DJ, Fortner JG (1975) Tumors of the liver demonstrated by angiography, scan and laparotomy. Surg Gynecol Obstet 141:409–410

73. Williamson BWA, Blumgart LH, McKellar N (1980) Management of tumors of the liver. Am J Surg 139:210–215

74. Blumberg BS, Larouze B, London WT, Werner B, Hesser JE, Millman I, Saimot G, Payet M (1975) The relation of infection with the hepatitis B agent to primary hepatic carcinoma. Am J Pathol 81:669–682

75. Linder GT, Crook JN, Cohn I Jr (1974) Primary liver carcinoma. Cancer 33:1624–1629

76. Fortner JG (1977) Current manageent of tumors of the liver. Surg Clin North Am 57:465–472

77. Morton DM (1974) Cancer immunotherapy: an overview. Semin Oncol 1:297–310

78. Rosenberg SA (1975) Future prospects for immunotherapy. Cancer 36:821–824

79. Bray AE (1978) The immunology in cancer. Surg Gynecol Obstet 147:103–108

80. Burnet FM (1970) Immunological surveillance. Oxford: Pergamon

81. Terry WD (1980) Immunotherapy of malignant melanoma. N Engl J Med 303:1174–1175

82. Attiyeh FF, Wanebo HJ, Stearns MW (1978) Hepatic resection for metastasis from colorectal cancer. Dis Colon Rectum 21:160–162

83. Foster JH (1978) Survival after liver resection for secondary tumors. Am J Surg 135:389–394

84. Pack GT, Brasfield RD (1955) Metastatic carcinoma of the liver: clinical problem and its management. Am J Surg 90:704–716

85. Brown CE, Warren S (1938) Visceral metastasis from rectal carcinoma. Surg Gynecol Obstet 66:611–621.

86. Grinnell RS (1953) Results of treatment of carcinoma of the colon and rectum; an analysis of 2,311 cases over a 35 year period with 5 year survival results in 1667. Surg Gynecol Obstet 96:31–42

87. Dukes CE, Bussey HJR (1941) Venous spread in rectal cancer. Proc R Soc Med 34:571–573

88. Dukes CE, Bussey HJR (1958) The spread of rectal cancer and its effect on prognosis. Br J Cancer 12:309–320

89. Willis RA (1952) The spread of tumors in the human body. London: Butterworth

90. Jaffe BM, Donegan WL, Watson F, Spratt JS (1968) Factors influencing survival in patients with untreated hepatic metastases. Surg Gynecol Obstet 127:1–11

91. Ramming KP, Sparks FC, Eilber FR, Morton DL (1977) Management of hepatic metastases. Semin Oncol 4:71–80

92. Watkins E Jr, Khazei AR, Nahra KS (1970) Surgical basis for arterial infusion chemotherapy of disseminated carcinoma of the liver. Surg Gynecol Obstet 130:581–605

93. Karakousis CP, Douglass HO Jr, Holyoke ED (1979) Technique of infusion chemotherapy, ligation of the hepatic artery and dearterialization in malignant lesions of the liver. Surg Gynecol Obset 149:403–407

94. Sundqvist K, Hafstrom LO, Jonsson PE, Ryden S, Forsberg L, Lunderquist A (1978) Treatment of liver cancer with regional intraarterial 5-FU infusion. Am J Surg 136:328–331

95. Cady B, Oberfield RA (1974) Regional infusion chemotherapy of hepatic metastases from carcinoma of the colon. Am J Surg 127:220–227

96. Grage TB, Vassilopoulos PP, Shingleton WW, Jubert AV, Elias EG, Aust JB, Moss SE (1979) Results of a prospective randomized study of hepatic artery infusion with 5-fluorouracil in patients with hepatic metastases from colorectal cancer: a Central Oncology Group Study. Surgery 86:550–555

97. Herbsman H, Hassan A, Gardner B, Harshaw D, Bohorquez J, Alfonso A, Newman J (1978) Treatment of hepatic metasases with a combination of hepatic artery infusion chemotherapy and external radiotherapy. Surg Gynecol Obstet 147:13–17

98. Taylor I (1978) Cytotoxic perfusion for colorectal liver metastases. Br J Surg 65:109–114

99. Patt YZ, Wallace S, Hersh EM, Hall SW, Menachem YB, Granmayeh M, McBride CM, Benjamin RS, Mavligit GM (1978) Hepatic arterial infusion of corynebacterium parvum and chemotherapy. Surg Gynecol Obstet 147:897–902

100. Taylor I, Rowling J, West C (1979) Adjuvant cytotoxic liver perfusion for colorectal cancer. Br J Surg 66:833–837

101. Weiss RB and DeVita VT Jr (1979) The dilemma regarding postoperative chemotherapy in primary carcinoma of the colon. Surg Gyncol Obstet 149:267–271

102. Ansfield FJ, Ramirez G, Davis HL, Wirtanen GW, Johnson RO, et al (1975) Further clinical studies with intrahepatic arterial infusion with 5-fluorouracil. Cancer 36:2413–2417

103. Jochnimsen PR, Zike WL, Shirazi SS, Pearlman NW (1978) Iatrogenic liver abscesses. Arch Surg 113:141–144

104. Mach JP, Jaeger Ph, Bertholet M-M, Ruegsegger C-H, Loosli RM, Pettavel J (1974) Detection of recurrence of large bowel carcinoma by radioimmunoassay of circulating carcinoembryonic antigen. Lancet 2:535–540

105. Minton JP, James KK, Hurtubise, PE, Rinker L, Joyce S, Martin EW Jr (1978) The use of serial carcinoembryonic antigen determinations to predict recurrence of carcinoma of the colon and the time for a second-look operation. Surg Gynecol Obstet 147:208–210

106. Cohen AM, Wood WC (1979) Carcinoembryonic antigen levels as an indicator for reoperation in patients with carcinoma of the colon and rectum. Surg Gynecol Obstet 149:22–26

107. Linder RM, Cady B (1980) Hepatic resection. Surg Clin North Am 60:349–367

108. Fortner JG, Yeh SDJ, Kim DK, Shiu MH, Kinne DW

(1979) The case for and technique of heterotopic liver grafting. Transplant Proc 11:269–275

109. Ong GB (1977) Techniques and therapies for primary and metastatic liver cancer. In: Curr Probl Cancer, vol 2. Chicago: Year Book

110. McDermott WV Jr (1979) Hepatic resection. In: Wright R, Alberti KGMN, Karran S, Milwood-Sadler GH (eds) Liver and biliary diseases. Philadelphia: WB Saunders, pp 1112–1120

111. Sawyer JL (1969) Discussion of 'Physiologic considerations in major hepatic resections' by HH Stone et al. Am J Surg 117:78

112. Priebe HJ, Skillman JJ, Bushell LS, Long PC, Silen W (1980) Antacid versus cimetidine in preventing acute gastrointestinal bleeding. N Engl J Med 302:426–430

113. Stothert JC, Simonowitz DA, Dellinger EP, Farley M, Edwards WA, Blair AD, Cutler R, Carrico J (1979) Randomized prospective evaluation of cimetidine and antacid control of gastric pH in the critically ill. Ann Surg 192:169–174

114. Zucker MB, Siegel M, Cliffton EE, Bellville JW, Howland WS, Grossi CE (1957) The effect of hepatic lobectomy on some blood clotting factors and on fibrinolysis. Ann Surg 146:772–781

115. Vajrabukka T, Bloom AL, Sussman M, Wood CB, Blumbart LH (1975) Postoperative problems and management after hepatic resection for blunt injury to the liver. Br J Surg 62:189–200

116. Starzl TE, Koep LJ, Weil R III, Lilly JR, Putnam CW, Aldrete JA (1980) Right trisegmentectomy for hepatic neoplasms. Surg Gynecl Obstet 150:208–214

117. Adson MA, Beart RW Jr (1977) Elective hepatic resection. Surg Clin North Amer 57: 339–360

118. Pack GT, Islami AH, Hubbard JC, Brasfield RD (1962) Regeneration of human liver after major hepatectomy. Surgery 52:617–623

119. McDermott WV Jr, Greenberger NJ, Isselbacher KJ, Weber AL (1963) Major hepatic resection: diagnostic techniques and metabolic problems. Surgery 54:56–66

120. Lin T-Y, Lee C-S, Chen C-C, Liau K-Y, Lin W-S-J (1979) Regeneration of human liver after hepatic lobectomy studied by repeated liver scanning and repeated needle biopsy. Ann Surg 190:48–53

121. Bucher NLR, Malt RA (1971) Regeneration of liver and kidney. Boston: Little, Brown

122. Hays DM (1974) Surgical research aspects of hepatic regeneration. Surg Gynecol Obstet 139:609–619

123. Karran S, Eagles C (1979) Regeneration, Part 1: physical agents. In: Wright R, Alberti KGMN, Karran S, Milwood-Sadler GH (eds) Liver and biliary diseases. Philadelphia: WB Saunders, pp 197–210

124. Leffert HL, Koch TM, Rubalcava B (1979) Hormonal control of rat liver regeneration. Gastroenterology 76:1470–1482

125. Mann FC (1940) The portal circulation and restoration of the liver after partial hepatectomy. Surgery 8:225–238

126. Whittemore AD, Kasuya M, Voorhees AB Jr, Price JB Jr (1975) Hepatic regeneration in the absence of portal viscera. Surgery 77:419–426

127. Bucher NLR, Swaffield MN (1975) Regulation of hepatic regeneration in rats by synergistic action of insulin and glucagon. Proc Natl Acad Sci 72:1157–1160

128. Guest J, Ryan CJ, Benjamin IS, Blumgart LH (1977) Portacaval transposition and subsequent partial hepatectomy in the rat: effects on liver atrophy, hypertrophy and regenerative hyperplasia. Br J Pathol 58:140–146

129. Clarke AM, Thomson RY, Fraenkel GJ (1968) Vascular factors in liver regeneration. Surg Gynecol Obstet 126:45–52

130. Karran SJ, Eagles C, Fleming J, Ackery D (1979) In-vivo measurement of liver perfusion in the normal and partially hepatectomized rat using Tc-99m sulfur colloid. J Nucl Med 20:26–31

131. Marchiora TL, Porter KA, Brown BI, Otte J-B, Starzl TE (1967) The effect of partial portacaval transposition on the canine liver. Surgery 61:723–732

132. Starzl TE, Francavilla A, Halgrimson CG, Francavill FR, Porter KA, Brown TH, Putnam CW (1973) The origin, hormonal nature, and action of hepatotrophic substances in portal blood. Surg Gynecol Obstet 137:179–199

133. Starzl TE, Porter KA, Kashiwagi N, Lee IY, Russell WJI, Putnam CW (1975) The effect of diabetes mellitus on portal blood hepatotrophic factors in dogs. Surg Gynecol Obstet 140:549–562

134. Starzl TE, Porter KA, Kashiwagi N, Putnam CW (1975) Portal hepatotrophic factors, diabetes mellitus and acute liver atrophy, hypertrophy and regeneration. Surg Gynecol Obstet 141:843–858

135. Starzl TE, Francavilla A, Porter KA (1978) The effect upon the liver of evisceration with or without hormone replacement. Surg Gynecol Obstet 146:524–532

136. Bucher NLR, Patel U, Cohen S (1978) Hormonal factors concerned with liver regeneration. Ciba Found Symp 55:95–107

137. Dugay LR, Skivolocki WP, Lee S, Orloff MJ (1977) Regulation of liver regeneration by pancreatic hormones. Gastroenterology 72:1053

138. Fisher B, Szuch P, Levine M, Saffer E, Fisher ER (1973) The intestine as a source of a portal blood factor responsible for liver regeneration. Surg Gynecol Obstet 137:210–214

139. Chandler JG (1976) Hepatotrophic activity in nonpancreatic, nonduodenal portal blood. Surg Forum 27:360–363

140. Griesler HP, Voorhees AB Jr, Price JB (1979) The nonportal origin of the factors initiating hepatic regeneration. Surgery 86:210–217

141. Holley RW (1975) Control of growth of mammalian cells in cell culture. Nature 258:487–490

142. Leffert HL, Moran T, Boostein R, Koch KS (1977) Procarcinogen activation and hormonal control of cell proliferation in differentiated primary adult rat liver cell cultures. Nature 267:58–61

143. Cohen S and Taylor JM (1974) Part I. Epidermal growth factor: chemical and biological characterization. Recent Prog Horm Res 30:533–550

144. Koch KS, Leffert HL (1979) Increased sodium ion influx is necessary to initiate rat hepatocyte proliferation. Cell 18:153–163

145. Terblanche J, Porter KA, Starzl TE, Moore J, Patzelt L, Hayashida N (1980) Stimulation of hepatic regeneration after partial hepatectomy by infusion of a cytosol extract from regenerating dog liver. Surg Gynecol Obstet 151:538–544

146. Starzl TE, Terblanche J, Porter KA, Jones AF, Usui S, Mazzoni G (1979) Growth-stimulating factor in regenerating canine liver. Lancet 1:127–130

147. Harris H (1968) Nucleus and cytoplasm. Oxford: Clarendon

148. Starzl TE, Koep LJ, Halgrimson CG, Hood J, Schroter

GPJ, Porter KA, Weil R III (1979) Fifteen years of clinical liver transplantation. Gastroenterology 77:375–388

149. Calne RY, Williams R (1979) Liver transplantation. Curr Probl Surg 16:3–44

150. Houssin D, Franco D, Corlette MB, Bismuth H (1980) Criteria for hepatic transplantation in cirrhosis. Surg Gynecol Obstet 151:30–32

151. Calne RY (1978) Transplantation of the liver. Ann Surg 188:129–138

152. Starzl TE, Putnam CW, Hansbrough JF, Porter KA, Reid HAS (1977) Biliary complications after liver transplantation: with special reference to the biliary cast syndrome and techniques of secondary duct repair. Surgery 81:212–221

153. Schroter GPJ, Hoelscher M, Putnam CW, Porter KA, Hansbrough JF, Starzl TE (1976) Infections complicating orthotopic liver transplantation. Arch Surg 111: 1337–1347

154. O'Keefe SJ, Carraher TE, El-Zayad AR, Davis M, Williams R (1980) Malnutrition and immunoincompetence in patients with liver disease. Lancet 2:615–617

155. Blackburn GL, Bistrian BR, Maini BS, Schlamm HT, Smith MF (1977) Nutritional and metabolic assessment of the hospitalized patient. J Parent Ent Nutr 1:11–22

156. Buzby GP, Mullen JL Matthews DC, Hobbs CL, Rosato EF (1980) Prognostic nutritional index in gastrointestinal surgery. Am J Surg 139:160–167

157. Martin DC (1980) Easy insertion of feeding tube. Am J Surg 139:728

158. Delaney HM, Carnevale N, Garvey JW, Moss CM (1977) Postoperative nutritional support using needle catheter feeding jejeunostomy. Ann Surg 186:165–170

159. Delaney HM (1980) An improved technique for needle catheter jejeunostomy. Arch Surg 115:1235–1237

160. Hoover HC Jr, Ryan JA, Anderson EJ, Fisher JE (1980) Nutritional benefits of immediate postoperative jejeunal feeding of an elemental diet. Am J Surg 139:153–159

161. Yeung CK, Young GA, Hackett AF, Hill GL (1979) Fine needle catheter jejeunostomy – an assessment of a new method of nutritional support after major gastrointestinal surgery. Br J Surg 66:727–732

162. Dudrick SJ, Wilmore DW, Vars HM, Rhoads JE (1969) Can intravenous feeding as the sole means of nutrition support growth in the child and restore weight loss in an adult? An affirmative answer. Ann Surg 169:974–984

163. Ota DM, Imbembo AL, Zuidema G (1978) Total parenteral nutrition. Surgery 83:503–520

164. Sapir DG, Walser M (1977) Nitrogen sparing induced early in starvation by infusion of branched chain keto-acids. Metabolism 26:301–308

165. Freund H, Yoshimura N, Lunetta L, Fischer JE (1978) The role of the branched-chain amino acids in decreasing muscle catabolism in vivo. Surgery 83:611–618

166. Blackburn GL, Moldawer LL, Usui S, Bothe A Jr, O'Keefe SJD, Bistrian BR (1979) Branched chain amino acid administration and metabolism during starvation, injury, and infection. Surgery 86:307–315

167. Freund H, Hoover HC, Atamian S, Fischer JE (1979) Infusion of the branched chain amino acids in postoperative patients. Ann Surg 190:18–23

168. Cerra FB, Siegel JH, Border JR, Wiles J, McMenamy RR (1979) The hepatic failure of sepsis: cellular versus substrate. Surgery 86:409–421

169. Dahn M, Kirkpatrick JR, Bouwman D (1980) Sepsis, glucose intolerance, and protein malnutrition. Arch Surg 115:1415–1418

170. Nakamura S, Tsuzuki T (1981) Surgical anatomy of the hepatic veins and the inferior vena cava. Surg Gynecol Obstet 152:43–50

171. Balasegaram M, Joishy SK (1981) Hepatic resection. Pillars of success built on the foundation of 15 years of experience. Am J Surg 141:360–365

172. Lefkowitch JH (1981) The epidemiology and morphology of primary malignant liver tumors. Surg Clin North Am 61:169–180

173. Joishy SK, Balasegaram M (1980) Hepatic resection for malignant tumors of the liver: essentials for a unified surgical approach. Am J Surg 139:360–369

174. Christou NV, Meakins JL, MacLean LD (1981) The predictive role of delayed hypersensitivity in preoperative patients. Surg Gynecol Obstet 152:297–301

175. Michel L, Serrano A, Malt RA (1981) Nutritional support of hospitalized patients. N Engl J Med 304:1147–1152

176. Shetty PS, Jung RT, Watrasiewicz KE, James WPT (1974) Rapid turnover transport proteins: an index of subclinical protein-energy malnutrition. Lancet 2:230–232

177. Nachbauer CA, Fischer JE (1981) The failing liver. Surg Clin North Am 61:221–230

178. Adson MA (1981) Diagnosis and surgical treatment of primary and secondary solid hepatic tumors in the adult. Surg Clin North Am 61:181–196

179. Rössner S, Johanasson C, Walldins G, Aly A (1979) Intralipid clearance and lipoprotein pattern in men with advanced alcoholic liver cirrhosis. Am J Clin Nutr 32: 2022–2026

180. Weigelt JA, Aurbakken CM, Gewertz BL, Snyder WH (1981) Cimetidine vs antacid in prophylaxis for stress ulceration. Arch Surg 116:597–601

181. Ukikusa M, Ozawa K, Shimahara Y, Asano M, Nakatani M, Takayoshi T (1981) Changes in blood ketone body ratio: their significance after major hepatic resection. Arch Surg 116:781–785

182. Moore EE, Dunn EL, Jones TN (1981) Immediate jejeunostomy feeding: its use after major abdominal trauma. Arch Surg 116:681–684

183. Starzl TE, Klintmalm GBG, Porter KA, Iwatsuki S, Schröter GPJ (1981) Liver transplantation with use of cyclosporin A and prednisone. N Engl J Med 305:266–269

INDEX

234